Quantitative Health Research

Quantitative Health Research

Issues and Methods

Edited by Elizabeth A. Curtis and Jonathan Drennan

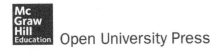 Open University Press

Open University Press
McGraw-Hill Education
McGraw-Hill House
Shoppenhangers Road
Maidenhead
Berkshire
England
SL6 2QL

email: enquiries@openup.co.uk
world wide web: www.openup.co.uk

and Two Penn Plaza, New York, NY 10121-2289, USA

First published 2013

A catalogue record of this book is available from the British Library

ISBN-13: 978-0-335-24573-4
ISBN-10: 0-335-24573-0
eISBN: 978-0-335-24574-1

Library of Congress Cataloging-in-Publication Data
CIP data applied for

Typeset by Aptara, Inc.

Fictitious names of companies, products, people, characters and/or data that may be used
herein (in case studies or in examples) are not intended to represent any real individual,
company, product or event.

Printed and bound by CPI Group (UK) Ltd, Croydon, CR0 4YY

Praise for this book

"Learning quantitative research is taken much for granted. This is probably why there are fewer generic books on quantitative than qualitative research. This book is long overdue. Clearly-written and well structured, it takes us through the whole journey of a research project from developing 'research questions' to 'presenting the findings', passing through philosophical underpinnings, recruitment of participants and ethical considerations. Written by an array of well-known researchers and teachers, this book will certainly appeal to new as well as seasoned researchers. Those who will use it, will not be disappointed."

Kader Parahoo, Professor in Nursing and Health Research, University of Ulster, UK

"The title of this text is somewhat misleading. It is not only an excellent and thorough guide to quantitative health research methods; it is also an excellent introduction to all forms of quantitative research. It takes the reader gently through theoretical and ethical concerns to the practicalities and benefits of utilizing quantitative approaches. As such it is that rare thing; a text that can be used by novice researchers to learn their craft, and a key reference resource for experienced research practitioners."

Dr. John Cullen, School of Business, National University of Ireland, Maynooth, UK

"This is a first-rate collection of essays that promotes an informed understanding of both underpinning principles and widely used techniques. A great deal of effort has clearly been invested in co-ordinating the contributions, and this has delivered clarity, complementarity and effective coverage. This is a welcome, carefully-crafted and very accessible resource that will appeal to students and researchers in healthcare and beyond."

Martin Beirne, Professor of Management and Organizational Behaviour,
University of Glasgow, UK

Contents

PART 3

Quantitative research designs

PART 4

Measurement and data collection

PART 5

Analysing and presenting data

Notes on contributors

Editors

Elizabeth A. Curtis MA, PhD, MEd, DMS, Dip Research Methods, RGN, ONC

Elizabeth Curtis is a Lecturer and Assistant Professor of Nursing in the School of Nursing and Midwifery, Trinity College, University of Dublin. She received her PhD and MEd degrees from the School of Education, Trinity College.

Elizabeth qualified as a general nurse in London and worked in the discipline of neurosciences in the NHS before moving to Ireland. During her time in clinical practice she always had an interest in education and this ultimately led to postgraduate study in this field. Completing a Master's in Education (MEd) provided a comprehensive background in the disciplines relating to the study of education and provided the impetus for her to move from the clinical environment to education.

Elizabeth has many years' experience of teaching research methods and in supervising research students at both undergraduate and postgraduate levels. Her research interests are varied and include job satisfaction, leadership and change. Elizabeth is currently collaborating with colleagues, both within and outside Trinity College, on a number of research initiatives and papers. Recent books include *Research Success in Nursing and Health Care: A Guide to Doing your Higher Degree* (2008) and *Delegation: A Short Primer for the Practising Nurse* (2009).

Jonathan Drennan PhD, MEd, BSc (Hons), PG Dip Statistics, RGN, RPN, RNID, RNT

Jonathan Drennan is a Lecturer at the School of Nursing, Midwifery and Health Systems at University College Dubin. He holds a PhD and Master's degree in Education from University College Dublin, a Postgraduate Diploma in Statistics from Trinity College Dublin and a Bachelor's degree in Nursing from the University of Ulster. Jonathan has had a number of papers published in the areas of ageing, education research, adolescent health and psychometrics in leading journals including *Ageing and Society, Journal of Advanced Nursing, Social Science and Medicine, Journal of Nursing Scholarship, Studies in Higher Education, International Journal of Nursing Studies* and *Journal of Nursing Management*. He has extensive experience of large-scale research projects, including: socialization of people with enduring mental illness, nurse and midwife prescribing, loneliness and social isolation in old age, and elder abuse.

Contributors

Ruth Belling BLib, PhD

Ruth Belling is a Reader in Evaluation Research with the Institute for Leadership and Service Improvement in the Faculty of Health and Social Care, London South Bank University, where she provides research advice and support to teaching staff in the faculty, leads the Service Improvement and Role Development research theme and is a doctoral supervisor. Her main research interests are: evaluation of leadership and management development, particularly in nursing; learning transfer; and service evaluation.

Michelle Butler BSc, MSc, PhD, RGN, RM

Michelle Butler is a Senior Lecturer at the School of Nursing, Midwifery and Health Systems at University College Dublin. She is a Registered Nurse and Registered Midwife, former Head of School and Dean of Nursing and Midwifery and is currently Head of Subject (Midwifery). She has been involved in the design and conduct of research since 1993 across a range of studies in nursing and midwifery, and in health services and public sector management. Her particular research expertise is in evaluation research, qualitative methods, mixed methods, systematic reviews and research ethics. Her research interests include: woman-centered care, maternity care outcomes, health outcomes, competence and learning, health policy, health service management, and nurse and midwifery staffing. Michelle is a Cochrane author and was an HRB Cochrane Fellow from 2007-2010. She lectures on advanced research methods, midwifery research, and health policy and planning and supervises graduate research students.

Catherine Comiskey BA (Mod) Mathematics and Philosophy, MSc Biomathematics, PhD Biomathematics, Statistics and Epidemiology

Catherine Comiskey holds a BA (Mod) degree in Mathematics and Philosophy from Trinity College, Dublin University, and MSc and PhD degrees in Biomathematics with Statistics and Epidemiology from Dublin City University. In 2007 she was appointed by the Minister of Education and Science to serve on the board of The Irish Research Council for Science, Engineering and Technology (IRCSET). Catherine has over 20 years' research experience in statistics and mathematics applied to health care. As Director of Research and Professor of Healthcare Statistics at the School of Nursing and Midwifery she is responsible for developing and implementing the School's strategic plan for research and for advising, directing and promoting research. Her personal research interest is in longitudinal modelling of treatment and intervention outcomes, with a special interest in substance use, infectious diseases and outcomes in children, young people and adults. In 2011, she was nominated to serve as the inaugural Chairperson of the Children's Research Network of Ireland and Northern Ireland (CRNINI) and the inaugural Director of the Centre for Practice and Healthcare Innovation (CPHI) at Trinity College Dublin.

Siobhan Corrigan PhD, MSc, BSc

Siobhan is a Senior Research Fellow in the School of Psychology, Trinity College, University of Dublin, with over 15 years of continuous and successful engagement with industry (e.g. aerospace, manufacturing, pharmaceutical, health and process) on action-based and applied human factors research. Her current research projects involve: developing, implementing and sustaining change; developing a prototype management system for identifying and actively managing systemic risks; and the role of reflective leadership in nursing practice and education.

Gloria Crispino PhD, B Econ, Cstat, Cmath, MIMA

Gloria Crispino is a member of the Royal Statistical Society, a Chartered Statistician, a Chartered Mathematician and Lecturer of Statistics and Mathematics in the School of Science and Computing at Institute Technology Tallaght, Dublin, Ireland. Gloria holds a PhD in mathematical biology and biostatistics from ITT Dublin and a degree in Economics with major in statistics from L. Bocconi University, Milan, Italy. She has been working in biostatistics and mathematical biology research for over 15 years, in academia and industry, both in Europe and the USA. Her areas of research include medical statistics, clinical research, epidemiology, environmental health and mathematical biology. Her most recent publications include design, analysis and interpretation of large clinical studies in neurology, emergency medicine and paediatrics.

Orla Dempsey PhD, BA

Orla holds a BA degree in Mathematical Studies from the National University of Ireland, Maynooth, and completed her PhD in 2011 at Trinity College Dublin on modelling the prevalence, incidence and geographical spread of opiate use. She has gained valuable experience through teaching statistics to health care providers and has also presented her work at international conferences and the Conference of Applied Statistics in Ireland. She is the Practice Lead at the Centre for Practice and Healthcare Innovation at Trinity College Dublin. Her research interests include: addiction; inherited risk of substance use; mathematical models for substance use; and modelling health outcomes of substance users.

Suzanne Guerin PhD, BA

Suzanne Guerin is a Lecturer in Research Design and Analysis with the School of Psychology at University College Dublin. Suzanne teaches in the areas of applied psychology and research methods and has extensive experience in the delivery of modules at both undergraduate and postgraduate levels. Dr Guerin is also the Director of the Centre for Disability Studies at University College Dublin. Research interests include disability, well-being and applied research. Suzanne has extensive experience of working on university research ethics committees.

Maree Johnson BAppSci, MAppSci, PhD

Maree Johnson is a Clinical Professor in the School of Nursing & Midwifery at the University of Western Sydney. Maree has extensive teaching experience within undergraduate and postgraduate research units and supervision of Honours, Masters and PhD students in nursing and health. Professor Johnson has experience of quantitative and qualitative methodologies, systematic reviews and in the development and implementation of clinical guidelines in practice. Maree has published widely in refereed journals in nursing and health and is currently undertaking research in the areas of women's and children's health and patient safety.

Carmel Kelly PhD, MSc, BSc, RGN

Carmel Kelly is a Nurse Consultant in sexual health for the South Eastern Health and Social Care Trust in Northern Ireland and a research associate at the School of Nursing and Midwifery, Queen's University Belfast. She has specific research interests in HIV nursing, sexual health nursing and sexual risk-taking behaviour. As part of her PhD research, Carmel examined men and women's experiences of pregnancy affected by HIV and her findings have been published in *Culture Health and Sexuality*, *Journal of Clinical Nursing* and *Midwifery*. In addition, Carmel is leading the development of a UK-wide web-based education programme for health professionals on caring for HIV affected women and their partners during pregnancy.

Elaine Lehane PhD, MSc, BSc (Hons), Dip Nursing Studies, RGN

Elaine Lehane is a college lecturer at the Catherine McAuley School of Nursing and Midwifery, University College Cork, Ireland, and holds a BSc (Nursing), MSc (Clinical Nursing) and PhD. She has practised in both acute general surgical and medical units, and her clinical background underpins her research interests, which include patient adherence to therapeutic regimens, medication/health literacy and quality of life in chronic illness. Her research methodological area of expertise is psychometrics: specifically, looking at developing tools for understanding behaviour related to medication adherence.

Maria Lohan BA, PhD

Maria Lohan is a Senior Lecturer in Health Sciences in the School of Nursing and Midwifery, Queen's University Belfast. She is co-author of two books *Sociology for Health Professionals in Ireland* (IPA) and *Social Theory Health and Health Care* (Palgrave Macmillan) and is keenly interested in how social theory can be applied to understanding the social dimensions of health and healthcare. Maria's research on men's health and in particular on men's sexual and reproductive health is published in leading international journals such as *Social Science and Medicine* and *Journal of Adolescent Health*. She is currently a guest editor for a special issue of *Journal of Family Issues* on 'Men preparing for parenthood' and is leading an *Economic and Social Research Council* funded study on teenage men and pregnancy entitled 'If I were Jack' (see www.qub.ac.uk/IfIWereJack).

Susan McLaren PhD, BSc (Hons), RGN

Susan McLaren completed her RGN training at the Royal Sussex County Hospital, Brighton, and following this specialized in acute medical, intensive care and coronary care nursing. At the University of Newcastle upon Tyne she read physiology and subsequently took up an appointment as a Lecturer in Nursing Studies at the University of Surrey. While at Surrey she completed a PhD investigating nutritional and metabolic problems following acute stroke, eventually becoming Senior Lecturer and Deputy Head of the Nursing Studies department. Following this she was appointed to a Chair in Nursing at Kingston University and St Georges' Hospital Medical School Joint Faculty, leaving in 2003 to take up a post at London South Bank University (LSBU). At LSBU she became Director of the Institute for Strategic Leadership and Service Improvement, Pro-Dean Research and Professor of Nursing. Her current research interests focus on health services research and neurorehabilitation.

Deirdre Mongan

Deirdre Mongan works as a Research Officer in the Evidence Generation and Knowledge Brokering Unit of the Health Research Board in Dublin, where her role is to generate and synthesize evidence, and promote the application of knowledge to support decision making by policymakers. Her research also focuses on the prevalence of alcohol use and the health and social harms associated with alcohol use in Ireland. Prior to this, she attended the National University of Ireland Galway, where she obtained her PhD on cerebral palsy epidemiology in 2006.

Corina Naughton PhD, MSc (Epidemiology), RN

Corina Naughton is a Lecturer at the School of Nursing, Midwifery and Health Systems, University College Dublin. Corina has a particular interest in evaluation research and implementation science with a broad range of experience in evaluative research, audit, epidemiological studies and randomized controlled trials. Corina has conducted research into elder abuse, older people's experiences in emergency departments, nurse and midwifery prescribing, the impact of academic detailing on prescribing practice and patient outcomes from cardiac and non-cardiac surgery. The research findings derived from these studies have been disseminated through the media and high quality peer-reviewed journals such as Age and Aging, Journal of Advanced Nursing and The European Journal of Cardiothoracic Surgery.

Rhona O'Connell PhD, Med, BA, RGN, RM, RNT

Rhona O'Connell is a Lecturer in Midwifery in the Catherine McAuley School of Nursing and Midwifery, University College Cork. She has a PhD from the University of Central Lancashire and a master's degree from Trinity College Dublin. She has extensive experience in both midwifery education and practice, which includes neonatal care. Her research and teaching interests are in normal childbirth, woman-centred care, midwifery education and neonatal care. She has methodological expertise in hermeneutic phenomenology and metasynthesis. Rhona has collaborated in publications with nursing and midwifery colleagues and she has presented her work internationally. Rhona is a reviewer for international journals and conferences and has been a member of national advisory bodies for midwifery with the Department of Health and An Bord Altranais (Nursing Board).

Elaine Pierce PhD, BSc (Hons), ILM (level 3), RCNT, RGN, RN (RSA), RM (RSA)

Elaine Pierce is a principal lecturer and director for short programmes in the Institute for Leadership and Service Improvement, London South Bank University (LSBU). She trained as a general nurse, midwife, nurse teacher, and thereafter as a neuroscientist. She has previously worked in the field of neurosciences as a researcher, a research and development manager and as head of a research and development support unit. At LSBU, she lectures to MSc and professional doctorate students on research philosophies and methods of enquiry, delivering an evidence-based service and clinical audit. She also delivers clinical audit training and clinical effectiveness training through study days and bespoke courses to doctors, nurses and professionals allied to health at various National Health Service trusts and primary care trusts throughout London.

Gary Rolfe PhD, MA, BSc, RMN, PGCEA

Gary Rolfe took a degree in philosophy at Surrey University before training as a mental health nurse in the early 1980s. After working for several years in a therapeutic community for people with alcohol problems and in a nurse-led acute admission unit, he became a Lecturer in Nursing at Portsmouth University. Since taking up a Chair in Nursing at Swansea, Gary has devoted much of his time to establishing the Wales Centre for Practice Innovation. Gary has written widely in the fields of action research, nursing philosophy and reflective practice, and has published over 100 papers and ten books. Gary has an honorary Chair in Innovation and Development with his local Health Board, and is Visiting Professor at Trinity College Dublin and Canterbury Christ Church University.

Eileen Savage PhD, MEd, BNS, RGN, RCN

Eileen Savage is a Professor of Nursing at the Catherine McAuley School of Nursing and Midwifery, University College Cork. She leads a programme of research on chronic illness management with a special interest in quality of life, self and family management. She is Principal Investigator of funded studies involving national and international interdisciplinary collaborators. Her research appears in scholarly journals such as *Journal of Advanced Nursing, Journal of Clinical Nursing, Social Science and Medicine*, as well as in the Cochrane Library.

P. Anne Scott PhD, MSc, BA (Mod), RGN

Anne Scott is Professor of Nursing, former Head of the School of Nursing and Deputy President and Registrar in Dublin City University. She has also worked as a Senior Lecturer in the Department of Nursing and Midwifery, University of Stirling and as a lecturer in Glasgow Caledonian University and the University of Glasgow. Anne trained as a nurse in the west of Ireland, in Sligo General Hospital, and took her primary degree in Philosophy/Psychology in Trinity College Dublin. She then moved to the University of Edinburgh for her MSc (Nursing Education) and University of Glasgow, for her PhD in Health Care Ethics. Anne has worked clinically and as an academic in Ireland, Scotland and Kenya. She is a Fellow of the European Academy of Nursing Science and a member of the Philosophy and Ethics Committee, Royal Irish Academy. Anne was also a founding member of the Irish Council for Bioethics. Her research interests are in the philosophy and ethics of health care and in clinical judgement and decision making. She has published extensively in these and related fields.

Emma Stokes MSc (Management), PhD, MSc (Research), PG Dip Statistics, BSc (Physio)

Emma Stokes is a Lecturer, Researcher and Fellow of Trinity College Dublin. She is a physiotherapist who has presented her work nationally and internationally since the mid-1990s. Her research interests include professional practice issues and rehabilitation. She supervises master's and PhD students. She is the Vice-President of the World Confederation for Physical Therapy.

Roger Watson BSc, PhD, RN, FFNMRCSI, FRSA, FHEA, FEANS, FSB, FRCN, FAAN

Roger Watson is Professor of Nursing, University of Hull, UK and Professor of Nursing, University of Western Sydney, Australia and Editor-in-Chief, *Journal of Advanced Nursing*. His first degree in Biological Sciences was obtained from The University of Edinburgh and his PhD in Biochemistry from the University of Sheffield. Roger trained as a nurse at St George's Hospital, London and holds Honorary and Visiting positions in the UK, Australia, Hong Kong and China; areas of the world to which he is a frequent visitor. He was the first European elected a Fellow of the American Academy of Nursing. Following clinical work with older people, Roger has focused his research on the assessment and alleviation of feeding difficulty in older people with dementia. As a result he has developed an interest in psychometrics and is experienced in the application of multivariate statistical methods and item response theory, especially Mokken scaling, to large databases. He is author and editor of several books including *Anatomy and Physiology for Nurses 13th edition* (2011) and *Nursing Research: Design and Methods* (2008 with McKenna, Cowman & Keady).

Acknowledgements

The successful completion of this book owes much to several people.

First, we wish to express our sincere thanks and gratitude to all our colleagues and fellow academics who wrote chapters. We are only too aware of the demands on their time and appreciate their interest and commitment in working with us to get this book written.

Second, we would like to thank all our postgraduate students who, through their persistence, finally convinced us that this book was needed.

Third, we wish to acknowledge the work of the academics selected by the Open University Press to review the book proposal. We appreciate their input, and the constructive feedback provided was useful in revising the proposal.

Finally, we would like to extend our heartfelt thanks to Rachel Crookes and Abigail Jones from Open University Press. Their kindness, expert advice and insights enriched our thinking and helped shape the book into reality.

List of tables

List of figures

Introduction

Elizabeth A. Curtis and Jonathan Drennan

Background and rationale for the book

The idea for this book emerged from several sources: teaching, research, postgraduate students, and academic colleagues. The editors have extensive experience of teaching quantitative research methods to students at undergraduate and postgraduate levels. This teaching experience convinced us that there was a need for a textbook on research methods that would meet the needs of the busy postgraduate student, enabling them to develop and apply the theory of research to their professional practice. In particular, we identified that when students are completing a research project they have to deal with practical problems such as negotiating with ethics committees, applying theory to research problems, using designs other than randomized controlled trials and identifying statistical tests that would be suitable for analysing their data. In addition to teaching, we have undertaken several evaluations of master's degree programmes, and in particular the research components of these programmes. This work identified that students required assistance with the practical problems of research such as questionnaire design and distribution, probability sampling, and increasing response rates. These ideas and observations were confirmed in our discussions with academic colleagues here in Ireland and abroad. The fact that we were able to acquire so many distinguished academics to write chapters acknowledges the need for this book.

Aims

This book addresses issues in quantitative research methods. Our intention in putting it together was to provide a set of resource chapters to help you undertake your research project, whatever its purpose, by providing knowledge about the concepts, theories and issues relevant to quantitative research. The book also aims to present that knowledge in a way that facilitates learning and encourages further reading. It is important to stress, however, that the contents provided are not exhaustive, but we have done our best to include the main issues we consider important for helping you with your research project.

Readership

This book is intended for all health care professionals who are undertaking a postgraduate research degree, as well as researchers. It is also intended for practitioners who have to complete research as part of their professional role in health care. Researchers working in the field of health services research will find the book useful. Students from social science and psychological disciplines will also find benefit as the book discusses issues that are relevant to all researchers using quantitative designs.

Structure

For this book a structured academic style was used and the *stages of the research process* were used as a guide for sequencing chapters. The book consists of five parts and contains 20 chapters. Each chapter provides an overview of the theory behind the topic that is being discussed as well as practical examples of how the theory is applied in practice.

Part 1: Philosophy, theory, research problems and research questions

Part 1 introduces the reader to various concepts and issues that are essential to understanding and planning a quantitative research study. It contains four chapters.

- **Chapter 1: Philosophical basis for research**
  This chapter provides an introduction to the philosophical ideas, theories and terminology needed for understanding the processes of research. Main sections include: science philosophy and the origins of social research; the emergence of quantitative health research; towards a philosophy of quantitative research; and problematizing quantitative research.
- **Chapter 2: The importance and use of social theory in health care research**
  In Chapter 2, Maria Lohan and Carmel Kelly examine how theory, and in particular social theory, can provide a framework for health care research. The authors provide an overview of the principal social theories and how these theories have been used in quantitative research. This is followed by a practical example of how social theory influenced the design of a quantitative research study, including the development of hypotheses, the selection of measures and the interpretation of results. The authors conclude by demonstrating how social theory can be used in research to provide insights in the complex world of health care.
- **Chapter 3: Identifying research priorities**
  In this chapter Michelle Butler describes how to identify research topics that are relevant to health care. Approaches to identifying priorities for research such as the Delphi technique, the nominal group method and the listening model are discussed. In addition, other approaches to identifying sources for relevant research topics are outlined, including using stakeholders and referring to systematic reviews. This chapter takes you step by step through the processes of identifying areas for research and developing research questions and topics that are researchable and relevant for health care today.
- **Chapter 4: Writing research questions and hypotheses**
  In Chapter 4, Maree Johnson discusses how well-developed research questions and hypotheses are essential to the development of a research design. Providing examples from the literature, the author explores definitions of research questions and hypotheses and how these are used to design the sampling technique and approaches to data collection, as well as the analysis

procedures. The relationship between the research topic, research question or hypothesis and design are also discussed. In addition, definitions and examples of the types of hypotheses that a researcher may use are outlined as well as examples of their applicability to health care research.

Part 2: Ethical considerations

Part 2 reiterates the importance of ethics in research and examines key issues that all researchers encounter and have to address. It contains three chapters.

- **Chapter 5: Ethical principles in health care research**
  In Chapter 5, Anne Scott discusses in detail how ethical principles guide and inform health care research. The chapter is presented around the values and principles that are central to the conduct of research. The researcher is introduced to the key concepts that inform ethical practice in research, including respect for the person, informed consent, beneficence and non-maleficence, and justice. Ethical issues as they pertain to each stage of the research process are also outlined, including ethics and data analysis, ethics and the relationship between the researcher and research participant, and ethics and the dissemination of research findings. The chapter concludes by demonstrating how good ethical practice is essential in ensuring the development of high-quality evidence-based research.
- **Chapter 6: Communicating with research ethics committees**
  In Chapter 6, Suzanne Guerin comprehensively outlines the steps that a researcher must take when applying for ethical approval to a research ethics committee (REC) or an institutional review board (IRB). Using a practical example, the researcher is taken step by step through the ethics application process, including how to avoid the pitfalls that can commonly occur. The chapter, drawing on a body of literature in this area, discusses the role of RECs and IRBs, how to prepare your submission, issues regarding methodology and data protection that may arise during the process, submitting documentation and negotiating with committees.
- **Chapter 7: Recruiting samples from vulnerable populations**
  Many important decisions have to be made regarding potential respondents since it is unlikely that everyone in a given population can participate and the success of a study will hinge on those selected. This chapter begins with an explanation of the term 'vulnerability', and provides information on key issues that researchers must consider when using samples from vulnerable populations. Main sections include: types of vulnerability, regulations and guidelines on vulnerability; ethical issues surrounding the use of samples from vulnerable populations; concerns and problems with recruiting samples from vulnerable populations; strategies for improving the recruitment of samples from vulnerable groups; and the role of research ethics committees in protecting vulnerable populations.

Part 3: Quantitative research designs

Part 3 explores the philosophy underpinning the quantitative methodology and examines sampling issues as well as some of the less frequently used research designs in health care research. It contains six chapters.

- **Chapter 8: Designing and conducting quantitative research studies**
  Quantitative research is systematic, empirical and utilizes various methodological approaches and techniques. Main sections in this chapter include: positivism; deductive and inductive approaches; empirical data; why a quantitative research design; experimental research; the quantitative research process; and quantitative and qualitative research.
- **Chapter 9: Sampling issues in health care research**
  Questions such as 'what size should my sample be?' and 'what type of sampling design should I use?' are two of the most frequently asked questions in quantitative research. In Chapter 9, Gloria Crispino takes the researcher through the steps needed to understand sampling designs and sample size calculations. Starting from the research question, the author takes the researcher through the research design and the statistical analysis plan and shows how they are all interrelated in accurately computing a sample size. This chapter also discusses the reasoning that informs sampling and how sampling is related to inference. Using practical examples, various approaches to sample size calculation are presented.
- **Chapter 10: Planning and conducting surveys**
  This chapter begins with a historical overview of survey design before addressing contemporary designs. Main sections include: the planning of a survey; probability and non-probability sampling; survey methods; validity and reliability; limitations and strengths of survey approaches; and sources of error.
- **Chapter 11: Quasi-experimental and retrospective pretest designs for health care research**
  Increasingly, health care interventions and treatments are becoming more complex and researchers need to have access to designs that will allow them to effectively measure and evaluate these innovations. In Chapter 11, Jonathan Drennan discusses designs that researchers can use when it is not feasible or ethical to use a randomized controlled trial (RCT). These designs are quasi-experimental designs and the retrospective pretest design. Both designs are approaches that can be used in the field and are increasingly being used in health care research. The first section discusses quasi-experimental designs. This design is similar in many respects to randomized controlled trials, the fundamental difference being that subjects are not randomly allocated to the intervention or control group. In the second half of the chapter the author reports on an approach that is increasingly being used in health care research to measure the extent to which patients change over the course of a treatment. This approach is known as the retrospective pretest design and is sometimes used in conjunction with a quasi-experimental design.

- **Chapter 12: Audit in health care**

  In Chapter 12, Corina Naughton provides a comprehensive overview of a growing field in health care – audit. Many clinicians in health care are required to develop and carry out audits as part of their practice. Increasingly, practitioners are drawing on research principles to design audits. This chapter provides definitions of audit and compares and contrasts the audit process with research. The chapter also examines the role of health care practitioners in relation to audit and provides practical examples of the audit process, taking the reader through the stages involved in planning and designing an audit.

- **Chapter 13: Evaluation research**

  This chapter introduces the reader to the concept and purposes of evaluation and its importance in health care research. It begins by defining the term 'evaluation research', before moving on to distinguish between evaluation, audit and research. Main sections include: the importance and purposes of evaluation in health care; the importance of key stakeholders; types of evaluation; design principles; planning and carrying out evaluation research; and report planning and feedback of findings.

Part 4: Measurement and data collection

Part 4 discusses methods associated with measurement and collecting data in health care research. It moves from designing and pretesting questionnaires through to the steps required to ensure the measurement tools used are both valid and reliable.

- **Chapter 14: Using cognitive interviewing in health care research**

  In Chapter 14, Jonathan Drennan introduces a structured technique for developing and pretesting questionnaires that are used in health care research. Starting from the premise that research instruments are developed from the perspective of the researcher rather than the respondent, the author takes the reader step by step through the cognitive interviewing process. This method helps researchers to understand the cognitive processes used by respondents when they complete questions on survey instruments. The benefit of this approach to health care research is outlined and, drawing on the literature, the chapter demonstrates how this approach is beneficial when developing and/or testing questions with vulnerable groups.

- **Chapter 15: Questionnaires and instruments for health care research**

  This chapter reinforces the importance of using well-developed and accurate instruments when conducting quantitative research in health care. It begins by explaining the types and uses of measurement instruments in health care research, before discussing the conceptual issues for measurement. Other key sections in the chapter include: psychometric considerations for measurement; methodological considerations for measurement; practicalities of using instruments; and review of measurement instruments.

- **Chapter 16: Issues and debates in validity and reliability**
  In Chapter 16, Roger Watson provides a comprehensive overview of the concepts reliability and validity. The chapter discusses the concepts of psychometrics and measurement and provides examples of measurement in health care research. Types of reliability and validity are defined as well as the statistical approaches used to ascertain the psychometric properties of instruments. The integration of reliability and validity in the testing of instruments used in health care research is discussed as well as techniques that are emerging in the field.

Part 5: Analysing and presenting data

Part 5 addresses a number of issues important to the quantitative researcher that are not often discussed adequately in many research texts that we have reviewed. It contains four chapters.

- **Chapter 17: Understanding probability**
  This chapter demonstrates the significance of probability to evidence-based decision making in health care by providing students with a step-by-step guide with practical-based examples on the key concepts, rules and calculations of probability in applied health care research. Main sections include: definition of probability; basic terminology; rules of probability; conditional and joint probabilities; applying probabilities to data analyses; and sampling methods.
- **Chapter 18: Analysing data from small and large samples and non-normal and normal distributions**
  In phase one clinical trials, smaller-scale studies or studies dealing with sensitive topics the number of cases can be quite small and the data obtained may not have a normal distribution. Also, data arising from a large study may have some key variables with a non-normal distribution. This chapter addresses the different data types and discusses a range of methods for analysing data from large- and small-scale studies.
- **Chapter 19: Secondary data analysis**
  Secondary data analysis uses pre-existing data to explore newly formulated research questions. It is rarely used by post-graduate students to as a method for conducting research. Several factors may contribute to this, and some of these are explored in this chapter. Main sections addressed include: advantages and disadvantages of secondary data analysis; locating datasets for secondary data analysis; ethical issues; how to determine the feasibility and suitability of using a dataset for secondary analysis; analysing secondary data; and examples of secondary datasets.
- **Chapter 20: Presenting your research findings**
  There is no point in conducting a thorough analysis of data obtained from a research study if the findings are then presented inadequately. Researchers must be able to transform raw data into findings that are meaningful and

be able to convey this information succinctly. Several approaches are available to the researcher for presenting data. The chapter addresses some of these approaches. Main sections include: presenting research findings in a dissertation or thesis; presenting research findings at conferences; presentation formats; poster presentations; and oral presentations.

Presentation

We hope that the style in which the content is presented in this book will help you plan and undertake your research project successfully as well as assist learning and encourage further reading. All chapters outline the key themes addressed using bulleted points. Diagrams and tables are used where appropriate to help explain concepts and illustrate points or examples being discussed. At the end of every chapter the author(s) summarize(s) the key concepts/points addressed, provide(s) key readings on the topic, give(s) examples of relevant research studies, list(s) useful websites and provide(s) a list of references.

PART 1

Philosophy, theory, research problems and research questions

1 Philosophical basis for research

Gary Rolfe

Chapter topics

- The origins and history of scientific research
- The emergence of quantitative social research
- Experimental design, statistics and evidence
- Direct and critical realism
- Problems and issues:
  - The problem of induction
  - Reductionism
  - Statistical and clinical significance

Introduction

There is a growing tendency nowadays to regard research simply as a procedure for which people can be 'trained', with rules and guidelines governing every aspect from submitting the research proposal to writing the final report. This can be seen even at the highest academic level, where doctoral programmes are often referred to as 'research training'. This is particularly true in the field of quantitative research, where the rigorous adherence to protocols is seen as the guarantor of validity, and where many journals now impose a regulation format on the presentation of findings, which can influence the design of the study. However, while it might be convenient to think of research as a more or less mechanical procedure, many experienced researchers consider it to be a *practice*, not dissimilar to the practice of nursing or medicine, in which every new situation throws up fresh challenges and where the standard procedures often need to be modified and improvised in order to take account of unexpected developments. It is therefore necessary for researchers to think on their feet: when faced with new and uncertain situations which cannot be resolved by applying established protocols, practitioners are forced to go back to first principles, and this requires an understanding of the fundamental philosophical assumptions which underpin research methods, methodologies and paradigms.

This introductory chapter therefore provides researchers with some of the basic philosophical ideas, theories and terminology necessary for an understanding of how research 'works' so that they are able to make informed decisions about how far and in which directions they are permitted to stray from the narrow path of protocol without compromising the validity and integrity of the project. As with most areas of philosophy, the philosophy of science needs to be set in a historical context to fully understand the current issues and recent innovations in the field. This chapter therefore begins by tracing the historical development of the scientific method, with particular emphasis on the emergence of the social sciences and quantitative research methodologies. It continues with a brief overview of the philosophical assumptions of the quantitative research paradigm and the 'direct realist' and 'critical realist' theories on which much contemporary thinking in quantitative research is founded. Finally, it examines some of the philosophical and practical issues and problems that quantitative researchers are likely to encounter at some time during their research careers.

Science, philosophy and the origins of social research

The origins of what we now think of as empirical scientific research are usually traced back to the seventeenth century and the work of Francis Bacon, Galileo Galilei and Isaac Newton. In a series of works beginning with *Novum Organum* (New Method) in 1620, Bacon outlined the founding principles of his 'new philosophy' based on a systematic form of inductive reasoning developed from Galileo's earlier work. The method of induction entails the collection of facts about the world to build up a picture based on past observations, which will then allow us to make predictions about what is likely to happen in the future. For example, Galileo observed and collated observations of the movements of the planets and stars to verify Copernicus's theory that the Earth revolves around the Sun, which also enabled him to predict future events such as solar eclipses. However, it was Bacon who formulated a scientific method which allowed the researcher to identify, and to some extent control, certain variables while observing and measuring the effects on others. This empirical method was later adopted so successfully by Newton and other prominent scientists in the late seventeenth century that it became the blueprint for experimental research for the next hundred years, and was largely responsible for initiating and driving the industrial revolution of the eighteenth and nineteenth centuries. Although we would now recognize this inductive method of data collection and analysis as the origins of modern science, the term was not used in this way at the time. Newton, Bacon and Galileo would have referred to themselves as 'natural philosophers', and the word 'science', which at the time simply meant 'knowledge', did not acquire its modern usage until the early years of the nineteenth century (Gower 1997; Okasha 2002).

The origins of the social sciences

In 1830, the French philosopher Auguste Comte first applied this scientific method to the newly established 'social sciences', a term coined by William Thompson six years earlier, referring to his attempts as the 'positive philosophy', 'a positive science of society', or simply as **positivism** (see Box 1.1) (Comte [1830] 1988). Comte argued that human knowledge passes through three stages: theological, philosophical and scientific. In the first two stages, the mind 'directs its researches mainly toward the inner nature of beings, and toward the first and final causes of all the phenomena that it observes – in a word, toward absolute knowledge' (Comte [1830] 1988: 2). However, this quest for 'absolute knowledge' is metaphysical rather than scientific, and the characteristic of the scientific or 'positive' state of mind is the recognition of the impossibility of obtaining absolute truth. The positivist method, then, 'endeavours now only to discover, by a well-combined use of reasoning and observation, the

---

Box 1.1   Positivism

The term 'positivism' is often used to describe the philosophy underpinning quantitative research. It was first used by Auguste Comte in an attempt to unite the natural and social sciences under a common philosophy and scientific method, and maintained that the aim and purpose of social research was the discovery of the natural laws governing human behaviour through the collection and analysis of empirical data. Comte believed that the search for first causes should be left to religion or metaphysics (literally, that which is *beyond* the remit of physics) and that positivism should restrict itself to simple associations between measurable variables. The term is nowadays used in a much wider and more general sense than Comte's original formulation, often to refer simply to the collection of quantitative data through the methods of science. It is also sometimes confused with the philosophical movement of logical positivism, to which it is related but from which it is substantially different (Stadler 2012).

---

actual laws of phenomena' (Comte [1830] 1988: 2). In other words, Comte's positivist science was concerned only with establishing observable empirical relationships or laws between phenomena, and abandoned completely any attempt to explore or explain the inner workings of people or societies. Thus:

> The fundamental character of the positive philosophy is to consider all phenomena as subject to invariable natural laws. The exact discovery of these laws and their reduction to the least possible number constitute the goal of all our efforts; for we regard the search after what are called causes, whether first or final, as absolutely inaccessible and unmeaning. (Comte [1830] 1988: 8)

The positivists approached the study of people in the same way that nineteenth-century physicists approached the study of inanimate materials. J.S. Mill, an early advocate of positivism, argued that 'the phenomena of human thought, feeling and action are subject to fixed laws' (Mill [1843] 2001: 572), and believed that, by discovering these laws, the social scientist would be able to predict and control human behaviour in the same way the physicist could predict and control the behaviour of inorganic matter.

Although positivism was developed in an attempt to emulate the successes being enjoyed at the time by the physical sciences, the positivist method was quite different from the experimental method of physics and chemistry. In the physical sciences, a single experiment is enough to establish or test a general law. For example, if we wish to discover the boiling point of a particular liquid, we need only heat a single sample and measure the temperature at which it boils. If we wish to discover how its boiling point varies with altitude, we need only conduct the experiment once at each of a variety of different locations. If the experiment *is* repeated, it will be to check for accuracy (reliability) rather than in the expectation that a second or third sample will behave differently from the first.

However, whereas samples of a particular liquid (or, indeed, any inorganic substance) are assumed to behave identically to one another, at least at the 'macro' everyday level,[1] the same principle cannot be applied to living beings, and particularly to people. If we wish to discover how *people* react to increased temperature, we cannot simply observe one individual and generalize to a population or a social law. Rather, we must measure the individual responses of a large number of people and calculate an *average* score, or else observe several individuals and collect their responses into general categories or themes. For example, the French sociologist Émile Durkheim used data on the average rates of suicide for a number of European countries to arrive at the general theory that suicide occurs (at least partly) as a result of weak levels of social control and low levels of social integration. Clearly, these conclusions could not have been derived from the observation of single cases or small numbers, but rely on large and statistically significant samples (Durkheim [1897] 2006).

While Durkheim, Mill and others embraced Comte's 'positive philosophy' and set about developing a quantitative human science paradigm modelled on the physical sciences, others reacted against it. For example, the German philosopher and historian Wilhelm Dilthey (pronounced *Dil-tay*) argued that the social sciences are *fundamentally* different from physics and chemistry, and suggested that whereas the aim of the physical sciences is to *explain* phenomena in terms of cause and effect (*Erklären*), the social sciences seek to *understand* (*Verstehen*) on a deeper and more personal level (Dilthey [1900] 1976). This alternative paradigm to positivist science was developed most notably by Max Weber (pronounced *Vay-ber*), who urged sociologists to go beyond scientific explanation to 'accomplish something that is never attainable in the natural sciences, namely the subjective understanding of the action of the component individuals' (Weber [1922] 1992: 13). While Mill and Comte adopted a more or less determinist view that human beings are subject to invariable laws which govern their behaviour, Weber, Dilthey and others took the opposing view that these so-called 'laws' were no more than narrative accounts of human activity; that is to say, social and psychological theories are *descriptive* rather than *causal*.

By the early years of the twentieth century, two distinct approaches could clearly be discerned in the rapidly developing discipline of social research. On one side stood hermeneutics, ethnography, phenomenology and other so-called 'qualitative' approaches, whose principal methods involved the collection and analysis of data in the form of *text*, in order to describe and understand human behaviour and social phenomena. On the other side stood the positivist methods which mostly involved the collection and statistical analysis of *numerical* data in order to explain the workings of the social world. And whereas the phenomenologists and ethnographers emphasized a subjective hermeneutic understanding of one human being by another, the positivists placed great value on objectivity and a detached 'scientific'

---

[1]At the molecular level many substances display random behaviour (for example, Brownian motion in gases and liquids), and at the atomic and subatomic levels they appear sometimes to defy the currently accepted physical laws of the universe.

perspective, to the extent that 'the first and most fundamental rule is: consider social facts as things' (Durkheim [1895] 1964: 14).

This quantitative positivist approach dominated the social sciences for most of the first half of the twentieth century. In the UK, the 1920s and 1930s saw large-scale social surveys being conducted in many industrialized towns and cities, including London, Tyneside, Sheffield, Southampton and Merseyside (Moser 1967: 18), culminating in 1941 with the establishment of the Government Social Survey, whose role (as its name suggests) was to carry out large-scale surveys on behalf of the state. The main exception to this trend towards a macro-level quantitative social research paradigm concerned with demographics, town planning and (increasingly) market research came from the discipline of anthropology, where small fieldwork studies employing an ethnographic methodology were the norm. While many early ethnographic studies were conducted in exotic overseas locations (see, for example, the work of Radcliffe-Brown 1948, Malinowski 1922 and Mead 1943), anthropology has more recently 'come home' as more and more researchers look towards aspects of their own cultures for social groups and issues to study. Although the Chicago School of sociologists had been conducting studies of their local area since the 1920s, it was only in the 1950s and 1960s that qualitative field study research began to offer a serious challenge to the dominant statistical paradigm. This, in turn, reignited an interest in phenomenology, hermeneutics, critical theory and other philosophical theories of social science, and a number of researchers set to work translating these theoretical positions into empirical research methodologies and methods.

In the last 30 years, other approaches to social research have been introduced from outside the mainstream philosophical and sociological traditions, including semiotics, post-structural literary criticism, feminist theory, postcolonialism and deconstruction, giving way to a so-called 'post-positivist' era (Sarantakos 1993: 6). Thus:

> Sociological methodology is no longer a uniform body of theory and research based on positivism only, as it was in the past, but a body of diverse methodologies with diverse theoretical backgrounds and diverse methods and techniques, all of which appear to be considered equally acceptable, equally valid and equally legitimate. (Sarantakos 1993: 6)

In the face of this enormous variety of methods, methodologies and competing paradigms, a growing number of researchers are now adopting what has come to be known as a 'mixed-methods' approach in which a number of qualitative and quantitative methods are integrated into a philosophically and methodologically coherent research design (Cresswell 2008; Cresswell and Plano Clark 2010).

The emergence of quantitative health research

The development of what we now think of as quantitative health research resulted from the coming together of two quite separate programmes of work, each of which predates the origins of sociological research in the mid-nineteenth century.

Descriptive statistics and public health

The first of these was the collation and interpretation of statistical (from the Latin *statisticus* – relating to politics and the state) information about the population. The German term *Statistik* was first used in the mid-eighteenth century and was introduced into the English language in 1791 by Sir John Sinclair with his *Statistical Account of Scotland*. One of the most notable of the early exponents of statistics in health research was Florence Nightingale, who pioneered the use of graphical representation of numerical data to illustrate both the effects of poor sanitation (for example, on mortality rates – see Figure 1.1) and also to demonstrate the improvements that her reforms brought about (Nightingale 1858).

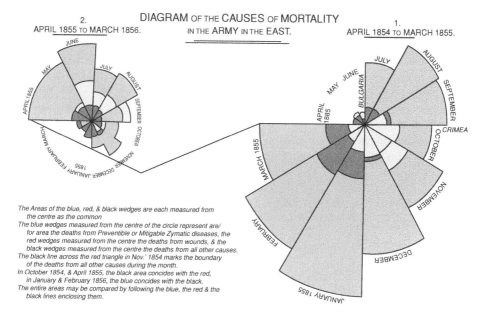

Figure 1.1 Nightingale's circular histogram of the causes of mortality in the Army in the East.

The early Victorians tended to treat the collection and display of statistics in a somewhat unsystematic and ad hoc way, and it was only after Comte had called for a 'positive science' based on careful reasoning and systematic observation that the idea of quantitative data collection and analysis developed from a descriptive account of the social world to an analytic tool for building theories and testing hypotheses. As we have seen, the collection and analysis of demographic and other descriptive statistical data came to prominence during the first half of the twentieth century, where it was employed in the planning of public and social services, as well as for commercial enterprises such as market research. As statistical tests became more and more sophisticated, the findings from surveys and censuses could be used not only to describe the demographic and other properties of a population, but increasingly to compare, predict and model the behaviour of subgroups within that population. Statistical tests can be used, for example, to determine the likelihood that a sample is representative of a larger population, to calculate the degree of association or difference between and within groups, and to make predictions or inferences based on limited or incomplete data.

Inferential statistics and controlled experiments

The second strand of thought leading to the development of modern quantitative health research was the theory of **experimental** design. Health-related **quasi-experiments** involving control and comparison have been an integral part of medical treatment throughout its long history, and gradually increased in sophistication. James Lind carried out a controlled experiment to determine the causes and treatment of scurvy as early as 1757. But it was the American philosopher and polymath C.S. Peirce (pronounced *Purse*) who, in the 1870s and 1880s, introduced and refined many of the experimental designs and methods of data analysis that led to the development of the modern idea of inferential quantitative research, in particular the double-blinded **randomized controlled trial** (RCT) (see Box 1.2). In two groundbreaking publications, Peirce ([1879, 1883] 1992) introduced the concept of blinded experiments, refined the idea of statistical confidence, and made an important contribution to data modelling and regression analysis.

Box 1.2 Experimental design

While the term 'experiment' is used rather loosely by scientists to describe a wide variety of work, social scientists usually employ the term more specifically to refer to a research design in which all variables apart from one are controlled or kept constant. Looser forms of experimental design are often referred to as 'quasi-experiments'. The experiment is the methodology of choice if the researcher wishes to establish causality (for example, to show that smoking causes lung cancer), since by only allowing a single variable to change over time any effect can be attributed solely to that variable. The most powerful and highly regarded experimental design used in health research is the randomized controlled trial (RCT). This design compares the measured outcomes from two or more groups (an experimental group and one or more control groups), to which subjects are randomly allocated. All variables are matched across all groups apart from the intervention, which is given to the experimental group but not to the control group(s). The design usually involves double blinding, in which neither the experimenters nor the subjects know which group they are allocated to. This often entails the administration of placebos to one or more control groups, thus ensuring that no one involved in the trial is aware of whether or not they are receiving the treatment (Campbell and Stanley 1963).

Although the RCT is nowadays most commonly associated with medical research, its first applications were in agriculture, where it was developed by the geneticist and statistician R.A. Fisher during the 1930s as a method for comparing crop treatments (Fisher 1935). The first published example of an RCT in the field of medicine appeared in the 1948 paper entitled 'Streptomycin treatment of pulmonary tuberculosis' (Streptomycin in Tuberculosis Trials Committee 1948). During the 1960s and 1970s a number of medical practitioners, including Archie Cochrane, became frustrated both at the paucity of RCTs on which to base their practice and also at the lack of any systematic collation and organization of them (Cochrane 1972). As a direct result of his work, the Cochrane Library was founded in the late 1980s as a database of systematic reviews and meta-analyses of RCTs. The launch of the evidence-based medicine movement, with the RCT as its 'gold standard' source of evidence (see Table 1.1), rapidly followed (Evidence-Based Medicine Working Group 1992) and has grown to become a dominant influence not only in medicine but across all of the health and social care disciplines.

Table 1.1 A hierarchy of evidence for therapeutic and preventative interventions (Oxford Centre for Evidence-Based Medicine 2009)

Level	Type of evidence
1a	Systematic review of RCTs
1b	Individual RCT
1c	All or none case-series
2a	Systematic review of cohort studies
2b	Individual cohort study (including low-quality RCT; e.g. <80% follow-up)
2c	'Outcomes' research; ecological studies
3a	Systematic review of case-control studies
3b	Individual case-control study
4	Case-series (and poor quality cohort and case-control studies)
5	Expert opinion without explicit critical appraisal, or based on physiology, bench research or 'first principles'

Towards a philosophy of quantitative research

What is quantitative research?

These two strands of descriptive, survey-based social enquiry and controlled experimentation together constitute what is now usually referred to as quantitative health research. However, although there is a general agreement that the term refers in some way to research that involves the collection, manipulation and analysis of numerical data, there remains some confusion about precisely what it means. Most simple descriptions of quantitative research define it almost exclusively in terms of the methods used to collect and analyse the data. For example, the evidence-based medicine online journal *Bandolier* states that 'Quantitative research generates numerical data or data that can be converted into numbers, for example clinical trials or the National Census, which counts people and households' (Bandolier 2012), while a nursing research text adds that 'Quantitative research is a formal, objective, systematic process in which numerical data are used to obtain information about the world' (Burns and Grove 2008: 27)

Many of these simple definitions point out that quantitative research methods are best suited to answering particular kinds of research question. For example, Shields and Twycross (2003: 24) suggest that 'At the most basic level, quantitative research methods are used when something needs to be measured, while qualitative methods are used when a question needs to be described and investigated in some depth'. They continue: 'Often, the two methods are used in tandem to provide measurements for comparison and evaluation and to give an in-depth explanation of the meaning of an idea'. These definitions regard quantitative and qualitative research as simply different tools for the collection of data, and the choice of which to use therefore depends almost entirely on the kind of data or information required to answer a particular research question. As Shields and Twycross point out, there is a growing tendency nowadays to employ both quantitative and qualitative tools in the same 'mixed-methods' study. Burnard et al. (2011) have summarized these simple descriptions and definitions into seven features of quantitative research, including the design of experiments to establish and test laws and hypotheses, the use of tests, scales and statistical methods to gather and analyse numerical data, and an emphasis on objectivity, validity and reliability.

Other writers take issue with the idea that quantitative research can be defined simply in terms of the methods it employs to collect data, and suggest that its defining features are *epistemological* rather than pragmatic. That is to say, the starting point when designing a research study is not with practical issues of how best to collect the data required to answer a particular research question, but with more fundamental concerns about the very nature of knowledge itself. This provides an altogether different perspective on the meaning of quantitative (and, of course, qualitative) research, and takes it into the realms of philosophical enquiry. From this perspective, quantitative research is not defined simply by its methods, but according to deeper considerations about the nature of knowledge and how it might most effectively be collected, analysed and disseminated. When making decisions about research methods and methodologies, the issue is not just a question of data collection or even of study design, but rather of what can be known about the world, what it means to know it, and how that knowledge can best be obtained.

The quantitative research paradigm

All researchers work within frameworks or paradigms of underpinning philosophical assumptions about the nature of knowledge (epistemology), the nature of reality (ontology) and the philosophy of science, even though they will not necessarily be aware of them, and might not even claim to hold them. Powers and Knapp (2006) define a paradigm as an organizing framework that contains:

- concepts, theories, assumptions, beliefs, values and principles that form a way for a discipline to interpret the subject matter with which it is concerned
- research methods considered to be best suited to generating knowledge within this frame of reference
- what is open to investigation – priorities and views on knowledge deficit areas where research and theory-building are most needed
- what is closed to enquiry for a time

Many disciplines and professions contribute to health care research, and each has one or more preferred or 'dominant' paradigms along with a number of other competing paradigms, each with its own assumptions, beliefs and values which it holds to be true. While ideas and definitions of quantitative research will vary from discipline to discipline, the epistemological values and beliefs held by quantitative researchers might include some or all of the following assumptions:

- The world is more or less directly observable and hence knowable.
- Accurate observation and measurement of the world is possible.
- Knowledge about the world is largely independent of the individual observer.
- Subjective internal states such as feelings, attitudes, perceptions and beliefs can be operationalized and objectified by translating them into numerical data.
- These numerical data are objective representations of those states rather than subjective constructs.
- These data can be combined, manipulated and displayed graphically while retaining an objective relationship to the internal states from which they originated.
- Knowledge gathered from artificially constructed and controlled environments can be more accurate and more useful than knowledge from observations of 'real life'.
- It is possible in certain controlled situations to generalize from relatively small samples to large populations, and subsequently to make accurate and meaningful assumptions about individuals based on those generalizations.

Put simply, the quantitative paradigm regards research as a sort of mapping or modelling exercise in which aspects of the world can be accurately represented in numerical form, and the resulting map or model is then deployed to make further discoveries and test new hypotheses, which can be used better to find our way around the real world (Toulmin 1953).

Not all quantitative researchers will hold all of these beliefs, nor will they necessarily be aware of them. Some might claim that these philosophical assumptions are irrelevant or insist that they do not subscribe to any of them. Others might strongly believe them to be true and take exception to them being referred to as merely beliefs or assumptions. However, whatever views about these philosophical beliefs are expressed, almost everyone brings with them some underlying ideas and concepts about the theory and practice of research in terms of beliefs about what counts as knowledge and how best to obtain it. In some cases these philosophical views will be apparent at the outset and will lead them to gravitate towards particular research paradigms, whereas in others the philosophical position of the researcher will only become evident as the study progresses.

A realist ontology

The choice of the research methods and methodologies we use to gain knowledge about the world depends to a large extent on what we consider to be our relationship to 'reality' – that is, to what extent we perceive the world as it really is. This is to some extent an ontological issue in so far as it is concerned with the question of 'being'.

The common sense view of our experience of the world is that we perceive it more or less as it really is; that is to say, the world and everything in it exists 'out there' independently of our experience of it. This view is known as 'realism', and in its simplest form it states that we can obtain accurate and direct knowledge of objects in the world (including people) through our senses. In other words, when I observe a tree or a person I am collecting accurate information about their various physical properties which I can use to build up a picture of them, and this picture corresponds more or less to what they are 'really' like. Research is therefore simply a matter of looking, measuring and recording our measurements (Cole 2002).

While this 'direct realist' idea of the world might on first sight seem appealing, it quickly becomes apparent that we do not have such a simple and direct access to reality, and that things are not always exactly as they seem to us. For example, we know that objects can appear to change colour depending on the ambient light, can seem hotter or colder to the touch depending on our own skin temperature, and seem to shrink in size as they move away from us. From a direct realist perspective, if the properties of objects appear to change over time, then either the objects really are changing or else we do not perceive the world directly and cannot rely entirely on our senses to provide us with accurate knowledge about the external world. Since very few people would concede that objects really do become smaller as they recede into the distance, direct realism is not often advanced as a serious philosophical position. In terms of the design of research projects, this suggests that direct observation of the world does not guarantee valid and reliable data, and so our methods of data collection have to take into account the fact that seeing is not always believing (Box 1.3).

The philosopher Roy Bhaskar (1979, 1989) addressed this challenge to empirical science in the 1970s and 1980s and proposed a 'critical realism' that combined realist experimentation (what he called 'transcendental realism') with an acknowledgement that research conducted on, with and by people occurred within social structures and communities ('critical naturalism') that influenced and distorted the straightforward collection and interpretation of data. Put simply, Bhaskar's combination of *critical* naturalism with transcendental *realism* states that there is an independent reality 'out there', but that certain aspects of it are not available or amenable to direct observation and can only be perceived indirectly. He therefore offers 'a coherent account of the nature of nature, society, human agency and philosophy' (Bhaskar 1989: 190)

Box 1.3 Example from the published literature: Durkheim's study of suicide

---

It might appear on first sight that rates of suicide would be one of the simplest and most objective variables to collate, compare and analyse. In Durkheim's famous study of suicide (Durkheim [1897] 2006), he compared rates in a variety of European countries and concluded that suicide rates in Catholic countries were lower than those in Protestant countries. From this analysis, he constructed an elaborate theory about social cohesion and anomie based on the premise that familial and social bonds were looser in Protestant countries, leading to greater alienation, less social support, and hence greater numbers of suicides. However, Durkheim's study was subsequently heavily criticized on the grounds that his primary data were not, in fact, measuring what he thought they were. Durkheim worked on the direct realist assumption that it is possible to gain direct and accurate access to the 'real' social world – that is to say, that published statistics for suicide are a direct measure of the number of people who had taken their own lives. However, it is clear that, in many cases, the only person who can know whether a death really was an intentional suicide is now dead, and so the suicide rate for a particular country is *not* a direct measure of death by suicide, but rather an *interpretation* by a coroner of the intent of a dead person, who cannot be called upon to verify its accuracy. Thus, Durkheim was not measuring what he thought he was, and the differences he found between recorded rates of suicide in Catholic and Protestant countries are usually attributed to the reluctance of Catholic coroners to attribute a mortal sin to a dead person.

---

as a framework to assist the researcher with this interpretive (re)construction of reality. Critical realism is therefore, at the same time, an acknowledgement of the limitations of direct realism and a strategy for overcoming them.

For example, early IQ (intelligence quotient) tests were considered to be objective and scientific measures of intelligence, and were used for many years to make important and often life-changing decisions, such as whether children in the UK were sent to grammar or secondary modern schools. Educationalists and psychologists would talk and act as though IQ scores and intelligence were the same thing, leading to beliefs that different social classes, nationalities, races and sexes had different mean levels of intelligence, and to various theories about why such differences might exist. In some cases, these theories would lead to negative discrimination and exclusion, and in other cases to positive discrimination and inclusion, but in all cases it was assumed that IQ scores were real and accurate measures of a real phenomenon.

However, whereas the direct realist would believe and act as if the IQ score was an objective and more or less accurate indication of intelligence, and whereas the qualitative researcher might suggest that intelligence is no more than a social or psychological construct which has no objective reality, the critical realist would accept the 'reality' of IQ but would bring into play a number of other influences and factors such as the vocabulary and language skills of the child, their class and cultural background, and any other prevailing social, psychological and environmental conditions. That is to say, critical realists would accept that IQ tests are flawed and biased towards certain groups and types and would make allowances for these extraneous variables. More generally, they would make the distinction between the map (the representation of reality) and the territory (reality itself) and would be careful not to confuse the numerical score from an IQ test with the actual level of intelligence. Furthermore, they would not wish to be seduced into thinking that a numerical score is necessarily more *objective* or *accurate* than a verbal account or some other non-numerical expression of intelligence, but would acknowledge that it is simply the most *convenient* way of thinking and acting when dealing with large groups (Gould 1996).

Problematizing quantitative research

Critical realism is nowadays considered to be the most common philosophical position of scientists, and particularly of quantitative scientific researchers, since it provides some useful middle ground between the direct or naive realism of 'what you see is what you get' and the out-and-out scepticism of the anti-realists, for whom the entire social world is a series of social and psychological constructs. However, a critical realist stance introduces a number of challenges and caveats into the process of designing, conducting, interpreting and applying research.

The problem of induction

Firstly, we must bear in mind the inherent limitations of the scientific method regardless of our chosen research approach. Chief among these is what has been known for centuries as the problem of induction, and which is usually associated with the Scottish empiricist David Hume (1711–76). Stated briefly and simply, the problem of induction points out that we cannot predict future outcomes based solely on observations of past occurrences. To take a commonly used example, just because each and every swan that I have ever observed has been white, I am not logically justified in predicting that the next swan I see will also be white, nor indeed that all swans are white. While this might not present a problem to me in everyday life (after all, there is a high probability that the next swan I see *will* be white), it nevertheless precludes me from generalizing from my observations of swans to the theory that *all* swans are white. Similarly, the fact that a new drug has been tested on a thousand (or even a million) people and has been found to produce no harmful side effects does not enable me to derive the general statement that this drug has no harmful side effects. Furthermore, Hume argued that the number of positive cases is irrelevant; it matters not whether the drug is tested on a hundred, a thousand or a million subjects, its effect on the next patient is equally uncertain. So, for example, the number of white swans in the world (and hence, the number available to be seen) is irrelevant to whether or not there are also black swans.

Hypothetico-deductivism and falsificationism

It could be (and has been) argued that the problem of induction exposes a fatal flaw in the logic of scientific discovery, since it implies that we can never know anything for certain. It would not matter how many apples Newton saw falling to the ground, he could never induce from these observations the universal law that all objects fall to the ground. It is notable, then, that the most famous response to the problem of induction was concerned less with refuting it than with distancing it from the scientific method. In his book *The Logic of Scientific Discovery*, the philosopher of science Karl Popper ([1935] 2002) did not deny that there is a problem with the method of induction, but insisted rather that induction plays no substantive part in the scientific method. In its place, Popper proposed the method of hypothetico-deductivism, in which hypotheses are formulated, consequences of these hypotheses are deduced, and experiments or observations are carried out to establish whether the proposed consequences occur. For example, Einstein hypothesized that light is subject to the force of gravity (Einstein [1916] 2001: 76). From this hypothesis, it was deduced that light travelling from distant stars would be bent as it passed through the gravitational field of the sun, and an experiment was later conducted to test out this prediction during an eclipse, when light from stars passing close to the sun could be observed.

As Popper points out, however, the fact that Einstein's hypothesis was confirmed does not *prove* his theory of gravity, but merely fails to disprove it. Thus, for Popper, science should not be concerned with attempting to prove theories, which is in any case impossible, but with trying our hardest to *disprove* them. The harder we try – and fail – to refute a hypothesis, the more confidence we can have in it. However, we can never have absolute faith in any theory, since it is always possible that the next experiment will disconfirm it. Thus, one of the more shocking consequences of Popper's hypothetico-deductivism is that there is no such thing as a scientific law; the best we have are theories which have so far resisted attempts to refute them. Thus, he cautions: 'we must regard all laws or theories as hypothetical or conjectural; that is, as guesses' (Popper 1979: 9).

This conjectural nature of scientific research is often forgotten. For example, we talk about the laws of physics as if they are immutable and fixed, forgetting that much of the 'certain knowledge' of previous ages has now been replaced by new and more up-to-date 'certain knowledge', which is likely in turn to be overturned by new 'certainties' as science continues its hypothetico-deductive project of refutation and falsificationism.

Reductionism

It could be argued that a great deal of quantitative health care research is not experimental and therefore falls outside of Popper's logic of scientific discovery. While few researchers are engaged in the exciting process of discovering new health care interventions, many others are involved in what Thomas Kuhn (1962) called 'normal science' – in this case, testing those interventions for efficacy and safety. This activity largely involves working with small samples and generalizing, through the logic of induction and the use of increasingly sophisticated statistical tests, to much larger populations, and it introduces a number of pitfalls for the unwary researcher. Firstly, it usually involves measurement and comparison, which means that outcome measures must be presented in a numerical format that is amenable to statistical manipulation and testing. Since not all variables can be enumerated in this way, quantitative researchers are immediately presented with a number of limitations on the scope of their work. Any translation of variables into numerical data inevitably entails a reduction and irretrievable loss of information. For example, asking respondents to express their attitudes on a five-point Likert scale reduces the vast range and richness of their responses to a number between one and five. While it might be possible to recover some of this information through a mixed-methods approach, almost all quantitative health and social research is, by its very nature, reductionist.

Distinguishing between what can be counted and what counts

This reduction of aspects of the social world to numerical data inevitably leads to other challenges. On the one hand, the researcher must constantly bear in mind that the numbers have no external reality outside of the research study. While it might be tempting to think and write about (say) an attitude score of four as referring to something concrete and objective, it should never be forgotten that this is simply a subjective and simplified interpretation of a complex and often volatile internal state. On the other hand, we must take care not to confuse what is most easily measurable with what is clinically important. Some variables, such as temperature and rates of suicide, appear relatively easy to convert into numerical form; others, such as attitudes and intelligence, are somewhat more problematic, while others present real and sometimes insurmountable difficulties. It is important that as health researchers we do not simply ignore or avoid areas of study and fields of research that might cost more in time and resources, in order to focus always on simple work that might have very limited impact on health and social care. As Albert Einstein is reported to have said, 'Everything that can be counted does not necessarily count; everything that counts cannot necessarily be counted' (cited in Garfield 1986: 156).

Statistical and clinical significance

In addition, the increasing sophistication of the statistical tests being used to ensure the internal and external validity of the research means that many researchers do not fully understand what those tests are indicating. To take a fairly simple example, the concept of statistical significance (usually expressed as a p-value) is often thought of as showing the effectiveness of a treatment, whereas it is merely an indicator of the probability that any measured differences between (say) a test group and a control group are the result of chance factors in the selection of the sample. For example, a p-value of 0.1 tells us nothing about whether or not the intervention is effective, but only that there is a one in ten chance that any difference in scores between the groups is due to non-random samples. Thus, an RCT to test the effects of an antidepressant drug might show a *statistically* significant difference between the experimental and control groups for scores on a depression inventory, but these differences might have very little *clinical* significance. In other words, the antidepressant effect of the drug might be real but so small as to render it of little practical use (LeFort 1993; Beyea and Nicoll 1997).

Conclusion

Most modern philosophers would agree that the purpose of philosophy is not to provide answers but to foreground problems, that is, to problematize issues and practices which are usually taken for granted. The purpose of this chapter has therefore been to signpost some of the conceptual and practical pitfalls that the quantitative researcher might fall into, and to equip the reader with enough understanding of the relevant philosophical underpinnings of research and the scientific method either to avoid falling in or else to climb out without too much harm being done.

Philosophers often warn of the dangers of scientism – the tendency to treat the methods and findings of science as the only truth. However, it seems fitting to end this chapter by warning the reader of the equally dangerous tendency to over-philosophize, or to treat philosophy as a similarly infallible method. Philosophy provides us with some extremely powerful analytic tools, but while the philosophical method tends to result in *logical* conclusions, it does not always guarantee the *truth*, and we must be aware of the dangers of placing too much trust in philosophical reasoning at the expense of common sense. For example, the philosophy of science distinguishes between association and causality, and warns that even if two events are consistently found to follow one after the other, it is not possible to make the logical inference that the second is caused by the first. Thus, night invariably follows day, but we would not want to say that night is *caused* by day.

This philosophical understanding of the difference between association and causality is often applied to quantitative health research findings to good effect. However, if it is allowed to override common sense it can also cause great harm. For example, it has been known for many years that smokers are more likely to develop certain illnesses than non-smokers, and several quantitative studies conducted in the 1950s demonstrated that the statistical correlation was so strong that there was little doubt that smoking was a major cause of lung cancer (Doll and Hill 1954, 1956). However, the statistician R.A. Fisher, who was possibly employed at the time as a consultant by the tobacco industry, compared the correlations in these papers to a correlation between the import of apples and the rise of divorce to demonstrate *ad absurdum* that correlation does not imply causation. While Fisher's argument is logically and philosophically sound, it nevertheless leads to a false conclusion which has been used over the years by the tobacco industry not only to sell cigarettes but also to avoid paying compensation to sufferers from lung cancer.

Key concepts

- The practice of research requires a philosophical understanding of its basic principles.
- Contemporary philosophical ideas and theories can only be understood fully in their historical context.
- Modern ideas and practices of quantitative health research emerged in the early years of the twentieth century.
- The paradigm of quantitative research is underpinned by the philosophical theory of critical realism.
- The quantitative researcher must be aware of a number of philosophical challenges and caveats, including the problem of induction, falsificationism, reductionism and significance.
- Researchers must also be aware of over-philosophizing at the expense of common sense.

Key readings in the philosophical basis for research

- D. Cardinal, J. Hayward and G. Jones, *Epistemology: The Theory of Knowledge* (London: John Murray, 2004)
  A simple introduction to some of the key ideas and terminology of the philosophy of knowledge. This text is an ideal starting point for readers who are new to the subject.
- B. Gower, *Scientific Method: An Historical and Philosophical Introduction* (London: Routledge, 1997)
  An introduction to the history and philosophy of ideas, focusing on the lives and work of some of the pioneers of the scientific method, including Galileo, Bacon and Newton.
- J. Hughes, *The Philosophy of Social Research* (London: Longman, 1990)
  A more advanced text, and one of the few books on the philosophy of social research to focus on the positivist, quantitative paradigm.
- S. Okasha, *Philosophy of Science: A Very Short Introduction* (Oxford: Oxford University Press, 2002)
  As the title suggests, this is a very short introduction to the philosophy of science, with a useful chapter on realism and anti-realism.

References

Bandolier (2012) *Qualitative and Quantitative Research*. Available at http://www.medicine.ox.ac.uk/bandolier/booth/glossary/qualres.html [Accessed 27 April 2012].

Beyea, S.C. and Nicoll, L.H. (1997) An overview of statistical and clinical significance in nursing research, AORN *Journal*, 65(6): 1128–30.

Bhaskar, R. (1979) *The Possibility of Naturalism*. Brighton: Harvester.

Bhaskar, R. (1989) *Reclaiming Reality*. London: Verso.

Burnard, P., Morrison, P. and Gluyas, H. (2011) *Nursing Research in Action*. Basingstoke: Palgrave Macmillan.

Burns, N. and Grove, S.K. (2008) *The Practice of Nursing Research: Conduct, Critique, and Utilization*, 6th edn. St. Louis, MO: Elsevier.

Campbell, D. and Stanley, J. (1963) *Experimental and Quasi-experimental Designs for Research*. Chicago: Rand McNally.

Cochrane, A.L. (1972) *Effectiveness and Efficiency: Random Reflections on Health Services*. London: Nuffield Provincial Hospitals Trust.

Cole, P. (2002) *The Theory of Knowledge*. London: Hodder and Stoughton.

Comte, A. ([1830] 1988) *Introduction to Positive Philosophy*. Indianapolis: Hackett.

Cresswell, J.W. (2008) *Research Design: Qualitative, Quantitative and Mixed Methods Approaches*, 3rd edn. Thousand Oaks, CA: Sage.

Cresswell, J.W. and Plano Clark, V.L. (2010) *Designing and Conducting Mixed Methods Research*, 2nd edn. Thousand Oaks, CA: Sage.

Dilthey, W. ([1900] 1976) The rise of hermeneutics, in H.P. Rickman (ed.) *Wilhelm Dilthey: Selected Writings*. Cambridge: Cambridge University Press, pp. 247–9.

Doll, R. and Hill, A.B. (1954) The mortality of doctors in relation to their smoking habits, *British Medical Journal*, 328(7455): 1529.

Doll, R. and Hill, A.B. (1956) Lung cancer and other causes of death in relation to smoking: A second report on the mortality of British doctors, *British Medical Journal*, 2(5001): 1071–81.

Durkheim, E. ([1895] 1964) *The Rules of Sociological Method*. New York: Free Press.

Durkheim, E. ([1897] 2006) *Suicide*. London: Penguin.

Einstein, A. ([1916] 2001) *Relativity*. London: Routledge.

Evidence-Based Medicine Working Group (1992) Evidence-based medicine: A new approach to teaching the practice of medicine, *Journal of the American Medical Association*, 268(17): 2420–5.

Fisher, R.A. (1935) *The Design of Experiments*. Edinburgh: Oliver and Boyd.

Garfield, C.A. (1986) *Peak Performers: The New Heroes of American Business*. New York: William Morrow.

Gould, S.J. (1996) *The Mismeasure of Man*. New York: Norton.

Gower, B. (1997) *Scientific Method*. London: Routledge.

Kuhn, T.S. (1962) *The Structure of Scientific Revolutions*. Chicago: University of Chicago Press.

LeFort, S.M. (1993) The statistical versus clinical significance debate, *Journal of Nursing Scholarship*, 25(1): 57–62.

Malinowski, B. (1922) *Argonauts of the Western Pacific*. London: Routledge & Kegan Paul.

Mead, M. (1943) *Coming of Age in Samoa*. Harmondsworth: Penguin (first published 1928).

Mill, J.S. ([1843] 2001) *A System of Logic*. London: Adamant Media.

Moser, C.A. (1967) *Survey Methods in Social Investigation*. London: Heinemann Educational.

Nightingale, F.N. (1858) *Notes on Matters Affecting Health, Efficiency, and Hospital Administration of the British Army*. London: Harrison and Sons.

Okasha, S. (2002) *Philosophy of Science: A Very Short Introduction*. Oxford: Oxford University Press.

Oxford Centre for Evidence-Based Medicine (2009) *Levels of Evidence*. Available at http://www.cebm.net/?o=1025 [Accessed 27 April 2012].

Peirce, C.S. ([1897, 1883] 1992) *The Essential Peirce: 1867–1893*, i: *Selected Philosophical Writings*. Chichester: Wiley.

Popper, K. (1979) *Objective Knowledge*, rev. edn. Oxford: Clarendon Press.

Popper, K. ([1935] 2002) *The Logic of Scientific Discovery*. London: Routledge.

Powers, B. and Knapp, P. (2006) *Dictionary of Nursing Theory and Research*, 3rd edn. New York: Springer.

Radcliffe-Brown, A.R. (1948) *The Andaman Islanders*. Glencoe, IL: Free Press. (first published 1922).

Sarantakos, S. (1993) *Social Research*. Basingstoke: Macmillan.

Shields, L. and Twycross, A. (2003) The difference between quantitative and qualitative research, *Paediatric Nursing*, 15(9): 24.

Streptomycin in Tuberculosis Trials Committee (1948) Streptomycin treatment of pulmonary tuberculosis. A Medical Research Council investigation. *British Medical Journal* 2 (4582), 769–82.

Stadler, F. (2012) The Vienna Circle, in J.R. Brown (ed.) *Philosophy of Science*. London: Continuum, pp. 53–82.

Toulmin, S. (1953) *The Philosophy of Science*. London: Hutchinson.

Weber, M. ([1922] 1992) *Economy and Society*. Los Angeles: University of California Press.

2 The importance and use of social theory in health care research

Maria Lohan and Carmel Kelly

Introduction

The purpose of this chapter is to examine the significance of social theories to quantitative health and health care research design. By focusing on the interconnectedness of society and individuals living in it, these theories can provide a framework for understanding the social world along with powerful insights into health and illness. The chapter is divided into two parts. First, we outline the philosophical principles of the main social theories: political economy, structural functionalism, feminist theory and critical realism, providing some examples of how they have been applied to quantitative or mixed-methods health and health care research. In doing so, the impact of social factors such as gender, socio-economic status, culture and educational attainment will be brought into focus. In addition, social processes such as professional boundaries, relationships and organizational contexts will also be central to our enquiry. Secondly, we draw on an example of a study on adolescent men and unintended pregnancy. While this quantitative research study drew on both social and psychological theories, we have chosen it to illustrate how social theory informed the development of hypotheses, the selection of measures and the interpretation of results.

Political economy

The origins of this theory are most closely associated with the writings of Karl Marx (1818–83), who maintained that society could only be understood through an examination of its economic system (capitalism, feudalism and so on). According to Marx, it was the configuration of the economy and class relations within it that laid the 'superstructure' that affects all other aspects of society. Marx's theory is referred to as *materialist* because in this theory it is the material conditions that dominate everyday life (rather than any cultural or ideological basis) that shape society. Marx was also known as a political thinker and, in particular, he believed that class consciousness, emerging from the class inequalities of the capitalist system of production, would lead to major 'contradictions' or conflicts in society. These contradictions would, in turn, result in the transformation of the capitalist system to a socialist-based economy.

The political economy approach is particularly important to understanding health and health care, because of its emphasis on the impact of socio-economic conditions on the health of groups and individuals. Centuries of political thought, dating back beyond Marx's studies of the working class in Victorian times, have highlighted the persistent relationship between social class and health – a person's socio-economic status is closely linked with the level of health they enjoy. For example, in most Western societies, those in the lowest socio-economic group have a life expectancy of between five and seven years less than that of individuals in the highest socio-economic group (for example, see Warren and Hernandez 2007; White and Edgar 2010).

Quantitative studies of health generally provide an analysis of class position and health outcomes. This can be done in an exploratory or comprehensive way, depending on the centrality of class issues to the hypothesis being tested. North American researchers tend to use a combination of income and education to measure social class; while British and Irish researchers tend to use occupational scales derived from the Erikson-Goldthorpe schema (E-G schema), such as the new UK National Statistics Socio-Economic Classification System (NS-SEC) (Office for National Statistics 2002).

A more in-depth way of studying social class and health outcomes requires carefully working through the social mechanisms linking social class and the health outcomes. A fuller understanding of political economy theories of health generally identifies three core approaches: a materialist versus cultural/behavioural approach; materialist versus psychosocial approach; and a 'life course' approach (see Box 2.1).

Box 2.1   Political economy: three core approaches

The materialist versus cultural/behavioural approach sets two opposing views against each other.

The materialist approach suggests that it is people's underlying economic conditions such as poverty, unemployment, housing, living in poor neighbourhoods and exposure to hazards that are directly related to poor health outcomes.

A cultural/behavioural approach focuses on individual behaviour rather than environmental conditions, and measures diet, tobacco and drug use and lack of exercise, for example. More 'holistic' approaches, however, tend to combine these hypotheses and measure both sets of variables and investigate links between them.

A psychosocial approach maintains that it is not simply poverty that causes ill health but *relative poverty* and, in particular, the psychological effects of poverty. Therefore, operationalizing this theory in quantitative research involves measuring psychological variables such as stress levels, relative self-esteem, self-efficacy in negotiating resources and/or individuals' sense of trust in their communities to provide services.

Finally, the life course approach to understandings of social class and health is very similar to the materialist approach, and arguably not a different theory but an extension of the timeline of the variables measured. The life course approach may involve measuring health outcomes and determinants of health outcomes at specific critical periods of the life course – the so-called 'critical periods approach' – for example, at birth and follow-up in adolescence or adulthood. Equally, the life course approach may involve the study of the accumulative effect of socio-economic and biological factors over regular intervals for longer periods – the cumulative periods model – such as longitudinal 'growing up studies' that capture the same individuals over time.

Structural functionalism

The development of structural functionalism as a sociological theory evolved from the work of the French sociologist, Émile Durkheim (1858–1917). The basic principle of Durkheim's theory is that society is a system, not unlike an organic system such as the human body. Health care professionals readily recognize the 'structure' and 'function' of systems in the human body and appreciate that, in order to maintain the viability of the body, many different systems must interact. In comparing society to a living organism, Durkheim put forward the theory that the cohesiveness and survival of society depends on the contribution or 'function' of a series of social subsystems (education, religion, formal labour markets). In essence, human behaviour is structured by a set of cultural rules which are co-opted and valued by the members of the society in which one lives. These social structures can either promote or curtail all human action, suggesting that health and illness 'are not simply matters of individual responsibility' (Porter 1998: 22). Structural functionalist theory contributes to our understanding of health and illness by elucidating cultural and institutional structures in society and examining how these structures impact on individuals' health and well-being.

Durkheim developed his theories of structural functionalism and social integration in modern societies with particular reference to suicide (Durkheim ([1897] 1951). He identified four types of suicide identifiable across a range of societies. In modern industrialized societies, he noted that the most prevalent types were 'egotistic' and 'anomic' suicides that he associated with low levels of social integration, high levels of individualism and rapid social change. Durkheim identified 'altruistic' and 'fatalistic' suicides as being dominant in traditional societies in which, he argued, there is overbearing social control, leading to feelings of individual oppression. Durkheim's theories of suicide were developed through quantitative analyses of rates of suicide and an analysis of the prevailing socio-economic conditions of nation states similar to those currently used in studies of suicide.

However, it should be noted that later theories, which question the impact of structure alone, criticized Durkheim's analysis of suicide on two accounts. One, because his theory prioritized how macro-level structures in society (religious cultures and economic conditions) determine individual levels of suicide without analysing individuals' own understandings and motivations for suicide. The second criticism relates to Durkheim's failure to take account of the human element of interpretation which leads to a death being categorized as a suicide in the first place. Later research showed how the recording of a suicide is contingent on a number of social factors, not least the stigma of a recording of suicide. See Chapter 1 for a further discussion of Durkheim's study of suicide.

Durkheim's broader theory of structural functionalism is also re-emerging in contemporary studies of social capital and health – the so-called 'neo-Durkheimian turn' (Blaxter 2000; Turner 2003) – in which scholars look at the relationships between an individual's sense of social cohesiveness and their health and well-being. The central hypothesis is (as it was in Durkheim's original study) that individuals gain a sense of social support from participating in positive social environments – that is, environments in which there is a strong sense of shared values and norms. Such environments help individuals feel integrated into a broader society and prevent 'deviant' behaviour (such as endangering one's life through high-risk activities). For example, one recent study identified a positive relationship between high degrees of social capital in the home environment and long-term health and well-being outcomes for infants and children (Stewart-Brown and Shaw 2004). Indeed, the broader National Institute for Clinical Excellence (NICE) report (Morgan and Swann 2004), from which this example is drawn, contains several examples of quantitative studies of social capital and health.

The renewed popularity of structural functionalist theory can also been credited with the resurgence of another highly influential theory in health care research: that of the 'sick role' associated with Talcott Parsons (1902–79). Parsons's concept of the 'sick role' (Parsons 1951) drew attention to the social dimension of illness: sickness is not only a biological concept but also a social concept that is defined by social rules and norms. In particular, Parsons drew attention to the concept of health as being associated with our ability to fulfil particular roles in society. In order to deter individuals from withdrawing from social obligations at any time because of perceived ill health, illness is subject to rule-bound forms of regulation (see Box 2.2).

Box 2.2   Structural functionalism: examples from the literature

Parsons drew attention to the ways the health professional–patient relationship has a crucial role in the corroboration and validation of an individual as being 'sick' (Koekkoek et al. 2011). The sick role is structured by social expectations – the ill person can be temporarily relieved of their social obligations on the condition that: 1) they actively seek medical attention; and 2) they cooperate fully with health professionals.

Parsons's concept of the sick role has been influential in studies of patient compliance and non-compliance (Macdonell et al. 2011), studies of health care encounters (Miczo 2004), and health professional–patient relationships (Lillrank 2003). For example, a recent study used a cross-sectional survey design to explore the factors influencing Dutch community psychiatric nurses' (CPNs) labelling of patients with severe non-psychotic mental illness as 'difficult' (Koekkoek et al. 2011). The researchers highlighted

a number of factors associated with both individual patient and professional characteristics as well as societal factors such as the patients' social background or the nurses'
professional system. The study concludes that although the 'difficult' label is socially constructed, it is founded on a combination of variables – relating to patients, professionals,
mental health services and larger social systems (Koekkoek et al. 2011: 511).

Feminist theory

Feminist theory emerged in *academic* literature in the 1970s as part of what is known
as 'second-wave feminism'. While the acquisition of women's rights was central
to first-wave feminism (for example in relation to the right to vote, own property
and work), second-wave feminism crystallized around an intellectual project that
engaged with social theory and empirical studies of women's lives. Widerberg (2000)
identifies three core concerns of this project. The first phase was theoretical critique
challenging the very content of social science research. Prior to this, social science
had been predominantly concerned with the study of the *public* realm: large social
systems of religion, capitalism, labour markets and industrialization, imperialism
and urbanization. While the discipline of anthropology had always been concerned
with the study of family life, it was most often the family life of 'others' (for example, tribal groupings in traditional societies). Feminist theory and feminist research
not only opened up the study of the hitherto ignored *private* worlds of, for example,
family life, but also explored women's struggles to enter the public realm. In addition to critiquing the content of the social sciences, feminist theory also aligned
itself to other schools of interpretive sociology in critiquing the *methods* of social
science, specifically challenging positivist theory and the notion of objectivity in
research. In particular, feminist theory argued that the so-called scientific and objective theories of the world were notably grounded in male or 'malestream' perspectives.

A further concern of second-wave feminism, according to Widerberg (2000),
was in relation to 'visibilizing' women's experiences. This agenda sought to develop
ways of understanding through research based on women's experiences, giving rise
to 'women's standpoint theory' (Stanley and Wise 1993; Harding 2004). A third element of second-wave feminism, according to Widerberg (2000), was the 'reflexivity
phase'. This 'turn' within feminism led to a fundamental critique of the very concept
of feminist theory – although some refer to this critical/reflexivity phase as leading
to a fracturing of feminist social science, similar to post-structuralist trends which
are present across the social sciences. For example, Black feminist theory emerged
to query the concept of 'women' and 'womanhood' and the nature of patriarchy as
experienced by white women. Black feminism (see, for example, Hill Collins 1990)
drew sharper attention to ethnic, class and gender differences that divide women.
Socialist feminism had similarly, prior to Black feminism, concentrated on the
intersections of class and patriarchy in the subjugation of women (see, for example, appraisals of writings of Christine Delphy in Barrett and McIntosh 1979). In

addition, the practice of focusing exclusively on women to understand gender was questioned. While women's experiences were theorized in relation to men's, men's experiences had been generally excluded or were not seen as dynamic and changing in response to feminism and women's changing lives. In the late twentieth century, men's studies and the pro-feminist Critical Studies on Men and Masculinities (CSM) emerged alongside feminist studies in redefining the object and method of feminist studies.

CSM primarily studies men's lives, aiming to explore how gender defines the way men live. CSM widens the relational view of gender and patriarchy, seeing them as structures that are constructed *within* the everyday lives of men and women as well as mediated *through* contemporary social structures (see Lohan 2009 for an overview). In response to these changes in feminist theory, academic 'women's studies' departments have begun to convert to 'gender studies' departments.

This leaves the question of how useful feminist theory is to quantitative social or health scientists. Whereas feminist social theory is part of a broader sociological critique of positivist social science (which is the basis for most quantitative research, as discussed in Chapter 1), feminist theorists have also been active in the development of quantitative methods, notwithstanding their primary focus on health as an issue of fairness and equality (see Box 2.3).

Box 2.3 Feminist theory: examples from published literature

A much cited study has explored the relationship between women's gender equality at the state level in the US and how this differently affected women's and men's health (Kawachi et al. 1999). The 'equality' status of women in each state was assessed using four composite indices measuring political participation, economic autonomy, employment and earnings, and reproductive rights. The main outcome measures were female and male mortality rates and the mortality rate based on average number of days of activity limitations reported by women during the previous month. The study showed a striking correlation between women's equality status at state level and women's health outcomes. Higher political participation by women was correlated with lower female mortality rates as well as lower activity limitations. A smaller wage gap between women and men was associated with lower female mortality rates and lower activity limitations. These findings also held when statistically controlling for the effects of other plausible explanations, such as income inequality and poverty rates. In essence, the gender inequality of women was found to be associated with gender inequities in health – women's poorer health relative to men's.

Feminist scholars have also examined the relationships between gender and men's health (see Lohan 2007 for an overview). A similar study to the one cited above examined the impact of patriarchy and rates of male mortality (Stanistreet et al. 2005). The research focused on the relationships between female homicide rates (as a proxy for patriarchy as the overwhelming majority of violent crime is perpetrated by men on women) and lower life expectancy in men across countries in Europe, America, Australasia and Asia. They concluded that male mortality was higher in societies with a high female homicide rate, and that 'oppression and exploitation harm the oppressors as well as those they oppress' (Stanistreet et al. 2005: 873). The authors also accepted that alternative or additional measures of patriarchy would have strengthened their theoretical link between patriarchy and men's mortality. However, obtaining valid comparable measures across a range of countries can be an enormous challenge in quantitative research, and for this reason the authors did not use other plausible measures, such as female participation in gainful employment, the proportion of women in decision-making positions, or the sex division of household labour.

In summary, the use of feminist theory in quantitative research does not simply require the inclusion of the variables 'male' and 'female' at a research design stage, but a deeper exploration of the factors (the *how* and *why*) that cause the differences in women's and men's health outcomes. Feminist theory can help social scientists to map out these explanations and to relate the results back to a body of knowledge of men's and women's lives.

Critical realism

Contemporary social theorists such as the British philosopher Roy Bhaskar reject notions of human behaviour as being predominantly determined by either structural rules or individual agency in favour of a *critical realist* explanation. The basic assumption of this approach is that there is an external reality that is independent of our experiences and our thoughts (McDonnell et al. 2009). The concept of 'causality' is central to this theory, but differs from traditional positivist views of cause and effect. Positivism, with its emphasis on classical experimental methods, asserts that there is a single observable reality that can be identified, isolated and measured using controlled experiments that separate the objective from the subjective in a 'closed' system. When it comes to understanding an 'open' system such as society, critical realists reject the artificial creation of a closed system which, they claim, is created by the experimental approach itself. Realists such as Bhaskar argue that reality is not limited to surface objects. Specifically, he points to the causal criterion for reality – the natural forces that cause events to occur. In an open system, these forces can include organizational, cultural, psychological and biological factors (McDonnell et al. 2009).

In health care research, critical realist approaches have been applied to evaluate complex health care interventions, particularly those which involve changing the behaviour patterns of professionals and/or service users. As a methodological tool, critical realism (most notably, 'realistic evaluation' as developed by Pawson and Tilly (1997)) aims to explore the social processes underlying the success or failure of the promotion of health (see Box 2.4).

Box 2.4 Critical realism: examples from the published literature

---

Blackwood and colleagues (Blackwood et al. 2010) examine the use of critical realist strategies in combination with randomized controlled trials (RCTs) in Blackwood's own research on developing, implementing and evaluating protocols for weaning patients from mechanical ventilation in intensive care units in the United Kingdom (Blackwood et al. 2006). The authors highlight the fundamental contradiction of combining RCTs (that create closed systems that can be controlled) with realist approaches, which embrace a very different notion of causality. They argue that this approach could bring us closer to answering two equally important questions of health care interventions: namely, does it work and, if so, how does it work? (Blackwood et al. 2010).

Demonstrating the use of social theory in quantitative research

Most social science studies of health involve testing the effect of social variables on health and health care outcomes and, as such, are informed by social theory. In the following example, we will make explicit how the aim of the study and the explanations or hypotheses developed for the study are informed by social theory. First, we briefly describe the aim and research design of the study and then we address how it was informed by social theory.

The research centres on adolescent men's attitudes and decisions involving unintended pregnancy (Lohan et al. 2011). The vast research on the topic of teenage pregnancy has been characterized by a very pronounced historical gender bias towards the women's experiences. While research has begun to emerge on the experiences of teenage fathers, very little research has been available to date on adolescent men's roles in, or perspectives on, an unintended pregnancy (Lohan et al. 2010). The purpose of this study was to explore how adolescent men would deal with an unintended pregnancy and how they would choose to resolve this situation in their lives. The outcome choices of the study were 'keep the baby', 'abortion' or 'adoption'. The research question posed in the study was thus hypothetical: how, if an unintended pregnancy happened in their lives, in the context of an ongoing relationship, would they choose to resolve it? It was not a retrospective study of how men who have been in that situation have chosen to deal with an unintended or 'crisis' pregnancy.

A key methodological challenge of the study was the need to generate a hypothetical scenario of an unintended pregnancy with which adolescent men could identify. Drawing on a previous research study conducted in Australia (Condon et al. 2006), the research team produced an interactive video drama (IVD) entitled *If I were Jack*, which sought to represent a week in the life of a young man (Jack) whose girlfriend is unintentionally pregnant. The IVD was designed to be used by participants sitting at individual computers, wearing headphones and following the filmed drama imagining *if he were Jack*. As the story unfolds, participants responded to questions about how he would think and feel about this situation and how he might communicate with his partner, friends, parents and counsellors. Finally, each participant also had to decide how he would choose to resolve the pregnancy. The choices adolescent men made in relation to a hypothetical pregnancy in their lives were the main outcome or 'dependent variable'. The possible explanations (hypotheses) for these outcomes which were proposed and tested were derived from social theory (see below) and were contained in a paper and pencil questionnaire distributed 'under exam conditions' at the outset of the study. The data were collected from a sample of male adolescents (n = 360) drawn from a stratified random sample of schools in Ireland. Data were analysed using a random effects logistic regression model allowing for between-school variation.

Social theory in the study

The overall question for this study is derived from feminist theory. In the first part of this chapter we described how feminist theory put gender (as in culturally generated differences between men and women) on the pages of social science. We also noted how feminist-informed scholarship of Critical Studies on Men and Masculinities (CSM) has brought attention to gender effects in men's lives. This study is principally derived from feminist theory because it challenges the gender norms in society, as well the gender bias in research, which have constructed teenage pregnancy as a woman's concern only, leaving important questions relating to men's roles and responsibilities unanswered. From a health policy point of view, a greater understanding of men's roles and perspectives opens up possibilities for more gender-inclusive approaches to preventing and dealing with unintended pregnancies (Lohan et al. 2011).

The study is also informed by social theory in terms of developing the hypotheses or explanations for the dependent variable: adolescent men's pregnancy outcome choices. From our systematic review of the literature on adolescent men and pregnancy (Lohan et al. 2010), it became apparent that three particular social explanations of adolescent men's attitudes to pregnancy resolution choices stood out in the empirical literature: religiosity, socio-economic status and masculinity. These social explanations, as we will describe in more detail below, are respectively linked to functionalist theory, political economy theory and feminist theory. However, explanations derived from psychology, and especially social cognitive theory, also featured large in the previous research on adolescent men and pregnancy. In particular, previous studies drew upon the Theory of Planned Behaviour (Ajzen and Madden 1986; Ajzen 2005). The Theory of Planned Behaviour suggests that a person's attitudes towards a behaviour (especially the perceived outcomes of the behaviour) and their perception of what significant others would want them to do (subjective norms) are essential elements that lead to behavioural intention and behaviour. As is common in health research, we decided to develop our hypotheses from both the social theory-derived explanations (social variables) and also incorporate the more individual-level explanations derived from the Theory of Planned Behaviour. We referred to the attitudinal and subjective norm variables derived from Theory of Planned Behaviour as proximal variables because, relative to social context variables, they tend to be specific immediate precursors of the behaviour – more proximate to the outcome (Carvajal and Granillo 2006). We then referred to the social theory-derived variables as distal explanations.

Once researchers decide what the plausible explanations are, the next question becomes how to operationalize those questions in a measurable form for quantitative research methods. How to measure gender by contrast to sex is a complex question which again brings social theories of gender into play. In this study, the focus was on understanding gender difference (differences in conceptualizations of masculinity) among men. For this purpose, *The Male Role Attitudes Scale* (MRAS) (Pleck et al. 1993) short eight-item scale was used. Participants respond using a four-point Likert-type response format, from 'strongly agree' (4) to 'strongly disagree' (1). Scores can range from 8 to 32, with higher scores representing higher levels of male role attitude. Items include: 'I admire a guy who is totally sure of himself' (Item 3) and 'It bothers me when a boy acts like a girl' (Item 6). This particular scale was chosen because it is based on a social constructionist theoretical understanding of gender. The social constructionist principle underlying the scale views masculinity not as a fixed dimension of personality (or biology), but rather as a set of culturally derived beliefs and expectations about what men are like and what they should do. The scale tests the extent to which participants identify with these cultural notions of masculinity.

Social class in the study

We turn now to the second major social variable in our study: social class. As noted earlier, an understanding of the salience of social class in affecting health outcomes and health care use is grounded in political economy understandings of the impact of late capitalism on contemporary societies. In this study the UK's current official National Statistics Socio-Economic Classification (NS-SEC) questions were used to measure social class. Responses were sought to the following:

> Please indicate which best describes the sort of work your father does (if he is not working outside the home now please tell me what he did in his last job) 1) professional or higher technical work, 2) manager or senior administrator, 3) clerical, 4) sales or services, 5) small business owner, 6) foreman or supervisor of other workers, 7) skilled manual work, 8) semi-skilled or unskilled manual work, 9) other, 10) never worked, 11) not applicable.

The same question was asked about the respondent's mother. However, in cognizance of criticisms of parental and occupationally based measures of social class in relation to adolescents (Currie et al. 2008), an additional measure of educational aspirations of adolescents was used as a measure of 'predictive' social class. In social theory terms, the criticism of the above measures, derived from political economy approaches, is that they present an overly structuralist approach to understanding the effect of social class on individuals, while an educational aspirations question helps to bring individual agency into play. Responses to the following question were used:

What do you think you will be doing when you leave school? (Please tick one box only):

1) Doing a university degree or equivalent, 2) Doing a diploma or certificate, 3) On a training scheme/apprenticeship, 4) Unemployed, 5) Other, please specify.

Responses to these questions allowed a dichotomous 'university' versus 'other' variable to be generated.

Social theory of structural functionalism in the study

Finally, in relation to religion, the social theory of structural functionalism, as discussed above, is the theory which is most concerned with how individuals are collectively bound by values and norms that govern social practice or behaviours. Durkheim, in his study of suicide (Durkheim [1897] 1951), examined membership of different types of religions and referred to levels of integration in those religions, religiosity, the extent to which people 'buy into' a religious code of practice, and its importance in relation to many sensitive health subjects – especially those relating to life and death choices. Levels of religiosity were predicted in this research example as being relevant to adolescent men's unintended pregnancy resolution choices. The following single item was used to measure religiosity:

> How important would you say religion is to you? Is it: very important, fairly important, fairly unimportant or very unimportant.

The current research opted to include this variable in analysis in preference to religious attendance, primarily because religious importance is more representative of an intrinsic (or personal) religious orientation, while attendance is viewed as more representative of an extrinsic (or external) religious orientation (see Allport 1959).

The following hypotheses were constructed: adolescent men's support for abortion versus continuation of the pregnancy (keep the baby or adoption) is associated with three social context (distal) variables:

- lower levels of religiosity
- higher socio-economic status of parents
- lower stereotypical masculine beliefs

Turning now to the proximal variables as derived from Theory of Planned Behaviour, and specifically to the influence of adolescent men's attitudes (men's own beliefs about the consequences of the pregnancy outcomes) and subjective norms (the perception of how they feel significant others would expect them to behave), this theoretical framework led to a further two hypotheses. These are: adolescent men's support for abortion versus continuation of the pregnancy (keep the baby or adoption) is associated with two sets of proximal variables:

- perceived favourable parental attitudes to abortion
- favourable respondent attitudes to the consequences of abortion

In brief, the results of the study showed that almost half (46.7 per cent) of the adolescent men would choose 'to keep the baby'. 'Abortion' was the next most preferred choice (18.9 per cent), closely followed by 'leave it up to her' (18.3 per cent), with 'adoption' being the least preferred option (16.1 per cent) of the sample. However, it was concluded that only one of the 'social' or 'distal' hypotheses could be supported: adolescent men's support for abortion versus continuation of the pregnancy is associated with low religiosity. Respondents with high religiosity were over twice as likely as respondents with low religiosity to choose to continue the pregnancy rather than choose abortion. In relation to the proximal variables derived from the Theory of Planned Behaviour, it was concluded that the findings support both hypotheses – that is, that perceived favourable parental attitudes to abortion (mother only), and favourable respondent attitudes in relation to the consequences of abortion are associated with choosing abortion over continuation of the pregnancy.

Overall, the above example drew on different social and psychological theories to derive specific variables, but the study, when looked at as a whole, is most clearly derived from feminist theory, and particularly Critical Studies on Men and Masculinities. Thus, the study can be seen to also 'feed back' into this area of social theory. In particular, the study is an example of the way feminist theory has begun to open up intimate areas of men's lives such as men's reproductive intentions – which have previously mainly been studied in relation to women. In addition, the study arises from the trend in feminist social theory to deconstruct the terms 'woman' and 'man' and look for gender difference in the expression of masculinity. Finally, the analysis of gender was not studied in isolation, but in relation to other mediating variables such as religiosity and social class, as well as attitudinal variables to the health outcome – in this case, attitudes and subjective norms relating to the pregnancy outcome choices. This situated analysis of gender demonstrates how gender is a social process which is cross-cut by other social factors.

Conclusion

In short, the advice to those seeking to include social theory in quantitative research is to 'think back' into the theoretical origins of their hypotheses and to 'think theoretically' in terms of how theoretical principles can be applied to empirical findings, and vice versa. Many researchers begin with an empirical question such as 'how do different health care organizations manage sickness absence of their labour force?' The next question researchers frequently ask is what methods might be useful to answer that question. Researchers then often move forward by reading relevant (empirical) literature to explore the topic more thoroughly, refining the research question and research methods as they progress. Increasingly common in health care research is the use of 'systematic reviews' of the literature, which tend to home the researcher in on a very specific question to be answered through rigorous (and rigid) procedures for analysing the literature. However, all these research steps will only give the researcher a richer sense of the empirical field of study (for example, absence management in health care organizations), whereas, by also reading social theory (for example, political economy theory and critical realism), perhaps through leads from the empirical literature, the researcher has the opportunity to think about how their developing hypotheses are conceived and how they relate to broader understandings of how health and health care are managed in society. Essentially it is about asking: what is the bigger picture? Why are particular hypotheses emerging? What are the general principles framing them? Asking these questions as part of the literature review will reap dividends in the analysis stages, where the overall objective is to move beyond a description of findings to making sense of findings. The use of social theory in research draws the researcher's attention to more general principles of why particular research findings may have emerged, and may allow the researcher to draw links with patterns of health and health care more broadly. In summary, it is worth the trouble!

Key concepts

- Social theories offer a framework for understanding the social world, and can provide powerful insights into health and illness by increasing our understanding of the nature of the society in which we live.
- Quantitative health care studies that draw on social theories can purposefully explore the impact of social factors such gender, socio-economic status and educational attainment on health and illness experiences.
- Political economy theory emphasizes the centrality of economic systems to shaping society. It can help to increase our understanding of the impact of socio-economic conditions on the health of individuals and populations.
- Structural functionalist theory contributes to our understanding of health and illness by increasing our understanding of the nature of cultural and institutional structures in the society in which we live and how these impact on individuals' health and well-being behaviours.
- Parsons's concept of the 'sick role' emphasized the social dimensions of illness, implying that sickness was not simply a biological concept but also a social concept that is defined by social regulation and involves role expectations.
- The use of feminist theory in quantitative research means not simply entering the variables 'male' and 'female', but a deeper exploration of the factors (the *how* and *why*) that lead to differences in women's and men's health status, through an exploration of the social context of men's and women's lives (for example, education, employment, domestic divisions of labour).
- In the late twentieth century, men's studies and the more explicitly pro-feminist Critical Studies on Men and Masculinities (CSM) emerged alongside feminist studies. CSM is primarily the study of men's lives as men – in other words, opening up the ways in which gender structures also define the way men live.
- Critical realist theory rejects the notion of human behaviour being solely determined by either structural rules or individual agency. For this approach, the focus of enquiry is the 'causal criterion for reality' – the forces that cause events to occur. These forces include organizational, cultural, psychological and biological factors.

Key readings in social theory

- S. Porter, *Social Theory and Nursing Practice* (London: Palgrave Macmillan, 1994)
  A great introduction to social theory and its applications to health and health care research, written in a melodic tone.
- O. McDonnell, M. Lohan, A. Hyde and S. Porter, *Social Theory, Health and Healthcare* (London: Palgrave Macmillan, 2009)
  Slightly biased here, but this is also a very good introductory text. The book comprehensively covers many different social theories, which are applied in all cases to both health and health care research.
- The journal *Social Theory & Health*, published by Palgrave, may also be of interest.

References

Ajzen, I. (2005) *Attitudes, Personality and Behaviour*, 2nd edn. Maidenhead: Open University Press.

Ajzen, I. and Madden, T. J. (1986) Prediction of goal-directed behavior: Attitudes, intentions and perceived behavioral control, *Journal of Experimental Social Psychology*, 22(5): 453–74.

Allport, G.W. (1959) Religion and prejudice, *Crane Review*, 2: 1–10.

Barrett, M. and McIntosh, M. (1979) Christine Delphy: Towards a materialist feminism? *Feminist Review*, 1: 95–106.

Blackwood, B., Wilson-Barnett, J., Patterson, C., Trinder, T. and Lavery, G. (2006) An evaluation of protocolised weaning on the duration of mechanical ventilation, *Anaesthesia*, 61(11): 1079–86.

Blackwood, B., O'Halloran, P. and Porter, S. (2010) On the problems of mixing RCTs with qualitative research: The case of the MRC framework for the evaluation of complex healthcare interventions, *Journal of Research in Nursing*, 15(6): 511.

Blaxter, M. (2000) Medical sociology at the start of the new millennium, *Social Science and Medicine*, 51(8): 1139–42.

Durkheim, E. ([1897] 1951) *Suicide*. New York: Free Press.

Carvajal, S.C. and Granillo, T.M. (2006) A prospective test of distal and proximal determinants of smoking initiation in early adolescents, *Addictive Behavior*, 31(4): 649–60.

Condon, J.T., Corkindale, C.J., Russell, A. and Quinlivan, J. (2006) Processes and factors underlying adolescent males' attitudes and decision making in relation to an unplanned pregnancy, *Journal of Youth and Adolescence*, 35(3): 423–34.

Currie, C., Molcho, M., Boyce, W., Holstein, B., Torsheim, T. and Richter, M. (2008) Researching health inequalities in adolescents: The development of the Health Behaviour in School-Aged Children (HBSC) family affluence scale, *Social Science & Medicine*, 66(6): 1429–36.

Harding, S. (ed.) (2004) *The Feminist Standpoint Theory Reader*. New York and London: Routledge.

Hill Collins, P. (1990) *Black Feminist Thought: Knowledge, Consciousness, and the Politics of Empowerment*. New York: Routledge.

Kawachi, I., Kennedy, B.P., Gupta, V. and Prothrow-Stith, D. (1999) Women's status and the health of women and men: A view from the States, *Social Science & Medicine*, 48(1): 21–32.

Koekkoek, B., Hutschemaekers, G., Van Meijel, B. and Schene, A. (2011) How do patients come to be seen as 'difficult'?: A mixed-methods study in community mental health care, *Social Science & Medicine*, 72(4): 504–12.

Lillrank, A. (2003) Back pain and the resolution of diagnostic uncertainty in illness narratives, *Social Science & Medicine*, 57(6): 1045–54.

Lohan, M. (2007) How might we understand men's health better? Integrating explanations from critical studies on men and inequalities in health, *Social Science & Medicine*, 65(3): 493–504.

Lohan, M. (2009) Developing a critical men's health debate in academic scholarship, in S. Robertson and B. Gough (eds) *Men, Masculinities and Health: Critical Perspectives*. London: Palgrave Macmillan, pp. 11–29.

Lohan, M., Cruise, S., O'Halloran, P., Alderdice, F. and Hyde, A. (2010) Adolescent men's attitudes in relation to pregnancy and pregnancy outcomes: A systematic review of the literature from 1980–2009, *Journal of Adolescent Health,* 47(4): 327–45.

Lohan, M., Cruise, S., O'Halloran, P. Alderdice, F. and Hyde, A. (2011) Adolescent men's attitudes and decision making in relation to an unplanned pregnancy: Responses to an interactive video drama, *Social Science & Medicine*, 72(9): 1507–14.

Macdonell, K.E., Naar-King, S., Murphy, D., Parsons, J. and Huszti, H. (2011) Situational temptation for HIV medication adherence in high-risk youth, *AIDS Patient Care STDS*, 25(1): 47–52.

McDonnell, O., Lohan, M., Hyde, A. and Porter, S. (2009) *Social Theory, Health and Healthcare*. Hampshire: Palgrave Macmillan.

Miczo, N. (2004) Stressors and social support perceptions predict illness attitudes and care-seeking intentions: Re-examining the sick role, *Health Communication*, 16(3): 347–61.

Morgan, A. and Swann, C. (eds) (2004) *Social Capital for Health: Issues of Definition, Measurement and links to Health*. NHS Health Development Agency. Available at http://www.nice.org.uk/niceMedia/documents/socialcapital_issues.pdf [Accessed 15 February 2012].

Office for National Statistics (2002) *National Statistics Socio-Economic Classification NS-SEC for England, Scotland and Wales*. London: Office for National Statistics. Available at http://www.statistics.gov.uk/ [Accessed 12 February 2012].

Parsons, T. (1951) *The Social System*. New York: Free Press.

Pawson, R. and Tilley, S. (1997) *Realistic Evaluation*. London: Sage.

Pleck, J.H., Sonenstein, F.L. and Ku, L.C. (1993) Masculinity ideology: Its impact on adolescent males' heterosexual relationships, *Journal of Social Issues*, 49(3): 11–29.

Porter, S. (1998) *Social Theory and Nursing Practice*. Hampshire: Palgrave Macmillan.

Stanistreet, D., Bambra, C. and Scott-Samuel, A. (2005) Is patriarchy the source of men's higher mortality? *Journal of Epidemiology and Community Health*, 59(10): 873–6.

Stanley, L. and Wise, S. (1993) *Breaking Out Again: Feminist Ontology and Epistemology*, 2nd edn. London: Routledge.

Stewart-Brown, S. and Shaw, R. (2004) The roots of social capital: Relationships in the home during childhood and later life, in C. Swann and A. Morgan (eds) *Social Capital for Health: Issues of Definition, Measurement and links to Health*. NHS Health Development Agency, pp. 157–86.

Turner, B. (2003) Social capital, inequality and health: The Durkheimian Revival, *Social Theory and Health*, 1(1): 4–20.

Warren, J.R. and Hernandez, E.M. (2007) Did socioeconomic inequalities in morbidity and mortality change in the United States over the course of the twentieth century?, *Journal of Health and Social Behavior*, 48(4): 335–51.

White, C. and Edgar, G. (2010) Inequalities in healthy life expectancy by social class and area type: England, 2001–03, *Health Statistics Quarterly*, 45: 28–56.

Widerberg, K. (2000) Gender and Society, in H. Anderson and L. Bo Kaspersen (eds) *Classical and Modern Social Theory*. Oxford: Blackwell, pp. 467–87.

3   Identifying research priorities

Michelle Butler

Chapter topics

- Research priorities
- Identifying research priorities for health care research
- The Delphi technique
- Nominal group technique
- Listening model
- Developing research questions

Introduction

There are many clinical, managerial and educational research issues of interest to health care professionals. Researchers often spend considerable time identifying the specific focus of their study or developing a case to present to project sponsors or research funders for the importance of the particular research topic that they have chosen. At the same time, funding agencies, health policymakers and governments are keen to ensure that funding that is allocated for research is focused on those topics that are most important and that are most likely to address the particular issues they face within their jurisdictions. As such, both researchers and research sponsors are concerned with identifying topics that are relevant to decision making in clinical practice, patient care and health care education and that will make a substantive contribution to knowledge and understanding. This chapter begins by examining a range of formal approaches to identifying and agreeing research priorities among stakeholders, before going on to consider how researchers can align their ideas with priority research areas in the selection of an appropriate research topic.

Background

For some time now there has been an emphasis on formal prioritizing approaches to identifying and agreeing topics for health care research. This occurs as governments and policymakers seek to identify which of the many possible treatments and services they can provide to their constituents within limited health care budgets, to target resources at health services that are most likely to improve health and health services delivery, to make the best use of limited resources for research, and to ensure the issues that are addressed through research are those that are most important (Lomas et al. 2003; Viergever et al. 2010). As such, formal prioritization processes 'necessarily' assign some measure of *value* to research, explicit or otherwise, so that topics can be ranked in order of importance (Fleurence and Torgerson 2004: 2) (see Box 3.1).

Box 3.1   Reasons for undertaking formal research prioritization processes (Smith et al. 2009; Viergever et al. 2010)

- Align research with particular issues in relation to the burden of disease.
- Ensure research activity is aligned with the interests, needs and values of the community.
- Ensure research is focused on issues that are relevant to health care for patients and societies.
- Increase harmonization of health research at a global level.

Research priorities can be identified at a macro level (national, policy), meso level (regional, organization, discipline), or micro level (local, service, project), and can be informed by priorities set at the other levels. They can be used to provide direction in relation to funding research, selecting topics for grant submissions, and selecting topics for graduate research.

Approaches to setting research priorities

There is no clear consensus on the most appropriate methodology for priority setting (Fleurence and Torgerson 2004). As with study design generally, the selection of an appropriate approach should depend on what the exercise aims to achieve, the stakeholders to be involved, and how this can be best achieved given the strengths and limitations of the various approaches. The generation of ideas is usually the starting point, and approaches tend to seek a balance between what is already known or published in relation to research priorities and priority issues within services and obtaining the views of key stakeholders about new or emerging issues. This may begin by examining the findings of previous studies to identify priorities. In the case of the prioritization study conducted by Doorenbos et al. (2008), additional items were identified by project team members and by asking survey participants to identify three additional topics. Alternatively, the exercise may begin with a review of the current literature and policy documents to identify important issues to be researched and gaps in the literature. Ross et al. (2004) complemented this approach by conducting focus groups with community health councils (as representatives of the wider community and client groups) and telephone interviews with a wider range of stakeholders, to identify gaps in nursing and midwifery services as well as in nursing and midwifery research. In another example, the Association of Community Health Nursing Educators (ACHNE) Research Committee (2010) examined the research priorities of funding agencies, undertook a comprehensive review of research abstracts to identify priority issues, and asked two nursing journal editors for their views of current priorities for nursing research. In comparison, Glasgow et al. (2001) undertook a different approach and engaged work groups to summarize pertinent literature and make recommendations for research priorities. In some cases, no reference is made to existing priorities or policy priorities, or the literature, with the emphasis solely on obtaining the views of stakeholders based on their experiences as providers (Vella et al. 2000; Dowsett et al. 2007; Henschke et al. 2007).

Formal prioritization approaches usually involve both the generation of ideas and the prioritization of the ideas generated among experts or stakeholders. The approaches used to identify priorities for research most often reported in the literature are Delphi and nominal group techniques and the listening model.

Delphi methods

Delphi methods have been used in many research prioritization studies at local and national level, and are a relatively straightforward and effective way to reach group decisions (Meehan et al. 2005). The Delphi method is 'a method for the systematic collection and aggregation of informed judgments from a group of experts on specific questions or issues' (Reid 1988: 232). The method involves a number of rounds until consensus is achieved among the group of experts.

The name 'Delphi' was taken from the oracle at Delphi, where ancient Greeks were said to be able to forecast future events (Williams and Webb 1994). The Delphi method was originally used in the 1940s to predict horse racing outcomes, but was first used in scientific research to obtain consensus from a group of experts about the course of future events to solve a problem of national importance (Dalkey and Helmer 1963; Meehan et al. 2005). It was specifically 'designed to minimise the biasing effects of dominant individuals, of irrelevant communications, and of group pressure towards conformity' (Dalkey 1969: v). There are three elements to the (classical) Delphi approach. Firstly, responses are obtained anonymously, using a formal questionnaire. Keeney et al. (2006) suggest that in the classical Delphi approach the first round is usually qualitative in nature. Secondly, the process is an iterative systematic exercise involving several rounds with carefully controlled feedback between rounds. The third feature is statistical group response, where the opinion of the group is defined as an appropriate aggregate of individual opinions. This is the format in which information is fed back to the group between rounds and in which the final results are reported.

The first round of a Delphi study can be used to generate ideas for research, which will then be developed further in subsequent rounds. Open-ended questions may be asked in the first round to identify topics, themes or questions to be researched, based on participants' knowledge or experience. In some cases, participants may also be asked to rate the importance of the items that they have suggested (see, for example, Meehan et al. 2005; Grundy and Ghazi 2009). In other cases, based on a review of the literature, potential topics for research may be presented in the questionnaire that participants are asked to rank, but participants will also be invited to identify additional topics (Grundy and Ghazi 2009). Box 3.2 outlines the benefits of using a Delphi approach to identify priorities for research.

Green et al. (1999) suggest the Delphi method is attractive because it preserves the interpretative aspects of qualitative research while allowing aggregate data to be analysed statistically.

A number of challenges have been identified with Delphi approaches. In principle, the process continues with a number of rounds until consensus is achieved on

---

Box 3.2   Advantages of using a Delphi approach to identify research priorities

---

The method enables participants to express their views without fear of intimidation.

Consensus can be achieved without bias associated with one member dominating the discussion, or 'groupthink'.

The items identified in the process will have high face validity and high concurrent validity.

The method allows the views of a large number of people to be canvassed without them having to come together in a meeting; this can reduce the impact on costs and respondents' time.

(Reid 1988; Williams and Webb 1994)

---

the priorities for research. However, this is rarely practical and the number of rounds undertaken is often constrained by the resources or time available. Also, there is the danger of response burden, especially if too many rounds are used (McKenna 1994; Keeney et al. 2006). Keeney et al. (2006) suggest that the provision of feedback and opportunity to revise earlier responses will require at least two rounds. However, if the first round is qualitative and no attempt has been made to rate or rank responses, a third round, if not more, may be required. Furthermore, it is also argued that during the feedback process participants may change their views on the basis of what they perceive to be right, rather than what they think, and so further validation of results may be required (Williams and Webb 1994). For this reason, a fourth round may be used to validate results. In Meehan et al.'s (2005) study on identifying research priorities for nursing and midwifery research, workshops were used following three rounds of the survey to validate results and to identify short-, medium- and longer-term priorities with a sample of Delphi participants and service users.

As stated previously, the central aim of the Delphi method is to achieve consensus among stakeholders, and it is argued that the method encourages consensus by affording participants the opportunity to reconsider their views on the basis of the responses of the panel (Keeney et al. 2006). However, there is no clear agreement on how to measure consensus in Delphi studies. Williams and Webb (1994) examined a number of Delphi studies and found that some authors did not set parameters for consensus in advance, but arbitrarily decided if consensus had been achieved following the inspection of results. In other studies, consensus may be understood as the majority view and can be set as low as 51 per cent of participants stating that an item is important. Alternatively, having at least 80 per cent of the respondents agree or disagree with a statement may be used as an indicator of success (Green et al. 1999). In other studies a mixture of consensus and importance measures may be used. For example, Hardy et al. (2004) deemed consensus to be where at least 75 per cent of responses lie within a two-point bracket on the Likert scale and the item receives a mean rating of 4.5 or more in terms of importance after round three. Meehan et al. (2005) used a similar mix of importance and consensus determinants. However, they also used a reduction of standard deviation over rounds as an indication of consensus.

Response rates can be problematic in Delphi methods. This is not surprising given the commitment required of participants over the rounds. Williams and Webb (1994) also highlight the impact of attrition between rounds on consensus, and there is some discussion in the literature about how response rates can be maximized (for example, Keeney et al. 2006). Meehan et al. (2005) used Dillman's (2000) tailored design method to enhance response rates. They still only achieved an initial response of 42 per cent (midwives) and 47 per cent (nurses). However, of those that initially took part in the survey, response rates of between 81 per cent and 90 per cent were maintained between rounds.

The nominal group technique

The nominal group technique can be used both to generate ideas for research and to develop consensus among participants on the ideas generated. It is a structured approach to promote a democratic style of group interview (Evans et al. 2004), and is particularly useful for sensitive topics or where the generation of ideas, discussion or feedback is best done anonymously. Various techniques can be used to enable participants to contribute ideas, views or comments in a non-threatening environment.

The first round of a nominal group technique may be used to generate ideas, or the group may be required to deliberate on ideas that were generated before the nominal group process begins. For example, Fevang et al. (2011) used the first round of a four-stage modified nominal group technique to ask participants to identify five areas of physician-provided pre-hospital care most in need of research. Evans et al. (2004) began their nominal group technique with GPs, nurses and pharmacists working in a primary care group in London, with the 'silent generation' of ideas. The approach may seek to limit prior preparation, to ensure that the ideas are generated within the group alone and reflect the particular needs of group participants (Corner et al. 2007). Alternatively, information may be collected through a survey of a 'target population', independent of the nominal group, on the issues around which consensus is required (Allen et al. 2004).

To achieve consensus, the results are presented to participants at the meeting for discussion and are rated by the group. Ratings are presented back to the group in terms of the median score, the mean absolute deviation, and the level of consensus for each item. The facilitator may invite each participant to explain the rationale for the scores they have assigned to each item, and in this way any ambiguities can be highlighted. Where there are ambiguities, items can be reworded to meet the consensus views of participants. Participants can then be asked to re-score items in confidence. Analysis is repeated to calculate median scores, mean deviation and consensus levels. Any changes in mean absolute deviation between the first and second rating are considered to be an indication of the impact of the nominal group meeting in promoting consensus (Vella et al. 2000).

Compared with the Delphi method, the nominal group approach is more limited in terms of the number of participants that can be involved in achieving consensus. The ideal size of the nominal group is between 9 and 12 participants to ensure it is manageable and to allow for a broad range of opinion (Allen et al. 2004). The process itself, involving highly structured facilitated discussion, requires significant moderation to ensure that all members are allowed to participate fully. However, the nominal group technique is particularly useful where consumer involvement is required and where it is important for different stakeholders to hear each other's understanding of the issues. The approach allows each person to express their views and reduces the risk of participants feeling they should agree with the views of the majority or of more powerful group members (Allen et al. 2004).

The listening model

Lomas et al. (2003) report that the listening model is a useful method for setting the agenda for user-driven research and that the approach fosters ongoing 'linkage and exchange' between researchers and research funders. The process involves six steps, as follows:

1 *Identify stakeholders.* The appropriate mix of stakeholders should be representative of the potential users of research; this should be decided by a group of experts.
2 *Identify and assemble any data needed for the consultation.* Data are collated on current problems in the system or existing research priorities to inform discussions during the consultation phases and to help participants to build on previous knowledge.
3 *Design and carry out the consultation with stakeholders.* This should focus on identifying issues that are likely to be, and remain, priorities for research over the next three to five years. This is to allow time for the design, conduct and completion of studies. Consultation could also seek to identify issues that are relevant in the shorter term and that could be subject to synthesis or meta-analysis.
4 *Validate the priority issues against similar exercises.* This can help to ensure the priorities are generalizable and not 'artifactual'.
5 *Translate priority issues into priority research themes.* Lomas et al. (2003) state that this phase should be carried out by research experts, who should translate pressing issues into priority areas which are both possible and feasible to research.
6 *Validate the priority research themes with stakeholders.* In this final step stakeholders are consulted again to ensure that the final research priorities truly reflect their expressed views.

Involving stakeholders in the research prioritization process

In recent years there has been a greater emphasis on involving a diverse range of stakeholders, including the public, in the research prioritization process. This is seen as key to ensuring priorities are relevant to the issues that health care providers and recipients experience, and that research is feasible. It is also suggested that including relevant stakeholders in the prioritization process will help to increase the likelihood that research knowledge will be used (Smith et al. 2009), and that it will enable the validity of initial areas of importance to be reinforced and areas of additional concern to be identified, as well as improving the uptake of the process (Pickard et al. 2009). Furthermore, it is suggested that the interaction between the various stakeholders in the prioritization process can enable stakeholders to learn about, and perhaps understand, the constraints and issues that exist in different research contexts (Smith et al. 2009). However, in all of this, it is suggested that the process of inclusion is the most important consideration (Lomas et al. 2003). The process must be transparent and also ensure that no particular interest dominates the process, so that all participants have a voice. While the aim may be to represent the range of stakeholders that are relevant in the priority-setting process, the number of stakeholders involved adds to the complexity of the process (Fleurence and Torgerson 2004).

Engaging 'experts'

Certain consensus techniques (such as Delphi) begin by establishing a panel of 'experts' among whom consensus will be sought. The term 'experts' in this case refers to 'individuals who (based on criteria) are perceived to have expertise in the subject under investigation' (Keeney et al. 2006: 208). Further, Keeney et al. (2006) suggest the panel of experts must be selected in advance and they should be selected carefully, as the exact composition of the panel will affect the results. However, they conclude that there is no 'magic formula' for the selection of participants and the process is often constrained by 'funding, logistics, and rigorous inclusion and exclusion criteria' (Keeney et al. 2006: 209).

Involving managers and policymakers

Lomas et al. (2003) emphasize the importance of managers and policymakers being involved in the research prioritization process, as well as patients, clinicians and other providers, on the basis that it is managers and policymakers who constantly strive 'to make the best possible decisions in an evidence-based health service' (Lomas et al. 2003: 362). Lomas et al. (2003) remind us that, although we may wish to privilege the views of various stakeholders in the process, the aim of research prioritization is to identify topics for investment in research that will improve service delivery and organization, and as such, participants who deal with service delivery and organization on a daily basis need to be included. Further, they argue that 'not only do they have specific knowledge of the issues in the system, but they also are the ones who will choose to apply or ignore the results for health services research. Having them identify the priorities thus increases their sense of ownership and the likelihood that they will adopt and apply the research findings' (2003: 370).

Involving patients and the public in the process

The inclusion of members of the public in research priority setting is aimed at including a subjective assessment of patient or public preferences in the process (Lomas et al. 2003). It is also believed that involving the public will mean research will have a greater impact on the overall health of communities and that it is more likely to be responsive and applicable (O'Fallon et al. 2003). Taking a different tack, Buckley et al. (2007) suggest a greater emphasis is required on the priorities of the public to counteract the predominance of research that is funded by industry (for instance, pharmaceutical companies) over publicly funded trials. They suggest there is a 'mismatch between what is researched and the information needed to inform every-day decisions when patients, carers and clinicians are considering how best to manage health problems' (Buckley et al. 2007: 3).

There is scope for the public to be involved in the range of methods discussed so far in this chapter; O'Fallon et al. (2003) identify a range of methods that the US National Institute of Environmental Health Sciences (NIEHS) uses to centre the prioritization process around public participation. A comprehensive approach is used to develop partnerships with communities to set research priorities and develop research programmes that are aligned with public health concerns. Box 3.3 outlines approaches that can be used to involve key stakeholders in the research prioritization-setting process. It is reported that this range of methods enables the NIEHS to obtain advice and input from a broad array of researchers, heath care professionals, advocates, policymakers and community members.

Box 3.3   Approaches to involve key stakeholders in the research prioritization process

Workshops, round tables and retreats with researchers, representatives of disease advocacy groups and community-based organizations, health care and public health professionals, and programme staff.

   Public interest liaison groups to seek input from the community and enhance communication and outreach around particular disease groups and groups that represent particular at-risk populations.

   Town meetings and brainstorming sessions at various locations to further develop and modify research, communication and education programmes.

Herbison et al. (2009) identified the range of methods reported in the literature to elicit the views of patients in relation to research priorities. They included ranking, rating and other choice-based approaches, interviews, participatory action research, Delphi technique, focus groups and citizen's juries. They suggest that patients' views are important as they can differ from those of health professionals, but it can be difficult to get informed patients' views on complicated issues such as research. They suggest citizens' juries can be useful in relation to this because they use a combination of education (presenting evidence) and deliberation and so their views are more informed in the process.

Citizens' juries

Gooberman-Hill et al. (2008) provide the following definition of citizens' juries:

> Based on the principle of 'deliberative democracy', citizens' juries aim at entailing decision making based on processes of 'careful deliberation', debate

and respect for different viewpoints. In brief, citizens' juries bring together members of the public (jurors), and provide structured fora for discussion of relevant information provided by 'expert witnesses'. Citizens' juries represent an attempt to bridge the gap between 'top down' consultations that entail little involvement, and 'bottom up' community participation based entirely on lay knowledge and interests. Citizens' juries share similar aims with community-based participatory research. Facilitators and moderators are present to guide the process and witnesses provide 'expert evidence'. The end result is a written report authored by the jurors. (Gooberman-Hill et al. 2008: 272–3)

Gooberman-Hill et al. (2008) also identify a number of issues in the literature to be considered in relation to the involvement of the public in setting research priorities and citizens' juries. These include:

- the extent of involvement of the public and the appropriate format
- the need for early involvement
- the context of involvement and how well participants represent the views and opinions of the wider public or of individuals
- the nature of deliberation itself and the ability of citizens to address complex scientific issues
- the resources required for public involvement initiatives
- the success of public involvement initiatives
- the degree to which the results are translated into policy or practice

Choosing an approach

A range of approaches has been outlined in the previous sections, and, as already suggested, there is no agreement on what is the best way to establish research priorities. Viergever et al. (2010) suggest the optimal approach to priority setting will vary from situation to situation and a standardized approach would not be appropriate. Instead, they propose a checklist that defines nine different elements that should be included in any approach. This checklist is provided in Figure 3.1. Five of the items in the checklist refer to decisions and plans to be made at the preparatory phase. Two elements relate to the process of deciding the priorities, and the remaining two elements relate to what happens after the priorities have been set.

Identifying priority research topics for your research

It is unlikely that a research student will be conducting a Delphi study or nominal group technique to identify priorities for research. However, a number of studies have been conducted, some of which have been identified in this chapter, which could prove useful in terms of research that is likely to be of benefit to patients, health care

Preparatory work:

1   Decide what contextual factors (e.g. focus of the exercise, health, research and political environment, resources, underlying values and principles) underpin the process.

2   Decide which approach is appropriate (e.g. a comprehensive approach or the development of bespoke methods).

3   Decide who should be involved in the process.

4   Decide what information should be gathered to inform the exercise.

5   Establish plans for the translation of priorities to actual research (e.g. policies and funding, who will implement the priorities?).

The process of deciding the priorities:

1   Select relevant criteria to focus discussions around setting priorities.

2   Choose a method for deciding on priorities (e.g. consensus-based approach, a metrics based approach, or both).

After the priorities have been set:

1   Define when and how the established priorities and the priority setting process should be evaluated.

2   To ensure transparency, a clear report should be produced which discusses who set the priorities and how exactly they were set.

Figure 3.1   A priority-setting checklist (adapted from Viergever et al. (2010)).

providers or particular disciplines. Even where such studies do not exist, a useful starting point in identifying a potential research topic is to consider which issues are most relevant to practice, education, management or research. This can be discerned from a review of professional or research literature, policy documents, conference papers or issues reported in the media, as well as through discussions with colleagues, managers and other stakeholders. It is also important to clarify how the proposed research topic will contribute to the existing knowledge base. Through this process, a researcher can strengthen the case that they make in their proposal to project sponsors or potential research funders.

Assessing what is currently known around potential research topics

The proposal to study a particular topic needs to be set out against what is already known about the topic and how the proposed research will add to this. This can draw on the fact that little is known about the phenomenon to be investigated. If the topic has been investigated before, the argument for additional research could be that the evidence generated to date is limited and further, more rigorous research is required. Where there is good evidence, a case can be made to build on or to extend this research, to test the applicability of findings to new contexts or populations, or to explore particular aspects in more depth. Therefore, a review of the literature is a vital part of the process in identifying a topic for your research. This should include a review of the quality of the evidence available and of gaps and areas for further research. Systematic reviews or systematic evidence reviews provide the most comprehensive analysis of the research conducted to date in relation to a specific topic.

Systematic reviews

A systematic review enables the researcher to conduct a more objective appraisal of the evidence than traditional literature reviews, and can therefore 'contribute to resolve uncertainty when original research, reviews and editorials disagree' (Egger et al. 2001: 23). A systematic review is 'a review that has been prepared using a systematic approach to minimising biases and random errors which is documented in a materials and methods section' (Egger et al. 2001: 5). A systematic review differs from a standard literature review in that it will involve the assessment of the eligibility and quality of each study identified. As such, only the results of studies that have met the criteria set out in advance of the review will be included in the analysis and the final conclusions of the review. Box 3.4 outlines the protocol required for a systematic review.

Box 3.4 Requirements for a systematic review

1 The review question
2 Inclusion and exclusion criteria for participants, interventions and comparisons, outcomes, study design and methodological quality
3 A search strategy to identify eligible studies
4 The process to assess potential studies and recording process
5 The process to assess the quality of eligible studies and recording process
6 The process to extract data
7 The process to analyse and present results
8 The process to interpret results

The protocol strictly limits the types of studies to be included in the review. This may be limited solely to randomized controlled trials (RCTs), and only those RCT studies that have been assessed and deemed to meet minimum quality criteria. Also, some studies may be given higher priority in the final conclusions, on the basis of their quality, over other studies.

Analysis in a systematic review may include a statistical analysis of data from more than one study. In this way, the results of more than one study can be pooled to increase the sample size and the power of the findings. However, this is only appropriate where the studies are similar in relation to design, participants, intervention and outcome measures. This analysis is referred to as a 'meta-analysis: a statistical analysis of the results from independent studies, which generally aims to produce a single estimate of a treatment effect' (Egger et al. 2001: 5). Where there is insufficient data to conduct a meta-analysis, the authors may draw conclusions from the results of individual studies, with reference to design and quality issues.

The findings of a systematic review can be used to make recommendations for practice or to revise practice protocols or guidelines. Conducting this type of review can also highlight the limited nature of the evidence, even where several studies have been conducted in the past. For example, a recent Cochrane Review (Butler et al. 2011) set out to explore the effect of hospital nurse staffing models on patient and staff-related outcomes. All studies conducted in all jurisdictions and in any language were considered. This study included randomized controlled trials (RCTs), controlled clinical trials (CCTs), controlled before and after studies (CBAs), and interrupted time series studies (ITSs). The review identified over 700 eligible studies related to the topic. On closer examination, this number was reduced to 60 studies that had used an appropriate design. Only 15 studies were included in the final review: the remaining 45 were excluded on the basis of issues relating to the conduct of the study or the quality of the data available. The findings of this review highlight the importance of choosing an appropriate research design when undertaking a study.

Another variation of the systematic review is a systematic evidence review. These include effectiveness and comparative effectiveness reviews and use rigorous methods to evaluate the extent to which existing research answers specific clinical questions (Gold et al. 2011). This process also identifies gaps in the literature, which is the 'logical starting place' when seeking to identify and prioritize future research questions (Gold et al. 2011: 2). For example, O'Connor et al. (2009) conducted a systematic evidence review of the benefits and harms of screening adult patients for depression in a primary care setting, the benefits of depression treatment in older adults, and the harms of depression treatment with antidepressant medications. They used a wide range of sources of evidence, including randomized clinical trials and controlled clinical trials judged to be of fair to good quality, and large observational studies. They also included systematic reviews and meta-analyses previously conducted. Building on a previous review, they sought to identify new evidence published on the benefits of screening for depression in primary care, or in areas where the evidence in the previous review was insufficient or was not examined, and to integrate this new evidence with the previously identified evidence. This approach enabled conclusions to be drawn around the key questions but also highlighted gaps that remain in the literature. For example, they identified the limited evidence base in relation to antidepressant treatments, where much of the evidence for serious suicide-related harms comes from short-term RCTs conducted for drug development and regulatory approval. They highlight several reasons why this evidence may not be generalizable to primary care and issues with high placebo effects. This suggests this issue is an area for further research and also highlight design issues to be considered in future research.

Systematic reviews of qualitative studies

A number of newer techniques have been developed to conduct systematic reviews that include qualitative studies. These include meta-narrative review and realist synthesis. Meta-narrative review involves mapping or tracing the historical development of concepts, theories and methods to identify the seminal theoretical materials, and analysing the conceptual and theoretical models proposed by authors considered to be experts in the field. The approach is systematic, similar to the systematic review approach described earlier, but will consider all studies relevant to the topic of interest. The approach will culminate in a summary of the overall messages from the research literature and key recommendations for practice, policy and further research (Greenhalgh et al. 2004).

Realist synthesis is promoted as a pragmatic approach to reviewing research evidence, which acknowledges the complexity of health care initiatives and the importance of contextual factors in whether they work or not. As such, the approach complements the more established approaches to systematic reviewing. Realist synthesis acknowledges the inflexibility of traditional systematic reviews and offers an alternative approach, which although more flexible is just as rigorous – 'and it should be possible to "look behind" the review and see how decisions were made, evidence sought, sifted and assessed, and findings accumulated and synthesised' (Pawson et al. 2004: iv). Once again, such an approach culminates in an assessment of the current state of knowledge and the identification of areas for further research.

Understanding the preferences of research stakeholders

In choosing a priority research topic, it is also helpful to consider which topics or questions are likely to be considered to be important to those funding or using research. Pickard et al. (2011) (see Table 3.1) report criteria developed by the US Federal Coordinating Council to evaluate potential topics and questions for comparative effectiveness research. In these criteria, there are particular emphases on

Table 3.1 Criteria for research priorities (adapted from Pickard et al. (2011))

Minimum criteria	*Further criteria*
Feasibility	Potential impact
Responsiveness to stakeholder needs	Focus on diverse populations and patient subgroups
Potential to inform decision making	
	Potential to address uncertainty/variability in the workplace
	Potential to address gaps in evidence otherwise unlikely to be addressed through other initiatives
	Potential for multiplicative effect

responsiveness to stakeholder needs and relevance to decision makers, likely impact, and the potential to address gaps in knowledge and understanding. The criteria also include feasibility, which is always an important consideration in identifying a research topic.

Identifying treatment uncertainties

Another approach to identifying a priority research topic is to look at gaps in the knowledge base in terms of treatment uncertainties. Buckley et al. (2007) suggest there can be mismatches between the research priorities identified by researchers, academia and industry and those that are important to patients, carers and practising clinicians. As a result, there is a mismatch between what is researched and the research needed to inform decisions made daily by clinicians and patients in relation to how best to manage health problems. They report on the establishment of the James Lind Alliance (JLA) in 2004 to encourage patients and clinicians to work together to identify and prioritize treatment uncertainties and unanswered questions. A partnership approach is adopted by the JLA, which involves the following iterative stages. Firstly, uncertainties about the effects of treatments, which have not been addressed through an up-to-date systematic review, are identified. Next, these uncertainties are assembled in the DUETs (Database of Uncertainties about the Effects of Treatments) database. In the final stage, uncertainties are prioritized through agreement among partners. One or more of the following consensus methods may be used to prioritize potential research questions: Delphi techniques, expert panels, nominal group technique, online voting, interactive research agenda setting, and focus groups. Buckley et al. (2007) report that a range of research funding organizations, including the Medical Research Council and the NHS Health Technology Assessment programme, has used the work of the JLA. To date, the JLA has identified priorities in relation to asthma; ear, nose and throat; prostate cancer; schizophrenia; stroke; type 1 diabetes; urinary continence; and vitiligo. A similar database has been established in the UK (UK DUETs). Uncertainties about the effects of treatments are identified through: questions submitted by patients, carers and clinicians; knowledge gaps identified in systematic reviews and clinical guidelines; and systematic reviews and new primary studies in progress. However, in this case there is no attempt to prioritize the items contained – the view being that prioritization is best undertaken by those who have 'intimate knowledge of the health problems and treatments concerned' (UK DUETs 2012).

Personal interest

The researcher should also consider his or her own personal interests when choosing a research topic. Researchers often become quite specialized in the topics they choose to study. In some ways this relates to personal interest, but also to selecting topics that align with a professional career, or subjects that they believe will make a meaningful contribution to a specific body of knowledge. Researchers accumulate expertise over time around specific topics or research designs. They also become more conversant with the knowledge base and where gaps still exist. Boyd and Munhall (2001) suggest this personal interest is an important 'strategic tool':

> It provides the energy and the motivation to persevere with the challenges and tedium inherent in any scholarly work. More importantly, however, personal interest can position the researcher to attend to the phenomenon under study in a certain way; it establishes figure and ground for the research endeavour in what can be highly personalized ways that make the research a passion, a preoccupation, an intimate companion. (Boyd and Munhall 2001: 615)

As such, the topic selected can set a researcher's career in a particular direction and therefore it is important that the researcher has a genuine personal interest in the topic selected.

Translating your idea into a research question

Once a topic is selected, the challenge for the researcher is to set this idea out in a form of words that defines the focus of the research and the parameters of the study. This is done in one or more research questions. O'Leary (2010) suggests the researcher consider the following when writing the research questions:

- What is your topic?
- What is the context for your research?
- What do you want to achieve?
- What is the nature of your question?
- Are there any potential relationships that you want to explore?

This exercise may lead to a number of questions, and the researcher will need to identify which is the main question, based on the researcher's interest, practicalities, and on advice. The research questions will need to be refined so that they are clear and unambiguous, and the literature around the topic will be an important resource in terms of what is already known and how the proposed study will contribute to the knowledge base. Where the research will examine one or more relationships, it may be appropriate to set these out as hypotheses to be tested in the study.

Conclusion

When selecting a topic for research, it is important that the researcher considers how their research will make a difference to patient care, clinical practice and health policy, and how it will contribute to the knowledge base. The range of resources available to the researcher to do this was identified in this chapter. For those charged with funding research, a range of approaches has been discussed for generating ideas for research and for achieving consensus among key stakeholders on the priorities among these ideas.

Key concepts

- Research priorities for health care research can be identified at a macro level (national, policy), meso level (regional, organization, discipline), or micro level (local, service, project).
- There are two approaches to formal research prioritizing – generating ideas and gaining consensus among stakeholders about the relative importance of these ideas.
- A Delphi study, nominal group technique or the listening model can be used to generate ideas for research.
- The Delphi technique is the most frequently used approach for research prioritization studies and is a relatively straightforward and effective way to reach group decisions.
- There is increasing emphasis on involving stakeholders, including the public, in the research prioritization process.
- Research priorities can be identified at different levels of abstraction depending on the aims of the exercise.
- When identifying a potential research topic it is best to consider which issues are most relevant to practice, education, management or research by reviewing professional or research literature, policy documents and conference papers, and through discussions with colleagues, managers and other stakeholders.
- Systematic reviews or systematic evidence reviews provide the most comprehensive analysis of the research conducted to date in relation to a specific topic.
- In choosing a priority research topic, consider which topics or questions are likely to be considered to be important to those funding or using research.
- The researcher should also consider their own personal interests when choosing a priority research topic.

Key readings

- Z. O'Leary, Chapter 4: Developing your research question, in Z. O'Leary (ed.) *The Essential Guide to Doing Your Research Project* (Los Angeles: Sage, 2010), pp. 46–60

Useful websites

- James Lind Alliance – http://www.lindalliance.org/index.asp
- NHS DUETs database – http://www.library.nhs.uk/DUETs/page.aspx?pagename= UNCERT

References

Allen, J., Dyas, J. and Jones, M. (2004) Building consensus in health care: A guide to using the nominal group technique, *British Journal of Community Nursing*, 9(3): 110–14.

Association of Community Health Nursing Educators (ACHNE) Research Committee (2010) Research priorities for public health nursing, *Public Health Nursing*, 27(1): 94–100.

Boyd, C. and Munhall, P. (2001) Qualitative research proposals and reports, in P. Munhall (ed.) *Nursing Research: A Qualitative Perspective*, 3rd edn. Boston, MA: Jones and Bartlett, pp. 613–38.

Buckley, B., Grant, A., Firkins, L., Greene, A. and Frankau, J. (2007) *Influencing the Research Agenda: Establishing and Evaluating a Partnership of Patients, Carers and Clinicians to Identify Research Priorities – A Protocol*. Southampton: James Lind Alliance. Available at www.lindalliance.org/pdfs/JLA%20WP%20UI%20Protocol.pdf [Aaccessed 28 February 2012].

Butler, M., Collins, R., Drennan, J., Halligan, P., O'Mathúna, D.P., Schultz, T.J., Sheridan, A. and Vilis, E. (2011) Hospital nurse staffing models and patient and staff-related outcomes, *Cochrane Database of Systematic Reviews (Online)*, 7, CD007019.

Corner, J., Wright, D., Hopkinson, J., Gunaratnam, Y., McDonald, J.W. and Foster, C. (2007) The research priorities of patients attending UK cancer treatment centres: Findings from a modified nominal group study, *British Journal of Cancer*, 96(6): 875–81.

Dalkey, N. (1969) *The Delphi Method*. Santa Monica: RAND.

Dalkey, N. and Helmer, O. (1963) An experimental application of the Delphi method to the use of experts, *Management Science*, 9(3): 458–67.

Dillman, D. (2000) *Mail and Internet Surveys: The Tailored Design Method*. New York: John Wiley.

Doorenbos, A.Z., Berger, A.M., Brohard-Holbert, C., Eaton, L., Kozachik, S., LoBiondo-Wood, G., Mallory, G., Rue, T. and Varricchio, C. (2008) ONS Research Priorities Survey, *Oncology Nursing Forum*, 35(6): E100–7.

Dowsett, M., Goldhirsch, A., Hayes, D., Senn, H.-J., Wood, W. and Viale, G. (2007) International web-based consultation on priorities for translational breast cancer research, *Breast Cancer Research*, 9(6): R81–8.

Egger, M., Davey Smith, G. and Altman, D. (2001) *Systematic Reviews in Health Care: Meta-analysis in Context*. London: BMJ Books.

Evans, C., Rogers, S., McGraw, C., Battle, G. and Furniss, L. (2004). Using consensus methods to establish multidisciplinary perspectives on research priorities for primary care, *Primary Health Care Research and Development*, 5(1): 52–9.

Fevang, E., Lockey, D., Thompson, J., Lossius, H. M. and TTR Collaboration (2011) The top five research priorities in physician-provided pre-hospital critical care: A consensus report from a European research collaboration, *Scandinavian Journal of Trauma, Resuscitation and Emergency Medicine*, 19: 57.

Fleurence, R. and Torgerson, D. (2004) Setting priorities for research, *Health Policy*, 69(1): 1–10.

Glasgow, R., Hiss, R., Anderson, R., Friedman, N., Hayward, R., Marrero, D., Barr Taylor, G. and Vinicor, F. (2001) Report of the health care delivery work group: Behavioral research related to the establishment of a chronic disease model for diabetes care, *Diabetes Care*, 24(1): 124–30.

Gold, R., Whitlock, E.P., Patnode, C.D., McGinnis, P.S., Buckley, D.I. and Morris, C. (2011) Prioritizing research needs based on a systematic evidence review: A pilot process for engaging stakeholders, *Health Expectations*, Preview 10.1111/j.1369-7625.2011.00716.x.

Gooberman-Hill, R., Horwood, J. and Calnan, M. (2008) Citizens' juries in planning research priorities: Process, engagement and outcome, *Health Expectations*, 11(3): 272–81.

Green, B., Jones, M., Hughes, D. and Williams, A. (1999) Applying the Delphi technique in a study of GPs' information requirements, *Health & Social Care in the Community*, 7(3): 198–205.

Greenhalgh, T., Robert, G., Macfarlane, F., Bate, P. and Kyriakidou, O. (2004). Diffusion of innovations in service organizations: Systematic review and recommendations, The *Milbank Quarterly*, 82(4): 581–629.

Grundy, M. and Ghazi, F. (2009) Research priorities in haemato-oncology nursing: Results of a literature review and a Delphi study, *European Journal of Oncology Nursing*, 13(4): 235–49.

Hardy, D.J., O'Brien, A.P., Gaskin, C.J., O'Brien, A.J., Morrison-Ngatai, E., Skews, G., Ryan, T. and McNulty, N. (2004) Practical application of the Delphi technique in a bicultural mental health nursing study in New Zealand, *Journal of Advanced Nursing*, 46(1): 95–109.

Henschke, N., Maher, C.G., Refshauge, K.M., Das, A. and McAuley, J.H. (2007) Low back pain research priorities: A survey of primary care practitioners, *BMC Family Practice*, 8(1): 40.

Herbison, P., Hay-Smith, J., Paterson, H., Ellis, G. and Wilson, D. (2009) Research priorities in urinary incontinence: Results from citizens' juries, *BJOG: An International Journal of Obstetrics and Gynaecology*, 116(5): 713–18.

Keeney, S., Hasson, F. and McKenna, H. (2006) Consulting the oracle: Ten lessons from using the Delphi technique in nursing research, *Journal of Advanced Nursing*, 53(2): 205–12.

Lomas, J., Fulop, N., Gagnon, D. and Allen, P. (2003) On being a good listener: Setting priorities for applied health services research, *The Milbank Quarterly*, 81(3): 363–88.

McKenna, H.P. (1994) The Delphi technique: A worthwhile research approach for nursing?, *Journal of Advanced Nursing*, 19(6): 1221–5.

Meehan, T., Kemple, M., Butler, M., Drennan, J., Johnson, M. and Treacy, M. (2005) *Nursing and Midwifery Research Priorities for Ireland*. Dublin: National Council for the Professional Development of Nursing and Midwifery.

O'Connor, E., Whitlock, E., Bell, T. and Gaynes, B. (2009) Screening for depression in adult patients in primary care settings: A systematic evidence review, *Annals of Internal Medicine*, 151(11): 793–803.

O'Fallon, L.R., Wolfle, G.M., Brown, D., Dearry, A. and Olden, K. (2003) Strategies for setting a national research agenda that is responsive to community needs, *Environmental Health Perspectives*, 111(16): 1855–60.

O'Leary, Z. (2010) Developing your research question, in Z. O'Leary (ed.) *The Essential Guide to Doing Your Research Project*. Los Angeles: Sage, pp. 46–60.

Pawson, R., Greenhalgh, T. and Harvey, G. (2004). *Realist Synthesis: An Introduction*. Manchester: ESRC Research Methods Programme, University of Manchester.

Pickard, A.S., Lee, T.A., Solem, C.T., Joo, M.J., Schumock, G.T. and Krishnan, J.A. (2011) Prioritizing comparative-effectiveness research topics via stakeholder involvement: An application in COPD, *Clinical Pharmacology & Therapeutics*, 90(6): 888–92.

Reid, N. (1988) The Delphi technique: its contribution to the evaluation of professional practice, in R. Ellis (ed) *Professional Competence and Quality Assurance in the Caring Professions*. New York: Chapman and Hall, pp. 230–62.

Ross, F., Smith, E., Mackenzie, A. and Masterson, A. (2004) Identifying research priorities in nursing and midwifery service delivery and organisation: A scoping study, *International Journal of Nursing Studies*, 41(5): 547–58.

Smith, N., Mitton, C., Peacock, S., Cornelissen, E. and MacLeod, S. (2009) Identifying research priorities for health care priority setting: A collaborative effort between managers and researchers, *BMC Health Services Research*, 9: 165.

UK DUETs (2012) *UK DUETs: Where uncertainties about the effects of treatment are collected and published*. Available at http://www.library.nhs.uk/duets/ [Accessed 10 February 2012].

Vella, K., Goldfrad, C., Rowan, K., Bion, J. and Black, N. (2000) Use of consensus development to establish national research priorities in critical care, *British Medical Journal*, 320(7240): 976–80.

Viergever, R.F., Olifson, S., Ghaffar, A. and Terry, R.F. (2010) A checklist for health research priority setting: Nine common themes of good practice, *Health Research Policy and Systems*, 8: 36.

Williams, P.L. and Webb, C. (1994) The Delphi technique: A methodological discussion, *Journal of Advanced Nursing*, 19(1): 180–6.

4   Writing research questions and hypotheses

Maree Johnson

Chapter topics

- Falsification as the basis of hypothesis testing
- The origins of the word hypothesis
- The structure of a hypothesis and a research question
- The relationship between the thesis argument and the hypothesis or research question
- Operational definitions
- The application of theory to research questions and hypotheses
- An overview of hypothesis testing and when and why we use research questions versus hypotheses
- Varying forms of hypotheses: null, directional/non-directional, and their application, with examples from contemporary nursing and midwifery research
- The relationship between questions/ hypotheses and research method and design

Introduction

A clearly articulated research question or hypothesis in the right form(s) can direct the design, sample, data-collection tools, and also the analysis procedures to be used. The close alignment of the question or hypothesis with the design and analysis approach is more likely to result in the question being answered as intended. However, to ask the right question or hypothesis, in the right form, presents a particular challenge to the researcher. This chapter will explore key aspects of the definition of research questions and hypotheses and the forms they may take, provide examples based on diverse research designs, and conclude with a decision-making approach to the selection of questions or hypotheses.

The scientific method has been embraced by contemporary society as a way of determining the 'truth' about what to believe about our world. We use the results of scientific studies to assess whether one treatment is better than another or to understand whether relationships exist among events in our world (Browne and Keeley 1994). As one author suggests, research methods are 'a tool for life' (Beins 2009). The fundamental approach to scientific method is falsification or the disproving of proposed hypotheses. Beins (2009) describes falsification as the testing of hypothesized relationships (between concepts) to see if they are wrong. A particularly difficult issue surrounding hypothesis testing is the tendency for the researcher to engage in confirmation bias, or the tendency to seek out and prove information that supports a particular hypothesis (Mercier and Sperber 2011). A well-reasoned argument, considering the strengths and weaknesses of the existing literature, should precede the development of any research question or hypothesis.

Hypotheses defined

The word hypothesis is derived from the Greek word *hypothesis* meaning 'base', 'basis of an argument' or 'supposition', with the scientific use of the term appearing in the 1640s.[1] Hypotheses are derived from propositions or premises. Premises are relationships between one concept and another concept. The hypothesis is a special form of describing a relationship between two (simple) or more (complex) concepts. The form or presentation of the hypothesis influences (or relates to) the study research design, method of data collection and analysis. Johnson and Hengstberger-Sims (2011: 33) define hypotheses as: 'statements about the relationship between two (or more) variables' and they may include relationships between variables or independent variables that change outcomes (dependent variables). A variable is defined as 'an element in a research project that when measured, can take on more than one value' (Bein 2009: 123). Hypotheses or research questions are the fundamental building blocks of any research study and the correct definition of these components will correctly connect the topic with the subsequent design and analysis procedures. There are several forms of hypotheses that are noteworthy. These include the null hypothesis, non-directional hypothesis and directional hypothesis.

Null hypotheses

The null hypothesis is used when the researcher believes there is no difference between the groups being studied: 'it assumes that the two groups being examined are the same' (Dunn 2010: 177). This means that there is no effect following the intervention or manipulation of an independent variable – for example, pharmacy students in small and large classes will do equally well on end-of-term examinations (based on Dunn's (2010) example). In health research, examples are more often seen in relation to patient safety research or where there is a small prevalence of the outcome:

> Similar numbers (proportion) of infants with Apgar scores less than 7 at 5 minutes will be demonstrated for low risk mothers receiving primary health midwifery care and [mothers receiving] standard hospital care. (Johnson et al. 2005: 23)

Directional hypotheses

Directional hypotheses are the most frequently reported in the research literature. On reviewing the literature, the researcher identifies the likely direction, either increase or decrease, in a dependent (outcome) variable (Houser 2008; Nieswiadomy 2008; Dunn 2010).

---

[1]http://www.etymonline.com/index.php?allowed_in_frame=0&search=hypothesis&searchmde=none

As Dunn (2010: 178) notes, the researcher has 'a good idea of the character of the relationship between the variables of interest':

> We hypothesized that declines in marital satisfaction would predict contemporaneous increases in depressive symptoms and that increases in depression symptoms would predict contemporaneous declines in marital satisfaction. (Poyner-Del Vento and Cobb 2011: 208)

Non-directional hypotheses

A non-directional hypothesis is used when it is unclear from the literature as to whether an intervention will increase or decrease a behaviour or change in the dependent variable or outcome. Houser (2008: 126) defines a non-directional hypothesis as 'a two-sided statement of the research question that is interested in change in any direction':

> Consistent with the TPB [theory of planned behaviour], we hypothesised that changes in underlying behaviour, normative or control beliefs would be accompanied by a change in the relevant TPB component (attitude, subjective norm or perceived behaviour control), interventions and behaviours. (Elliott and Armitage 2009: 114)

Finally, Dunn (2010) suggests that hypotheses should fulfil the following criteria:

- identify specific relationships among concepts or variables
- be based on a theory or existing knowledge
- be to the point (approximately one to two sentences long)
- be capable of being tested
- be readily understood by others

Confidence intervals and hypothesis testing

In exploring whether a significant difference exists between variables, hypothesis testing is usually undertaken by calculating a p-value. Normally, if the p-value is ≤0.05 the difference is said to be statistically significant (see Chapter 10 for further details). However, in health care research the *size* of the difference is also required (Gardner and Altman 1986). Gardner and Altman challenge the approach of simply statistically testing the null hypothesis, due to its limited application in clinical practice for medicine and other health professions. They argue that simply knowing whether a treatment works or not is of limited value. Clinicians need to know by how much a patient improved using treatment A versus treatment B or treatment C. These authors conclude that confidence intervals should be presented and 'have a link to the outcome of hypothesis tests, [and] should become the standard method for presenting the statistical results of major findings' (Gardner and Altman 1986: 748). For more on the calculation and interpretation of confidence intervals see Gardner and Altman (1986) and Weathington et al. (2010).

Research questions defined

Research questions are less difficult to describe than hypotheses but the term itself is sometimes misleading. Often students assume that the research questions are the questions that you are going to ask a study participant, rather than the specific question(s) the study will answer. Research questions are defined as 'specific queries researchers want to answer in addressing the research problem' (Polit and Beck 2010: 46). Research questions can be used in a wide variety of studies, whereas hypotheses are slightly more limited in their application. By the very nature of the definition of a hypothesis, it is evident that hypotheses are not used in qualitative research, whereas research questions are frequently used in conjunction with qualitative designs as well as quantitative designs.

Although hypotheses or research questions are the most specific form of the study question, there are several other aspects of a research study that require clear articulation by the researcher that allow for the meaning or origins of the questions posed to be understood.

Other aspects of defining the study related to hypotheses and research questions

Several major aspects of the definition of the research study are interrelated. These include:

- the problem statement
- the aim or purpose of the study
- the specific objectives of the study
- the research questions
- the hypotheses

Other important components of the definition of these aspects include the use of a frame of reference and the formation of operational definitions. The researcher has initially synthesized the literature and would have presented an argument in relation to the scope of the study, that is, as follows:

- the population or sample concerned: for example, children with cystic fibrosis
- the phenomena of interest: for example, supportive care for children with cystic fibrosis or the intervention: for example, twice-daily physical therapy
- whether there is any comparison group: for example, children with cystic fibrosis receiving only daily physical therapy
- what outcomes are expected: for example, incidence of chest infections

The problem statement

The *problem* identification and *statement* is the first aspect of defining the scope of the study. A problem statement 'describe[s] what the situation is that requires changing or understanding and how the study will address these problems' (Francis et al. 1979: 27; Johnson and Hengstberger-Sims 2011). Box 4.1 demonstrates examples of problem statements in health care research.

Box 4.1   Examples of problem statements in health care research

---

An example of the problem statement is provided in a case of physical therapy for children with cystic fibrosis.[2] Initially, the researcher outlines areas for further research on a topic and states the problem statement. The problem statement is often a complex set of connected sentences that reflect the problem. For example: *high rate of chest infections in children with cystic fibrosis and known effectiveness of approaches to physical therapy for children with cystic fibrosis.* In addition, how this study specifically addresses some lack of knowledge in the area: *this study will compare twice-daily versus daily physical therapy not previously tested,* and the likely outcomes of the study: *to reduce incidence of chest infections.* An example of how these concepts are brought together is outlined below:

> Although there is a known high incidence of chest infections in children with cystic fibrosis and the effectiveness of daily physical therapy has been demonstrated, there is no study that has examined the effectiveness of twice-daily physical therapy in reducing the incidence of chest infections. This study will compare two approaches to home physical therapy to determine the best approach to reducing chest infections in children with cystic fibrosis.

Another example of a problem statement:

> There is considerable research comparing intermittent versus continuous naso-gastric feeding of patients with brain injury. However, there is little research comparing these feeding methods in stroke patients within the first 24 hours. This study will use a randomized controlled trial design to compare health outcomes (incidence of aspiration pneumonia) of intermittent versus continuous naso-gastric feeding in stroke patients.[2]

A critical aspect that often receives less attention until the proposal is fully developed is the issue of feasibility of a research study and problem. A study is considered feasible when there are sufficient participants to test the hypothesis, the technical expertise to complete the study, adequate funding and time to undertake the processes required (Houser 2008). The study scope is then limited to a manageable problem for the researchers (Houser 2008). Chapter 3 provides examples of research problems and how they are identified in practice.

Theoretical or conceptual frameworks

Another important aspect of defining the research is the application of theoretical and conceptual frameworks or models or classification systems to drive the research

---

[2] This is a fictitious example and will be used throughout the chapter as an example of the concepts discussed.

(see Chapter 2). The practical aspects of the application of theory in research are well outlined by Meleis (1997: 20), who states: 'the theory sets limits on what questions to ask and what methods to use' and also defines relationships between variables for testing and subsequently contributes to the theory's evolution (Meleis 1997). Theories or conceptual understandings from psychology, sociology, nursing and health have all been applied to research to more precisely define the scope of the study. Dunn (2010: 8), on citing Kurt Lewin, noted that 'good psychological theories foster explanation, organize facts, predict observations and guide new exploration of a topic'. Examples of theoretical frameworks used in research include:

- Bandura's theory of self-efficacy (Bandura 1982, 1986, 1987)
- Ajzen's theory of planned behaviour (Ajzen 1991)
- Aronson's taxonomy of medication error

Our first example of a theoretical framework uses the theory of self-efficacy by Bandura to explore the relationship between grandparents' perceived efficacy and their subsequent involvement with their grandchildren:

> Based on self-efficacy theory, we hypothesize that individuals who feel efficacious as a grandparent will play a larger and more active role in the lives of their grandchildren than grandparents who feel they have little influence. Although we expect judgments of self-efficacy to be related to behavior, a number of factors can affect the strength of this relationship. Social environments such as physical distance, poor health, or strained relations with adult children may place 'constraints' on what people do or may aid them to behave optimally. Similarly, individuals may lack the resources or equipment needed to perform the behaviour (Bandura 1982, Bandura 1986, 1987). (King and Elder 1998: 251)

The second example of a conceptual framework uses a taxonomy by Aronson to examine medication errors in nursing:

> Aronson (2009) states that the best approach to understanding how medication errors occur is to use a classification system that is contextual (specific time, place, medication, people), modal (way errors occur, omission, substitution), and more importantly psychological (explains events) (Ferner and Aronson 2006). Ferner and Aronson (2006) propose that a classification system that takes a preventive approach (psychological) is the most desirable and define their taxonomy as being made up of mistakes (knowledge-based and rule-based errors) and skill-based errors (action-based errors [slips, including technical errors] and memory-based errors [lapses]) . . . This study applies for the first time Aronson's behavioural-focused taxonomy to classifying medication errors in nursing and uses this information to propose strategies to reduce such errors. (Johnson and Young 2011: 129)

Both these approaches use existing theory or frames of reference to influence the research study questions.

As noted above, a theory or conceptual framework can be used to define the scope of the study, relationship between variables, domains within instruments, and in some cases data analysis. An example can be taken from Cowin's and others work on self-concept in nursing.

The self-concept theory has its origins in educational psychology (Marsh and Hattie 1996), however Cowin used this theory to explore nurses' professional self-concept. First, an instrument was designed using the known theoretical domains of nurses' self-concept (Cowin 2001), then relationships between nurses' self-concept and job satisfaction and retention of nurses were examined using this instrument (Cowin et al. 2008). Structural equation modelling, where simultaneous relationships can be statistically examined, was used to answer the hypotheses posed. Then further work by Cowin and Hengstberger-Sims explored new nursing graduates' self-concept and retention, also using this instrument (Cowin and Hengstberger-Sims 2006). In this example, the theory of self-concept has guided development of tools, the research hypotheses based on the relationships between variables in the theory, and new variables such as satisfaction and retention. Following this, the theoretical constructs were applied to another context, of new graduate retention. In this example of knowledge and theory development and evolution, the practical aspects of applying theory to shape a problem are highlighted.

Many studies, particularly clinical research, do not require a conceptual framework. However, all studies require the definition of specific terms or concepts used in the study. The precise definition of the terms or key concepts in a study allows for replication of the work and minimizes misinterpretation of the study concepts.

Operational definitions

Dunn (2010: 23) describes the development of operational definitions of the terms in a hypothesis: 'operational definitions change the conceptual elements from a research hypothesis into concrete, testable terms that can be observed, understood, agreed upon, and even used by other researchers'.

Terms or definitions of constructs, concepts, or biological measures should be defined in simple language. Sources of definitions vary from existing literature, dictionaries to technical glossaries (Francis et al. 1979). Operational definitions are often reported in terms of how the construct is measured. The following are examples of psychosocial constructs and biological measures from research:

> In a study of ethnically diverse older women, Lagana et al. (2011) sought to test measures of social quality of life for older women. All three measures – Older Women's Social Quality of Life Inventory (OWSQLI), Single Item Measures of Social Support (SIMSS) and the Medical Outcomes Study 36-item Short Form Health Survey (MOS SF-36) – represent an operational definition of social quality of life for older women i.e., social quality of life for older women as measured by the OWSQLI, SIMSS, and the MOS SF-36 (Lagana et al. 2011). Participants were administered the following: 50 items from which the final items of the new Older Women's Social Quality of Life Inventory

> (OWSQLI) were to be chosen; the Single Item Measure of Social Support (SIMSS); and the Medical Outcome Study 36-item Short-Form Health Survey (MOS SF-36). (Lagana et al. 2011: 1)

Another example of the use of an operational definition is highlighted in a study of the risk factors of autism. The definition of autism was described by the authors using the International Classification of Diseases (ICD) version 8 and 10 codes, as follows:

> A diagnosis of infantile or atypical autism (ICD-8 diagnosis codes 299.00–299.01 or ICD-10 diagnosis codes F84.0–F84.1x). (Larsson et al. 2005: 918)

In a quasi-experimental study of warming interventions for surgical patients with mild and moderate hypothermia, the following terms were defined:

> Heat gain (°C) refers to the number of degrees of temperature the subject had to gain to reach 36°C (i.e. 36°C minus arrival temperature at recovery). (Stevens et al. 2000: 270)

Research aim

A research aim is a statement about what the study is going to do. Often this is confused with the expected outcome of the study, such as provide knowledge about the best approach. An example of an aim for a quantitative study is presented below:

> The aim of this study is to examine the efficacy of two approaches to physical therapy in a group of children with cystic fibrosis.

Characteristics of 'good' research questions or hypotheses

According to Johnson and Hengstberger-Sims (2011: 34), research questions and hypotheses should have the following components:

- the participants
- the clinical context
- the phenomenon of concern
- intervention
- comparison group
- outcomes

A quantitative example of hypothesis/questions is presented below and in Table 4.1 to demonstrate these characteristics:

> Mild (35.5–36.0°C) or moderate (34.5–35.4°C) hypothermic patients who have undergone surgery for greater than 20 minutes, and who received Bair-Hugger™ warming, will achieve normothermia in less time (increased rewarming rate) than hypothermic patients receiving only warmed cotton blankets. (Stevens et al. 2000: 270)

Table 4.1   Characteristics of hypotheses

Participants	Mild (35.5–36.0°C) or moderate (34.5–35.4°C) hypothermic patients who have undergone surgery for greater than 20 minutes
Intervention	Bair-Hugger™ warming
Comparison group	Hypothermic patients receiving only warmed cotton blankets.
Outcome	Normothermia in less time (increased rewarming rate)

Table 4.2   The relationship between the research topic, research question or hypothesis and design

Study focus	Type of quantitative design	Study example
Descriptive research Defining the characteristics of people, places or events	Descriptive/ exploratory	What are the coping styles of pregnant adolescents? (Myors, Johnson and Langdon 2001)
Correlational research The literature, including theoretical or conceptual relations, suggests that one or more independent variables are related to one or more dependent variables	Correlational	We hypothesized that declines in marital satisfaction would predict contemporaneous increases in depressive symptoms and that increases in depression symptoms would predict contemporaneous declines in marital satisfaction (Poyner-Del Vento and Cobb 2011)
Intervention or treatment The literature suggests that one treatment or intervention is likely to have outcomes better than or similar to another	Experimental	Mild (35.5–36.0°C) or moderate (34.5–35.4°C) hypothermic patients who have undergone surgery for greater than 20 minutes, and who received Bair-Hugger™ warming, will achieve normothermia in less time (increased rewarming rate) than hypothermic patients receiving only warmed cotton blankets (Stevens et al. 2000: 270) (Directional hypothesis)
		Community-living clients, receiving a short course of intravenous antibiotic therapy with reinsertion of cannulae every 96 hours, will have a similar incidence of thrombophlebitis as clients having their cannulae replaced every 48 hours or when required (Johnson and Hengstberger-Sims 2011: 35) (Non-directional hypothesis)

The relationship between the question/hypothesis and the design of the study

The major research designs – descriptive, association, experimental (quantitative) and a range of qualitative or mixed methods – all have a role to play in the developing research questions and hypotheses. The final consideration of a researcher is the relationship between the design and the question or hypothesis posed. A framework within which to consider whether a research question or hypothesis should be used for a particular study, based on three levels of understanding, is presented in Table 4.2.

As can be seen from Table 4.2, the hypothesis or research question is consistent with the design or may indicate the design required. In addition, the design itself will dictate the likely data analysis approach to be taken.

Conclusion

Throughout this chapter the refinement of the research topic into testable research questions or hypotheses has been explored. The importance of the researcher clearly stating other aspects directly related to the question or hypothesis, such as the problem statement, aim, operational definition and the use of theory or frames of reference were also described. Characteristics of hypotheses or research questions, and criteria for their evaluation are presented. The various types of hypotheses and when they are to be used are outlined and examples provided. Finally, the relationship between the topic, the hypothesis/research question and the design and statistical method is detailed. Additional considerations, such as confidence interval testing, are emphasized to the reader but a comprehensive discussion on this topic is beyond the scope of this chapter.

Key concepts

- Hypothesis testing uses an approach known as falsification or the disconfirming of the proposed relationship between concepts.
- A well-reasoned argument should precede the development of any research question or hypothesis.
- A frame of reference or theory can be used to explore key relationships, predict outcomes, or further develop theory or analysis methods.
- Operational definitions of terms or concepts allow the research to be clearly understood, appropriately observed or measured, and ultimately replicated.
- The selection of a hypothesis or research question is contingent upon the type of topic: descriptive, correlational, experimental (quantitative) or exploratory (qualitative).
- There are various types of hypotheses, and the chosen type is related to whether there is no change (non-directional) or change (directional) expected in the dependent variable (outcome).

Key readings

- H. Hamilton and J. Clare, Reviewing the literature: Making 'the literature' work for you, *Collegian: Journal of the Royal College of Nursing Australia*, 11(1) (2004), 8–11
  This paper gives the researcher information on how to summarize the literature and present an argument or the foundation of the developing hypothesis of any study.
- D.F. Polit and C.T. Beck, *Essentials of Nursing Research: Appraising Evidence for Nursing Practice* (Philadelphia: Wolters Kluwer Health/Lippincott Williams & Wilkins, 2010)
  This textbook provides numerous examples of research questions and hypotheses applicable to nursing and midwifery practice.
- H. Mercier and D. Sperber, Why do humans reason? Arguments for an argumentative theory, *Behavioral and Brain Sciences*, 34(2) (2011), 57–74
  This article provides an extensive discussion on the use of argument, and particularly confirmation bias.

References

Ajzen, I. (1991) The theory of planned behaviour, *Organizational Behavior and Human Decision Processes*, 50(2): 179–211.

Aronson, J.K. (2009) Medication errors: definitions and classification, *British Journal of Clinical Pharmacology*, 67(6): 599–604.

Bandura, A. (1982) The self and mechanisms of agency, in J. Suls (ed.) *Psychological Perspectives on the Self*. Hillsdale, NJ: Lawrence Erlbaum, pp. 3–39.

Bandura, A. (1986) Self-efficacy, in A. Bandura (ed.) *Social Foundations of Thought and Action: A Social Cognitive Theory*. New Jersey: Prentice Hall, pp. 390–5.

Bandura, A. (1987) Perceived self-efficacy: Exercise of control through self-belief, in J.P. Dauwalker, M. Perrez and V. Hobi (eds) *Controversial Issues in Behavioral Modification*. Amsterdam: Swets & Zeitlinger, pp. 27–59.

Beins, B.C. (2009) *Research Methods: A Tool for Life*. Boston, MA: Pearson Education.

Browne, M.N. and Keeley, S.M. (1994) *Asking the Right Questions: A Guide to Critical Thinking*, 4th edn. Englewood Cliffs, NJ: Prentice-Hall.

Cowin, L. (2001) Measuring nurses' self-concept, *Western Journal of Nursing Research*, 23(3): 313–25.

Cowin, L.S. and Hengstberger-Sims, C. (2006) New graduate nurse self-concept and retention: A longitudinal survey, *International Journal of Nursing Studies*, 43(1): 59–70.

Cowin, L., Johnson, M., Craven, R. and Marsh, H.W. (2008) Causal modeling of self-concept, job satisfaction, and retention of nurses, *International Journal of Nursing Studies*, 45(10): 1449–59.

Dunn, D.S. (2010) *The Practical Researcher: A Student Guide to Conducting Psychological Research*. West Essex: McGraw-Hill.

Elliott, M.A. and Armitage, C.J. (2009) Promoting drivers' compliance with speed limits: Testing an intervention based on the theory of planned behaviour, *British Journal of Psychology*, 100(1): 111–32.

Ferner, R.E. and Aronson, J.K. (2006) Clarification of terminology in medication errors: Definitions and classification, *Drug Safety*, 29(11): 1011–22.

Francis, B.J., Bork, E.C. and Carstens, P.S. (1979) *The Proposal Cookbook: A Step by Step Guide to Dissertation and Thesis Proposal Writing*, 3rd edn. New York: Action Research Associates.

Gardner, M.J. and Altman, D.G. (1986) Confidence intervals rather than P values: estimation rather than hypothesis testing, *British Medical Journal*, 292(6522): 746–50.

Houser, J. (2008) *Nursing Research: Reading, Using and Creating Evidence*. Sudbury, MA: Jones & Bartlett Publishers.

Johnson, M. and Hengstberger-Sims, C. (2011) Introducing the research process, in S. Jirojwong, M. Johnson and A. Welch (eds) *Research Methods in Nursing and Midwifery: Pathways to Evidence-Based Practice*. Melbourne: Oxford University Press, pp. 23–51.

Johnson, M. and Young, H. (2011) The application of Aronson's Taxonomy to medication errors in nursing, *Journal of Nursing Care Quality*, 26(2): 128–35.

Johnson, M., Stewart, H., Langdon, R., Kelly, P. and Yong, L. (2005) A comparison of the outcomes of partnership caseload midwifery and standard hospital care in low risk mothers, *Australian Journal of Advanced Nursing*, 22(3): 22–8.

King, V. and Elder, G.H.J. (1998) Perceived self-efficacy and grandparenting, *The Journal of Gerontology: Social Science*, 53B(5): S249–57.

Lagana, L., Bratly, M.L. and Boutakidis, I. (2011) The validation of a new measure quantifying the social quality of life of ethnically diverse older women: Two cross-sectional studies, *BMC Geriatrics*, 11(1): 60.

Larsson, H.J., Eaton, W.W., Madsen, K.M., Vestergaard, M., Olesen, A.V., Agerbo, E., Schendel, D., Thorsen, P. and Mortensen, P. B. (2005) Risk factors for autism: Perinatal factors, parental psychiatric history, and socioeconomic status, *American Journal of Epidemiology*, 161(10): 916–25.

Marsh, H.W. and Hattie, J. (1996) Theoretical perspectives on the structure of self-concept, in B.A. Bracken, *The Handbook of Self-Concept*. New York: Wiley, pp. 38–90.

Meleis, A.I. (1997) Theory: Who needs it? What is it?, in A.I. Meleis (ed.) *Theoretical Nursing Development and Progress*. San Francisco: Lippincott-Raven Publishers, pp. 8–22.

Mercier, H. and Sperber, D. (2011) Why do humans reason? Arguments for an argumentative theory, *Behavioral and Brain Sciences*, 34(2): 57–74.

Myors, K., Johnson, M. and Langdon, R. (2001) Coping styles of pregnant adolescents, *Public Health Nursing*, 18(1): 24–32.

Nieswiadomy, R.M. (2008) *Foundations of Nursing Research*. Upper Saddle River, NJ: Pearson/ Prentice Hall.

Polit, D.F. and Beck, C.T. (2010) *Essentials of Nursing Research: Appraising Evidence for Nursing Practice*, 7th edn. Philadelphia: Lippincott Williams & Wilkins.

Poyner-Del Vento, P. and Cobb, R.J. (2011) Chronic stress as a moderator of the association between depressive symptoms and marital satisfaction, *Journal of Social and Clinical Psychology*, 30(9): 905–36.

Stevens, D., Johnson, M. and Langdon, R. (2000) Comparison of two warming interventions in surgical patients with mild and moderate hypothermia, *International Journal of Nursing Practice*, 6(5): 268–75.

Weathington, B.L., Cunningham, C.J.L. and Pittenger, D.J. (2010) *Research Methods for the Behavioral and Social Sciences*, Hoboken, NJ: John Wiley & Sons.

PART 2

Ethical considerations

5   Ethical principles in health care research

P. Anne Scott

Chapter topics
- The history of the evolving recognition of the need to regulate research involving human subjects
- Consideration of some key ethical principles relevant to the research process
- Applying ethical understanding in the practice of research

Introduction

Recognition of the need to regulate research on human beings can be traced back to reactions against the abuses associated with German and Japanese research during World War II. However, as the twentieth century rolled out it was increasingly recognized that a number of abuses, in terms of research on human subjects, continued into the post-war period in both democratic and Eastern Bloc countries (Mason and McCall Smith 2010). Revelations during the Nuremberg Trials, for example, of the atrocities committed in the name of medical experimentation during World War II, combined with other twentieth-century medical research scandals such as the Tuskegee Syphilis Study 1932–72 (Adams 1996), and the New Zealand cervical cancer inquiry (Cartwright 1988; Paterson 2010) have helped develop widespread resolve regarding the need to protect participants in human research projects and to continue to monitor the conduct of such research internationally. The first internationally accepted set of ethical guidelines with regard to these issues was the Nuremberg Code published in 1947 (for further comment see Annas and Grodin 1992). The World Medical Association (WMA) publicly endorsed the principles expressed in the Nuremberg Code by drawing up the Declaration of Helsinki in 1964 (WMA 1964). This declaration has been revised a number of times since its first publication.

The past 30 years have seen a number of countries and organizations highlight issues surrounding the ethics of research on human subjects: for example the Belmont Principles (National Commission 1979) and the Irish Council for Bioethics (2004). In the nursing arena, the International Council of Nurses (ICN 1996), An Bord Altranais (the Irish Nursing Board) (2007), the Royal College of Nursing (RCN 2009) and the Northern Nurses' Federation (1995) all published new or revised guidelines for nursing research. Issues regarding the human rights of research participants have also been underlined by the Council of Europe (Council of Europe 1997).

Guided by such international instruments as the Nuremberg Code (1947), the United Nations Declaration on Human Rights (United Nations 1948), especially articles 1, 3, 5, 12 and 19, the United Nations Convention on the Rights of the Child (1989), the Belmont Report (National Commission 1979), and the Declaration of Helsinki (WMA 2008), in addition to various ethical theories that have become influential in health care ethics in general, such as Kantian ethics and the principle-based framework of Beauchamp and Childress (2013), a conceptualization of appropriate ways to treat and protect human beings, both fully functioning adults and vulnerable human beings such as children, older people, the terminally ill, has emerged and continues to be modified over time.

However, as we move into the middle of the second decade of the twenty-first century there are certain ethical principles that are seen as fundamental to the framework of ethics that guides decisions regarding the morally appropriate consideration and treatment of human beings during research activities. For example the Irish Council of Bioethics in 2004 commented as follows:

> Research involving human participants should be based on a fundamental moral commitment to the individuals concerned and to advancing human welfare, knowledge and understanding. A number of guiding moral principles govern the ethical review of research proposals. These principles aim to protect the well-being and rights of research participants/volunteers. (Irish Council for Bioethics 2004: 6)

Some important considerations

Human beings are deserving of respect and protection as inalienable rights (United Nations 1948). This is equally the case during research activities as it is in any other circumstances. Based on the work of the philosopher Immanuel Kant, such values are expressed in the principle of respect for persons, sometimes translated as respect for autonomy. Such expressions, of course, raise questions of the definition of person and autonomy, and of when and in what set of circumstances such concepts are and are not applicable. However, for the purposes of this chapter we will take it that respect is applicable to all human participants in health care research. The question then arises regarding what this actually means in the case of individual participants in a particular research project. At a minimum, the considerations explored below are relevant.

Respect for the human person

In the context of research activity the principle of **respect for persons** is frequently articulated in terms of rights – both rights to autonomous participation and welfare rights – that is, the right to have one's support and protection needs respected. Some such rights are the following:

- the right not to be injured or mistreated
- the right to give informed, un-coerced consent to participate in the particular piece of research
- the right to privacy, confidentiality and/or anonymity

In terms of protecting the participant's right not to be injured or mistreated, it is normally the duty of the research team not to expose the research participant to significantly burdensome, unreasonable, known or predictable risk. On occasion, however, when significant burden or predictable material risk is unavoidable, it is the duty of the research team to provide appropriate information on the likely burden and/or risk involved, so that the participant can determine if they fully understand and accept that burden or risk. Thus, for example, in drug trials and trials involving medical devices, the trials are phased and normally commence with non-human (laboratory and animal) trials. Such measures help to provide insight into likely effects of the particular drug or device – at least on non-human subjects. Thus, by the time clinical trials (trials using human participants) commence, previous phases give insight into the actions of the agent (drug or device, for example). This provides a certain level of confidence that the agent will either not cause significant physical risk to the trial participants or that any such risks, which will be explained to the participant prior to participation, can and will be managed and/or mitigated by the research team. Where discomfort, burden and/or risk cannot be avoided, it must be proportionate to the anticipated gain, either directly to the individual participant and/or to humanity or society. Such considerations are directly linked to the discussion of the principles of beneficence and non-maleficence below.

Informed consent

Respect for the individual's right to make decisions about themselves and their life (respect for autonomy) requires that research participants are adequately and properly informed regarding the nature of the research project. For example, potential participants must be informed with regards to what will be required of the individual participant, including the approximate time requirement, any procedures that will be performed on him or her, any known or predictable risks or side effects, the nature of the trial (where a clinical trial is part of the research design), whether a placebo is being used, whether the trial is blinded and so forth. Such information enables the potential research participant to give **informed consent** to participate in the particular research activity or project.

There are two other crucial elements that must be in play to ensure that consent is not only informed but also voluntary – and thus autonomously exercised. These elements are:

- The participant must have both the capacity to understand the information being provided regarding the particular piece of research, including the implications of participation for the individual, and the (cognitive) ability to exercise consent.
- The participant must be free from coercion. Thus the participant must be assured and accept, for example, that refusal to consent will not affect her/his current care and treatment if the individual is being cared for by any member of a health care team, either in hospital or in the community. The individual should also be free from any other form of duress related to the research in question – from the research or health care team or from relatives

or significant others (see Doyal and Tobias (2001)) for a detailed discussion of the principal requirements of informed consent).

In instances where the potential research participant is a patient, practitioners should be aware of the profound influence that they may have on patients to whom they suggest participating in research. For example Kass et al. (1996: 4), in a study on participant consent to involvement in cancer clinical trials, express it thus:

> Clinicians should be mindful of the tremendous influence they have over their patients, given that the mere suggestion of enrolment in research by a patient's personal physician was interpreted by many patients to be endorsement.

Some research, in the context of health and developing the appropriate evidence base for health care provision, will require the participation of individuals who are incompetent or temporarily not competent to give consent to participate in the research activity. Such people should only be involved in research under very clearly articulated and strictly monitored conditions. If it is impossible to carry out the particular research project with competent participants (or, for example, to wait for the unconscious person to regain consciousness, or where this would invalidate the study), consent must be sought from the legally authorized guardian of the individual involved. As a general rule of thumb, incompetent individuals or members of other vulnerable groups should only be involved in research when it is reasonable to expect that the individual, or the group of which she/he is a member, will ultimately benefit from the research in question, and where the potential participant is exposed to minimal risk and burden. This is part of protecting the welfare of such individuals.

Should the potential participant, identified as incompetent to consent, be able to give assent to participation in research, such assent should be sought – in addition to the consent of the legal guardian as described above. In such circumstances a decision to withhold assent should be acknowledged and respected; thus this individual will not be included in the research project in question.

A corollary of informed consent is that the individual should be assured that her/his participation, responses, tissue samples and so forth are being used for the purposes of the identified research project only. Personal information and/or donated material, such as tissue samples, will then be destroyed under properly regulated mechanisms that are fully protective of the autonomy and privacy of the participant. If this is not the case, the potential participant should be made aware, explicitly, that it is intended to use the material for another, future study or studies. This enables the potential participant to knowingly consent, or withhold consent, to any potential future study. It clearly protects against a recurrence of cases such as those reported over the past decade in both Ireland and the UK (The Royal Liverpool Children's Inquiry Report 2001; The Dunne Inquiry 2005; Government of Ireland 2006), where human organs were retained, post mortem, for potential use in current or future research projects.

In some, perhaps many, health research projects, private, intimate information may be sought from the research participant during data collection: for example, information on previous medical history, information on personal behaviours and habits or information on the participant's children, siblings and so forth. Intimate, personally significant information may also be discovered as a result of interventions designed into the particular research initiative – i.e. genetic screening, chromosome studies, screening for risk of cancer and cardiac disease, alcohol use, sexual activity, patient satisfaction surveys and so forth. Research participants, in order to be properly protected from unwarranted risk of this personal information becoming available publicly, and thus potentially being used to the detriment of the research participant, (and to enable the participant to feel safe to participate in the particular study) should be assured that such **personal information will be kept private and confidential**. Where strict confidentiality cannot be assured, appropriate mechanisms should be designed into the study to protect participants. Participants can thus be assured that their identity will not be divulged – the **data-collection, handling and storage processes protect anonymity**. In this latter case, for example, participants are normally not asked to divulge their names on self-completed questionnaires – such as when completing patient satisfaction questionnaires or when a staff member completes a staff survey.

Beneficence and non-maleficence

Two of the internationally accepted, fundamental core principles underpinning both health care practice and research are the **principle of beneficence** (do good) and the mirror **principle of non-maleficence** (do not harm). Thus one should do good to and should not harm one's patients, clients or research participants. Clearly some interventions (for diagnostic, therapeutic and/or research purposes) may be uncomfortable, burdensome or painful. Some may cause a degree of harm – for example surgical intervention. However, the basic stance is that the core function of the health care professional is to work for the benefit of the patient or client from a health perspective. Thus the practitioner or the researcher must not cause unnecessary or avoidable harm or distress to their patients, clients or research participants. Article 6 of the Declaration of Helsinki states this position with particular clarity: 'In medical research involving human subjects, the well-being of the individual research subject must take precedence over all other interests' (WMA 2008).

To continue to develop the evidence base for health care practice, relevant, well-designed research is both important and essential. Conversely, the results of poorly designed research may, at worst, seriously harm participants or, at best, waste their time, while at the same time making misleading or detrimental contributions to the evidence base. This means that significant time and effort should be invested into research training and research oversight and governance.

At the level of the individual participant, the duty to do good, and prevent harm, warrants equal vigilance. In instances where the participant is likely to experience discomfort, burden and/or risk, it must be proportionate to the expected gain from the research study – either directly to the participant and/or to society as a whole. In the context of clinical trials, particularly drug trials for example, this gives rise to a number of issues. In the first instance, in order to warrant the use of a clinical trial there must be genuine doubt with regard to the efficacy of the drug or treatment intervention being considered. This is often referred to as a state of **equipoise.** Such conditions exist either when the evidence is not available from which to make a judgement regarding the impact of a particular intervention, or in situations where the evidence that does exist is inconclusive and/or contradictory. (For a useful discussion of this concept in particular, and ethical issues underlying intervention studies in general, see O'Mathúna 2012.)

As indicated above, when moving to set up clinical trials the relevant groundwork must be completed and verified before introducing human trials. Appropriate oversight of the trial, including close monitoring of participant responses, must be assured (see Chapter 6 for an outline and discussion of research governance). Furthermore, when patients are participating in experimental drug trials they must be fully aware of this, including being made aware of the very high chance of the experimental intervention not 'working'. From the perspective of the ethical conduct of the clinical trial it is good ethical practice for the research team to have a protocol in place to help determine when participation in the trial should be terminated. Such a protocol is particularly pertinent in experimental trials of new anti-cancer agents. The lack of such a protocol can lead to unnecessary hardship for very ill, vulnerable patients and for the staff who care for them. (For a detailed description and discussion of these and related issues see Hobson 2003.)

A corollary of the principles of beneficence and non-maleficence, in terms of clinical trials, is that a study must be stopped immediately when the risks are found to outweigh the potential benefits. A similar imperative exists when there is conclusive evidence of positive and beneficial results from one of the agents under investigation.

Justice

In the context of research activity the principle of justice can be conceptualized as fairness (Rawls 1985). In Rawlsian terms, fairness is achieved if the principles guiding distribution of capabilities and resources, for example, are applied so as to ensure that the 'least advantaged' are benefited and not harmed or forgotten. Thus research participants should be treated fairly. For example, if participants are being put at considerable discomfort, inconvenience or risk (given the discussion of the ethical principles providing an appropriate framework for ethically acceptable research activity it is assumed that participants are fully aware of the demands being made of them), then it may be completely reasonable to compensate a participant for such inconvenience and any expenses they may incur due to their participation in the particular research project. However, that compensation should not be such as to induce financially vulnerable individuals to place themselves at significant risk for financial gain.

Another issue that emerges during discussion of the principle of justice, in the context of research activity, is who should participate in research activity? Should certain groups be excluded on grounds such as vulnerability? Over the past number of years it has been recognized that all patient/client groups, including those identified as especially vulnerable, have the right to participate in – indeed may be necessary participants in – investigations to improve health care and to generate a sound evidence base for such care. For example the fifth article of the Declaration of Helsinki (WMA 2008) stated the following:

> Medical progress is based on research that ultimately must include studies involving human subjects. Populations that are under-represented in medical research should be provided appropriate access to participation in research.

However, article 17 qualifies this in the following manner:

> Medical research involving a disadvantaged or vulnerable population or community is only justified if the research is responsive to the health needs and priorities of this population or community and if there is a reasonable likelihood that this population or community stands to benefit from the results of the research.

Groups that come to mind are children, the terminally ill, those who are physically disabled or cognitively impaired. It is a matter of justice that such individuals are enabled to participate in relevant research as fully as possible. Such participation assists in developing our understanding of the health and illness experience of certain vulnerable groups. It helps gain insight into their perceptions of, responses to, and requirements of, interventions provided by health care practitioners (and the health service they encounter) over the course of their lives or their illness trajectory.

However, special considerations need to come into play to ensure appropriate support and protection of such individuals. In particular, specific mechanisms must be put in place to ensure that the welfare rights of vulnerable groups are recognized and protected. For detailed discussion of research with vulnerable groups please see Chapter 7.

Working it through: ethical issues and the stages of the research process

As indicated above, ethical issues and considerations permeate the entire research process. This begins with the research questions that are asked (and that receive research grant funding – as against those questions which do not get asked and those projects which, through lack of funding, do not proceed) and continues right through to reporting of research findings and terminating the researcher/respondent contact.

Researchers need to be sensitive to the nature of particular research agendas and the motivations, personal, political, institutional and sociocultural, that drive them. For example, the current drivers of evidence-based practice in health care are at least tripartite – political, economic and professional. As practitioners we are becoming more convinced that our practice must be evidence-based – and there are numerous clinical studies going on attempting to develop our evidence base. However, it is interesting to note that we are a lot less clear on what we mean by evidence, or what should count as evidence in health care practice (Scott 2006).

It seems reasonably clear that answers to the latter question are crucial in informing the former question. Despite this, little work is currently being carried out, or being funded, in relation to questions regarding the nature of the evidence base appropriate for health care and nursing practice. This problem has philosophical, moral and professional implications. One of the most serious is the potential impact that our lack of knowledge and understanding regarding the nature of an appropriate evidence base will have on patient care.

However, once the researcher has decided on the appropriate research question (see Chapter 3), it is a moral and professional requirement to ensure that the selected piece of research is necessary. Thus the researcher needs to be sure that the knowledge is required, and does not already exist in a sufficiently comprehensive state. This indicates the need for the researcher to be equipped to do the required literature searching. To do otherwise is not only likely to lead to a poorly refined research question and consequent poor research design, but is also wasteful of resources and shows a lack of respect for the study respondents and those who provide support for the researcher.

Assuming that the research question is a legitimate and useful one, the researcher must draw on personal or outside expertise in designing an appropriate study that will provide a real possibility of gaining answers to the research question posed, or which will provide a firm basis for further work. This is not only a methodological issue. Sound study design is required in order to ensure that the study is ethically sound. Lack of appropriate expertise in study design is again, at a minimum, wasteful of time and other resources and indicates a lack of respect for respondents and those supporting the work of the researcher. At worst, such a lack of expertise may be positively damaging to the research respondents. Given that health care researchers frequently carry out research with respondents already made vulnerable through illness, this is particularly unacceptable practice from an ethical perspective.

Once the researcher is confident that the design of the study is appropriate and that the data-collection methods or tools will obtain the data required, ethical considerations, we would argue, again concern notions of respect, with a focus on the following issues:

- The role of the practitioner/researcher and the implications of the researcher identifying him or herself as a nurse, doctor, physiotherapist, clinical psychologist and so forth. The implications are potentially both positive and negative. Such self-identification may make recruitment to a study much easier. However, it may also confuse or set up false expectations in patient participants. Conflicts of interest are likely to arise where a practitioner is using his/her own patient group in research. Such confusion of roles should normally be avoided. Where a self-identified, qualified practitioner is carrying out a piece of research (for postgraduate work, for example), it should be made clear to participants that the researcher is not responsible for the participants' care and that refusal to participate in the research will not have any impact on care provision. This should also be expressed clearly either on the written information participants receive regarding the research study and/or on the consent form.
- The balance of potential inconvenience or risk to participants over potential benefit to participants and/or others.

- Appropriate and sufficient information should be given regarding the nature of the study to enable the potential participant to make an informed choice, and to give or withhold informed, voluntary consent. In instances where the participants are unable to receive the information or to make informed decisions, for whatever reason, clear transparent processes which aim to ascertain and protect participants' interests, throughout the period of their participation, must be instituted. The continued right of competent participants to withdraw from the study, without any negative consequences to the participant, must be made clear at the commencement of the study and thereafter, as the study unfolds, as required.
- Issues of anonymity and confidentiality must be given careful consideration, and detailed information on these notions given to participants. As de Raeve (1996: 114) points out, this may be particularly pertinent for health practitioner/researchers who may, for example, be used to the rather broader notion of confidentiality which is used in the health care team.

In empirical studies, data collection is a crucial area for research ethics. Ethical issues can be identified in the following areas:

- obtaining permission for data collection from the organization in question
- obtaining permission for data collection from the participants (patients, professionals)
- guaranteeing appropriate ethical behaviour from researchers during the data-collection period

As discussed above, in obtaining permission from individual participants, the issue of informed consent is central. It should be noted that normally practitioners directly involved in care giving do not obtain participants' consent to participate in research as clear conflict of interest issues may arise. However, clinical nurses in particular may have a significant role in supporting patient participants in making informed decisions regarding participation in a particular piece of research (see, for example, Pranulis 1997; Watts 1997; Sadler et al. 1999; An Bord Altranais 2007).

In line with the principle of respect for persons, participants' anonymity, confidentiality and willingness to participate must be ensured. Risks, benefits and burdens to respondents must be explored. The risk or burden to the participant must be weighed against the potential benefits of the research findings to the general population or specific patient populations. Participants in clinical trials must be as fully informed as possible regarding the nature and objectives of the trial. It should be made clear to the participants the nature of any specific risks or benefits that may accrue to trial participants. It is also important to bear in mind that informed consent is an ongoing process. Research participants may have questions that arise during the data-collection process in particular that should be addressed. Participants must also be informed and assured that they may withdraw their consent and cease participation at any point during the research process, without this negatively impacting on them or their care.

Ethics and data analysis

Analysis of data is an interesting issue from an ethical perspective. At a minimum, the researcher and/or his or her research advisers need to have a good grasp of both the strengths and limitations of the method of analysis or any analytical tools used. This is important from an ethical perspective to ensure that no inappropriate claims are made, based on the analysis. The relevance of this point in terms of clinical practice and patient care is clear. A significant reason for carrying out empirical research in health care is to improve patient care and develop sound policy and practices. Inappropriate analysis is likely to lead to inaccurate results and thus potentially to poor policy and practice.

Ethics and the relationship with research participants

De Raeve (1996: 115) highlights the lack of attention to ethical issues surrounding 'leaving the field' or termination of the relationship between researcher and participant. This is likely to be a particularly complex issue for researchers involved in some forms of qualitative research and in some psychosocially focused intervention trials. The researcher needs to be aware of the potential problems in this type of researcher–participant relationship. Steps should be taken to ensure that the participant does not confuse the research relationship with a therapeutic, counselling-type relationship or a friendship. Insight and personal integrity is actively required from the researcher throughout the data-collection period to guard against misuse or abuse of the researcher–participant relationship. (See O'Mathúna 2012 for a wide-ranging and helpful analysis of the importance of researcher integrity throughout the research process.)

Ethics and dissemination of research

From an ethics perspective, if the researcher is to value and respect the contributions made by participants, funding bodies and others supportive of the research effort, it is incumbent on the researcher to report and disseminate the findings of the particular study – positive and negative – in the most effective ways available to the researcher.

In reporting the study results, the ethical issues include continued protection of the rights of, and honouring promises made to, participants (for example, confidentiality, protection of privacy, anonymity), reporting findings truthfully, accurately and completely, citing appropriately the work of others and ensuring the authorship credits and acknowledgements are stated accurately. To do otherwise once again indicates lack of respect for the various actors in the research process. It is also wasteful of valuable resources, including those of future researchers who might have gained from the signposting of 'blind alleys' and from insights into the findings, strengths and weaknesses of the unreported study.

Conclusion

A number of the key ethical principles relevant to research with human participants are explored in this chapter. The ethical understanding thus gained is then applied to the component elements of the research process. High-quality, ethically sound research is important in developing the evidence base for health care practice and in the provision of effective, humane patient care. Understanding the principles guiding ethically sound research activity is thus a key component in evidence-based health care delivery.

Key concepts

- Respect for persons: in the context of research, this refers to ensuring, for example, that participants are adequately informed about the research project. Such information should enable participants to give informed consent to participate in the piece of research in question. Respect for persons also requires that participants are assured of confidentiality or anonymity and that their privacy is protected.
- Beneficence and non-maleficence: literally this means, respectively, do good and do no harm. In the research context, participants should be adequately protected and researchers should avoid exposing participants to unnecessary and undue discomfort, burden or risk.
- Justice: research participants should be treated fairly. All sectors of the population including, where relevant, vulnerable groups and individuals, should be enabled to participate in research initiatives. Such participation may require additional protections to be in place.
- Ethical issues permeate the entire research process, from question identification and selection to dissemination of findings.

Key readings

- T.L. Beauchamp and J.F. Childress, *Principles of Biomedical Ethics*, 5th edn (New York: Oxford University Press, 2001)
  This is a classical text in health care ethics. The authors are the originators of what has become known as the Georgetown principles: respect for autonomy, beneficence, non-maleficence and justice. There are many interesting case applications of the principles, including research-relevant cases.
- J.K. Mason and R.A. McCall Smith, *Law and Medical Ethics*, 8th edn (London: Butterworth, 2010)
  This text provides a detailed discussion of ethical principles relevant to the health care context including the health research context.
- D.P. O'Mathúna, Ethical considerations in designing intervention studies, in B. Mazurek Melnyk and D. Morrison-Beedy (eds) *Intervention Research: Designing, Conducting, Analyzing, and Funding: A Practical Guide for Success* (New York: Springer Publishing, 2012), pp. 75–89
  O'Mathúna's chapter provides a comprehensive discussion of the research ethics issues involved in the design and implementation of intervention studies. The chapter includes a very useful discussion of the issue of researcher integrity.

Useful articles

- I. Coyne, Research with children and young people: The issue of parental (proxy) consent, *Children and Society*, 24(3) (2010), 227–37
  The author explores the implication of blanket requirements for parental consent on the moral agency and respect accorded to children and young people (under 18 years) in the research context.
- N.E. Kass, J. Sugarman, R. Faden and M. Schoch-Spana, Trust: The fragile foundations of contemporary biomedical research, *Hastings Center Report* (New York: Hastings Center, September–October 1996)
  This article highlights the very specific ethical issues that can underpin patient participation in anti-cancer experimental drug trials.
- J. Leaning, Ethics of research in refugee populations, *Lancet*, 357(9266) (2001), 1432–3
  The author explores the delicate balance to be maintained between the desire and the need to involve refugees in relevant research projects with the potential to exploit often very vulnerable individuals.

Useful websites

- Irish Council for Bioethics (2004) *Operational procedures for research ethics committees: Guidance*. Dublin: Irish Council for Bioethics – http://www.drugsandalcohol.ie/5889/1/Bioethics_Ethical_guidelines_for_research.pdf
- The National Institutes of Health (NIH) offers an online tutorial, 'Human Participants Protections Education for Research Teams' – http://phrp.nihtraining.com/users/login.php
- World Medical Association, *Declaration of Helsinki: Recommendations Guiding Physicians in Biomedical Research Involving Subjects* (1964, 1975, 1983, 1989, 1996, 2000, 2002, 2004, 2008) – http://www.wma.net/en/30publications/10policies/b3/

References

Adams, M. (1996) Final Report of the Tuskegee Syphilis Study 1932–1972. Available at http://www.hsl.virginia.edu/historical/medical_history/bad_blood/report.cfm [Accessed March 2013].

Annas, G.J. and Grodin, M.A. (eds) (1992) *The Nazi Doctors and the Nuremberg Code: Human Rights in Human Experimentation*. New York: Oxford University Press.

An Bord Altranais (2007) *Guidelines for Nurses and Midwives Regarding the Ethical Conduct of Nursing and Midwifery Research*. Dublin: An Bord Altranais.

Beauchamp, T.L. and Childress, J.F. (2013) *Principles of Biomedical Ethics*, 7th edn. New York: Oxford University Press.

Cartwright, S. (1988) *The Report of the Committee of Inquiry into Allegations Concerning the Treatment of Cervical Cancer at National Women's Hospital and into Other Related Matters*. Auckland, New Zealand: Committee of Inquiry. Available at http://www.nsu.govt.nz/current-nsu-programmes/3233.aspx [Accessed 27 November 2012].

Council of Europe (1997) *Convention for Protection of Human Rights and Dignity of the Human Being with Regard to the Application of Biology and Medicine: Convention on Human Rights and Biomedicine*, Oneda, 4.IV, European Treaty Series. Available at http://conventions.coe.int/Treaty/en/Treaties/Html/164.htm [Accessed March 2013].

de Raeve, L. (ed.) (1996) *Nursing Research: An Ethical and Legal Appraisal*. London: Ballière-Tindall.

Doyal, L. and Tobias, J.S. (eds) (2001) *Informed Consent in Medical Research*. London: BMJ Group.

Government of Ireland (2006) *Report on Post Mortem Practice and Procedures*. Chair Dr Deirdre Madden. Dublin: Stationery Office.

Hobson, D. (2003) Moral silence? Nurses' experience of ethical decision making at the end of life. Unpublished PhD thesis, City University, London.

International Council of Nurses (1996) *Ethical Guidelines for Nursing Research*. Geneva: ICN.

Irish Council for Bioethics (2004) *Operational Procedures for Research Ethics Committees: Guidance*. Dublin: Irish Council for Bioethics. Available at http://www.drugsandalcohol.ie/5889/1/Bioethics_Ethical_guidelines_for_research.pdf [Accessed 22 November 2012].

Kass, N.E., Sugarman, J., Faden, R. and Schoch-Spana, M. (1996) Trust: The fragile foundations of contemporary biomedical research, *Hastings Center Report*, September–October 1996. New York: Hastings Center.

Mason, J.K. and McCall Smith, R.A. (2010) *Law and Medical Ethics*, 8th edn. London: Butterworth.

National Commission for the Protection of Human Subjects of Biomedical and Behavioral Research (1979) *The Belmont Report: Ethical Principles and Guidelines for the Protection of Human Subjects of Research*. Washington, DC: US Government Printing Office. Available at http://www.hhs.gov/ohrp/humansubjects/guidance/belmont.html [Accessed 21 November 2012].

Northern Nurses' Federation (1995) *Ethical Guidelines for Nursing Research in the Nordic Countries*. Oslo: Sykepleiernes Samarbeid i Norden. Available at http://www.sykepleien.no/Content/337889/SSNs%20etiske%20retningslinjer.pdf [Accessed 27 November 2012].

Nuremberg Code (1947) *Trials of War Criminals before the Nuremberg Military Tribunals under Control Council Law*, 2(10): 181–2, 28, 29.

O'Mathúna, D.P. (2012) Ethical considerations in designing intervention studies, in B. Mazurek Melnyk and D. Morrison-Beedy (eds) *Intervention Research: Designing, Conducting, Analyzing, and Funding: A Practical Guide for Success*. New York: Springer Publishing, pp. 75–89.

Paterson, R. (2010) The Cartwright legacy: Shifting the focus of attention from the doctor to the patient, *The New Zealand Medical Journal*, 123(1319): 6–10.

Pranulis, M. (1997) Nurses' role in protecting human subjects, *Western Journal of Nursing Research*, 19(1): 130–6.

Rawls, J. (1985) Justice as fairness: Political not metaphysical, *Philosophy and Public Affairs*, 14(3): 223–51.

Royal College of Nursing (2009) *Research Ethics: RCN Guidance for Nurses*, 2nd edn. London: Royal College of Nursing. Available at http://www.rcn.org.uk/__data/assets/pdf_file/0007/388591/003138.pdf [Accessed 27 November 2012].

Sadler, G., Lantz, J., Fullerton, J. and Dault, Y. (1999) Nurses' unique roles in randomized clinical trials, *Journal of Professional Nursing*, 15(82): 106–15.

Scott, P.A. (2006) Philosophy, nursing and the nature of evidence, in J. Atkinson and M. Crow (eds) *Interdisciplinary Research: Diverse Approaches in Science, Technology and Society*. Chichester: John Wiley and Sons, pp. 175–90.

The Dunne Inquiry (2005) The Dunne inquiry into organ retention in paediatric hospitals in the Republic of Ireland. Unpublished report submitted to the Tánaiste and Minister of Health.

The Royal Liverpool Children's Inquiry Report (2001) *Report on the Removal, Retention and Disposal of Human Organs and Tissues at Alder Hey Children's Hospital*. Chair Mr Michael Redfern, QC. London: HMSO.

United Nations (1948) *The Universal Declaration of Human Rights*. Available at http://www.un.org/en/documents/udhr/index.shtml [Accessed 21 November 2012].

United Nations (1989) *Convention on the Rights of the Child*. Available at http://www2.ohchr.org/english/law/crc.htm [Accessed 21 November 2012].

Watts, D. (1997) Informed consent in emergency research: What every emergency nurse should know, *Journal of Emergency Nursing*, 23(1): 70–4.

World Medical Association (1964, 1975, 1983, 1989, 1996, 2000, 2002, 2004, 2008) *Declaration of Helsinki: Recommendations Guiding Physicians in Biomedical Research Involving Subjects*. Available at http://www.wma.net/en/30publications/10policies/b3/ [Accessed 22 November 2012].

6   Communicating with research ethics committees

Suzanne Guerin

Chapter topics

- Research ethics committees and institutional review boards
- The need for research ethics committees and institutional review boards
- Engaging with research ethics committees and institutional review boards
- Applying to research ethics committees and institutional review boards

Introduction

Engaging with research ethics committees (RECs) or institutional review boards (IRBs) is a core part of the research process for most, if not all, researchers in the health field. While the principles of research ethics have a long history, the development of formal review processes is a much more recent phenomenon. Central to ensuring success in these interactions is knowledge of the relevant REC or IRB's policies and procedures. Equally important is identifying and addressing the key ethical issues raised by the proposed research.

Health research covers a broad range of topics, research methods and therefore ethical issues; however there are a number of key elements that RECs and IRBs will typically focus on. These include several of the issues discussed in the previous chapter, such as consideration of vulnerable groups, potentially invasive or distressing research procedures, and issues regarding data protection. It is essential that researchers consider these issues carefully and outline how these will be addressed as part of the process of seeking approval.

Research ethics committees are a forum for safeguarding the rights of patients and clients who may be involved in research projects. However, students and early-stage researchers may be unaware of the complexity and importance of applying to a hospital or university research ethics committee. This chapter addresses the steps needed in applying for ethical approval. Using a standardized research ethics application, it takes the student step by step through the process and identifies the level of information needed to apply to a research ethics committee. It explains in clear and accessible language the type of information required by an ethics committee and how to ensure that patients are protected throughout the research process.

The Development of RECs and IRBs

Before focusing on the challenges of REC/IRB review and possible solutions, it is important to reflect on the factors influencing the development of these structures.

Being aware of the contextual factors that influence committees can inform the process of securing approval. While a comprehensive and critical discussion is beyond the scope of this chapter, this section provides an overview of the contextual factors influencing the development of RECs and IRBs.

Many writers discussing the early foundation of RECs and IRBs describe the process as a reactive one, with structures developing following key events such as human experimentation in Nazi Germany (Hamilton 2005; Kramer et al. 2009). Indeed the development of these committees is described as necessary to avoid or curb abuses that may occur during the research process (Hayes et al. 1995). In addition, Shuster (1997) suggests that research ethics after Nazi Germany also reflect the growing importance of a human rights framework. Other important steps in the development of RECs and IRBs were the Declaration of Helsinki (Rid and Schmidt 2010) and the National Commission for the Protection of Human Subjects in Biomedical and Behavioral Research, which resulted in the publication of The Belmont Report (National Commission 1979). An interesting shift over the course of these changes is the move from ethical practices to ethical principles, which several writers identify as an important factor in making the ethical requirements of research more universal (Fisher 2007; Devettere 2010).

An aspect that can be considered in relation to RECs and IRBs is the context in which these committees work. A key issue considered in the literature is the distinction between individual institution-based committees and centralized systems. While many institutions, be they academic or medical, have developed individual procedures and structures, the variation evident across settings can represent a challenge for researchers. Gold and Dewa (2005) reflect on the implications of individual committees for multisite studies in health services research. They highlight the lack of standardized forms, variations in the experience and knowledge of REC/IRB members, and institutional factors as key challenges, which they report can result in delays and unnecessary costs. For a sense of the extent of the challenge, a paper by Vaughan et al. (2012) estimates that securing ethical approval for their multisite study involved 3261 hours of work by the research team. A report by Smith et al. (2004) illustrates some of the difficulties experienced by multisite studies in Ireland when attempting to secure ethics approval for research in health settings. Interestingly, Loh and Meyer (2004) explored the view of US medical schools on the topic of centralized RECs and IRBs. Following a survey of accredited US medical schools they reported that the majority of respondents had no experience of centralized committees. Common concerns about such a procedure included a lack of representation and possible issues of liability. More than half of the respondents reported that they did not plan to use a centralized committee in the future. However, among the small group that had used such a system, the experience was predominantly positive, suggesting that once exposed to the process of a centralized REC or IRB the benefits followed.

Clearly the growth of multisite studies, particularly in health, highlights the need to consider the impact of individual systems involved in ethical approval, and the system in many contexts is responding to the challenge. In the UK the development of the Integrated Research Application System (IRAS – for more information see www.myresearchproject.org.uk) has created a centralized system for applications to a range of medical, health and social RECs and IRBs. The online nature of the process, as well as the use of a centralized system, offer numerous benefits to researchers, not least those conducting multisite studies and trials. The use of a centralized system or common application procedures is evident in a number of countries internationally, including New Zealand, where health and disability-related research is governed regionally by four Health and Disability Ethics Committees (see www.ethics.health. govt.nz) with shared procedures, and Australia, in the form of the National Ethics Application Form (see www.neaf.gov.au). In Ireland a standard application form exists for clinical trials, and since 2009 work has been ongoing on the development of a similar system for health-related studies (other than clinical trials), referred to as the Research Ethics Committee Standard Application Form (RECSAF) (Standard Application Form Consultation Group – Pilot Form Sub-Group 2010). While applications for clinical trials can only be submitted to approved committees, a range of health and academic RECs and IRBs are using or reviewing the suitability of the non-trial standard form (see www.molecularmedicineireland.ie/research_ethics for more information).

This brief consideration highlights the changing context for RECs and IRBs during the last 20 years. Indeed, one paper by Rosnow et al. (1993) offers a reflection on some of the changing issues faced at the time by these committees as they respond to changing norms and standards. Issues highlighted include the implications of research on the topic of communicable disease for expectations of confidentiality and the demands of public health legislation, the changing views of placebos in clinical trials, and also the growing importance of design issues in the deliberations of committees. Understanding the context and history of the REC/IRB system is an important step in engaging with the process.

In considering the process of engaging with RECs and IRBs a key feature, and one which stays with researchers, is their experience of the process. It is necessary to reflect on and perhaps deconstruct the views and experiences that may influence the way in which researchers will engage with the process. Anecdotally, researchers often use the phrase 'getting through' the ethics review process, and refer to tensions and difficulties throughout the process. However there are a number of interesting studies that explore researchers' experiences more systematically. Box 6.1 provides examples of researchers' perceptions of the process of dealing with ethics committees.

Box 6.1   Researchers' perceptions of research ethics committees

For the interested reader a paper included in the special issue of the *Journal of Applied Communication Research* (Vol 33(3), 2005) provides a broad insight into the views of one group of researchers through a series of narratives submitted for the issue. Koerner's (2005) analysis of these narratives highlights themes that will not be unfamiliar to researchers in health research. It is interesting to note that while there was evidence of both positive and negative experiences, the negative were expressed more frequently. While the dominance of negative experiences may hold intuitive appeal to some researchers, empirical studies have identified that this may not be reflective of the general experience of engaging with committees.

For example, an early survey by Ferraro et al. (1999) gathered the views of 337 staff and graduate students. Interestingly the experiences were predominantly positive, with only small percentages of staff and students reporting that they could not conduct their research as a result of problems with the review process, or that they had not been treated fairly. Indeed, this study reported that the majority of participants felt the process had improved the quality of their research. More recently Dyrbye et al. (2008) surveyed clinician educators on their experience of obtaining REC/IRB approval for medical education research. As these studies involve the participation of medical and health programme students in research, there are some unique ethical considerations that would not extend to other health research (for example many projects were considered exempt from review or minimal risk). Nevertheless, the findings are interesting in that they highlight moderate levels of satisfaction with the process and the importance of knowledge of the system for success, an issue this chapter will return to later.

Applying for REC/IRB approval

The remainder of this chapter focuses on the process of applying for approval to an REC or IRB. A central emphasis will be the challenges that arise during the process and possible solutions that will guide researchers. Given the variation in documentation and procedures evident in different countries, it is necessary to structure this consideration around common issues. However, before considering the content of the form, researchers must be familiar with the policies and procedures of the specific committee they are applying to.

Procedural knowledge

The first practical step in preparing a submission to an ethics committee is to *gather any available information on the specific committee that holds jurisdiction over the research*. Typically this will be the researcher's place of work or the setting through which potential participants will be contacted. While this appears somewhat obvious, anecdotally it is a common complaint by RECs and IRBs that those submitting for review have not familiarized themselves with the process. Work by Kotzer and Milton (2007) highlights the importance of researchers' knowledge of relevant procedures. They frame the committee structure as a resource, while stressing the need for researchers to be familiar with the relevant procedures and for RECs and IRBs to streamline those procedures. They go on to report an evaluation of an initiative designed to increase staff knowledge of committee guidelines. Worryingly, they report no significant improvement over time and in some cases a decline, though they do raise concerns about the effectiveness of the design and cite poor response rates and small samples as possible influences.

Time frames

In gathering information it is important that researchers *pay particular attention to the time frames* indicated by the committee. Key elements include the scheduling of committee meetings, the deadline for submission of information in advance of the meeting, and the expected time taken to review and feed back to researchers. Masterton and Shah (2007), in a very pragmatic paper on approaching RECs and IRBs, stress the importance of incorporating these time frames into the planning process. Another important part of the preparation is to *be aware of your role in the decision process*. Some committees will call the researcher to answer questions on the proposal (thus allowing for clarification), while others will make the final decision on the basis of the documentation submitted. Researchers should note that decisions made on the basis of documentation only serve to reinforce the need for familiarity with the process and procedures to avoid unnecessary delays.

Possible outcomes

Researchers should also *be familiar with the possible outcomes of the process*. For example, some committees may simply reject incomplete applications without information on the material that was included. Clearly this has the potential to impact on the time frames mentioned above. Possibly the most common response from an REC or IRB is to stipulate issues to be addressed by the researchers before approval can be confirmed (Hunter 2011). A paper by Sansone et al. (2004) reports on a review of the responses by one REC over a five-year period (the committee in question was a hospital committee in a suburban part of the Midwestern US). They found that in almost 85 per cent of cases there was at least one stipulation to be addressed. The nature of the types of stipulations that are common will be considered later (particularly as they represent a very useful list of 'dos' and 'don'ts' for researchers); however researchers will need to be aware of the implications of stipulations. RECs and IRBs may distinguish between major stipulations, which may require a repeat of the review process (with all of the associated delays), and more minor stipulations that represent areas for clarification. These clarifications can commonly be approved by the Chair of the committee rather than requiring a full review – clearly a more positive outcome from the researcher's perspective.

Procedures for low-risk research

Before considering the process of applying for REC or IRB approval, researchers should explore whether the committee from which they are seeking approval has procedures for consideration of research that meets criteria for low-risk review or exemption from full review. This refers to procedures by which studies that meet key criteria regarding the nature of the research and the level of risk may be entitled to an expedited review, or indeed may only require that the committee be notified. An examination of practice in other countries conducted as part of a review of REC/IRB structures and processes in Ireland (Research Ethics Committees Review Group 2008) highlighted the presence of procedures for 'expedited review' in the US, Canada, Australia, New Zealand, the UK and Ireland. Expedited procedures generally include a shorter application form and one or two members of the committee conduct the review. Criteria that may be considered low risk or exempt include:

- the use of existing and publicly available data
- data from standardized assessments
- research that involves topics and procedures that do not represent a risk to participants
- research that had been approved by another committee with responsibility for the research

Preparing your submission

Central to the ethics process is the ethics application form. Whether the REC/IRB decision-making programme is based on documentation only or not, it is essential that the researcher *fully and clearly completes the ethics application form* and provides all necessary supporting documentation. While these forms can be complex and are often detailed, it is important to recognize that the information is being requested to assist the committee in making their decision. Masterton and Shah (2007) stress the importance of clear communication, which avoids technical terms and jargon that may not be common to all members of the committee (an important consideration if the REC or IRB is a multidisciplinary one). Researchers should remember that the decision to be made by the committee is whether the appropriate standards of practice have been met, and if elements of the study are not clear then the REC or IRB cannot form an opinion on this issue. Greaney et al. (2012) stress the implications of such a lack of care for the timely completion of the review process.

While there is significant variation in the structure, language and requirements of research ethics application forms, it is possible to identify a number of common sections for completion. These include (but are not limited to):

- general information, which will often request details of the research team members, partners and collaborators
- cost and resource implications, funding and insurance/indemnity
- methodological details, i.e. a description of the study (possibly in plain language), study participants and research procedures
- medical information (for example the use of human biological material, medical devices and medicinal products)
- data protection and security considerations
- ethical issues, where the application is required to identify the study's main ethical concerns and detail the solutions to these issues

In addition, researchers are generally required to provide supporting documentation such as samples of materials, information and consent documentation.

The first point to note for researchers completing an application is that some sections of ethics application forms are mandatory and must be completed for all applications. These generally include the general information and study details and key sections such as data protection, costs and ethical issues. Most application forms will come with comprehensive guidance notes that will assist the novice or unfamiliar researcher. While this may not be the case for all RECs and IRBs, the researcher should note if a particular committee provides templates or sample documents to aid the process of securing review.

Consideration of methodology

Anecdotally, a significant source of tension between researchers and RECs or IRBs, and indeed within committees, is the debate regarding the consideration of research methodology as part of the review process. Masterton and Shah (2007) refer to the debates regarding the need for RECs and IRBs to comment on research design. Clearly if a committee is to consider the appropriateness of the proposed research they must also examine aspects of the methods used.

Key methodological issues that may be requested by the REC or IRB include the proposed population, the planned sampling techniques, and the data-collection procedures. However, Masterton and Shah also refer to concerns regarding competence and supervision, particularly for research conducted by less experienced researchers. In order to avoid difficulties it is important that applications describe the methodology of the study clearly and concisely, remembering that the committee will, more than likely, be made up of members from different disciplines as well as lay members. With this in mind the researcher should consider the need to provide a clear rationale for particular choices, for example the use of deception where the scientific rigour of the study demands it. Sharkey et al. (2011) describe in some detail the rationale behind many of the choices made in their study of an online discussion forum for young people who self-harm, including conducting the study anonymously so as to encourage participation and respect the centrality of anonymity to online social interactions.

Sample size and methodology

Another important area, which is highlighted by Masterton and Shah, is the area of data analysis. Some researchers may feel that the inclusion of questions regarding sample size and power reflect a more quantitative framework; however, central to these questions is the competence of the researcher to oversee the analyses needed. Whether the research is qualitative or quantitative the researcher should be able to provide a rationale for the sample size, whether this is based on statistical power, previous research, or in the case of more qualitative studies the demands of data saturation. Again, in these sections, a clear rationale for the choices made can address any concerns the REC or IRB may have about the ability of the study to draw a credible conclusion.

Data protection

As highlighted earlier, the issue of data protection is one where legislation has had a significant impact on the research process. A particular challenge in this area is the scope for interpretation of the relevant legislation. In the case of the UK, Parry and Mauthner (2004) report that the use of data for research purposes falls under an exemption that allows its use without explicit consent, though researchers are required to consider the potential for 'harm' and the sensitivity of the data. In Ireland this is not the case, though central to the legislation is the principle that data can be used as long as the use is not at odds with the initial reason for collection. Another key aspect of data protection is the level of identification possible from data, suggesting that anonymous data and its use is more in line with the requirements in this area. A final concern for many RECs and IRBs is the procedures for accessing existing data. Masterton and Shah (2007) highlight this in the context of databases of medical information. All data protection legislation considers the responsibility of data controllers to manage access to existing information, and researchers need to consider the extent to which they legitimately have access to this type of information. For example, a researcher who works as a practitioner in a particular setting may have access to patient records *as a practitioner*, however accessing this information *for the purpose of research* may not be acceptable to a committee, and in these situations researchers should consider the possible role of gatekeepers in supporting the process of accessing data.

Anonymity and confidentiality of data

There is no doubt that the key to addressing these issues to an REC or IRB's satisfaction is to *consider the nature of the data gathered* for the purpose of the research, particularly the sensitivity of the data, the procedures for accessing existing data and the level of identification necessary. In reflecting on data protection issues while preparing an application a researcher might consider *the need for data to be identifiable* and the associated *demands for security* depending on this and the sensitivity of the data. Related to this, it is also important to consider the distinction between anonymity and confidentiality. While many researchers may consider these terms to be interchangeable, there is an important difference between information that cannot be identified (anonymous) and data for which the researcher protects the identity and/or contributions of the participants (confidentiality). Scott (2005) presents an interesting consideration of issues of anonymity and confidentiality (though in relation to communication research), and considers some of the challenges of addressing this issue. From a practical perspective, Scott stresses the need for researchers to be clear on the level of protection being proposed for participants and how it is ensured. This detail will be important in the preparation of the application for review.

Limits of confidentiality

One point to note here is the concept of the *limits of confidentiality*. In Ireland and the UK the application of child protection guidelines typically means that researchers may have to breach confidentiality where there is a concern for the well-being of the child. Sieber (2004) describes the variation of requirements by state in the US and the extent to which RECs and IRBs will require researchers to warn potential participants of these requirements. Harbour (1998) considers this along with other issues that place constraints on guarantees of confidentiality, including having information relevant to the commission of a crime. A final point on the limitations of confidentiality relates to the impact of particular methods of data collection. For example, a researcher offering confidentiality to participants in a study that uses focus groups has perhaps not thought through the fact that in a group setting all members of the group will hear the contributions of other members, thus undermining the idea of confidentiality in these settings. Greaney et al. (2012) state that the implications of this type of method for privacy must be communicated to potential participants in advance.

Identifying ethical issues

An essential element in successfully securing ethics approval is the researcher's ability to identify and respond to key ethical issues and dilemmas in the research. The previous chapter considered a number of specific issues common in health research. However, this section focuses not on the issues themselves but the problem-solving process by which researchers consider these issues and present them to an REC or IRB. Figure 6.1 presents one framework within which researchers might reflect on their study in preparing an application. The figure highlights that the researcher must consider issues that arise as a result of the setting in which the research takes place, the people involved in the research (importantly the participants and the research team), the specific topic of the study, and finally the research process.

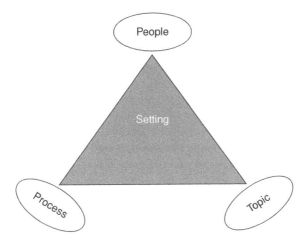

Figure 6.1   A framework for problem solving in preparation for seeking REC/IRB approval.

Box 6.2 provides an example of how the framework can be applied in seeking ethical approval.

Box 6.2 A framework for problem solving in preparation for seeking REC/IRB approval

A staff member based in a local health clinic is planning a piece of research as part of a postgraduate course they are completing. They propose to conduct the research in the clinic (*the setting*). The researcher must consider whether there are any issues relevant to the setting that must be considered in the application for approval, such as the procedures for organizational approval.

Moving to consider *the people*, the researcher may be targeting members of vulnerable groups receiving services and the REC or IRB will want to see evidence that the recruitment and consent procedures have taken this into consideration. Remembering that the researcher is also part of this element, the committee may consider if the researcher (as a student completing a programme) has the skills needed to complete the project as designed and that appropriate supervision is in place. A final issue that can regularly arise in relation to the people involved in the research is the presence of a pre-existing relationship between the researcher and the potential participants. Any REC or IRB will consider whether this impacts on the participants' freedom to consent or decline, and the committee will want to see that the researcher has put arrangements in place to manage this issue.

Moving on to ethical issues relevant to *the topic*, clearly the focus for many researchers is on sensitive topics. Here the challenge is for the researcher to be open to the participants' and the committee's views on whether a topic is sensitive or potentially distressing. In preparing the application for approval it is important that the researcher reflects on the possibility and the probability that the topic may be distressing and, in the application, clearly describe the procedures they will introduce to ensure that any distress is managed. The need to develop procedures for the management of distress is discussed in Vass et al. (2003) with reference to a study of communication patterns in people with Alzheimer's and their carers. While the topic would not necessarily be considered sensitive, the nature of the engagement between the researchers and the participants, and the particular vulnerability of the participants, could result in anxiety on the part of the participants. Recognizing this, the authors describe the procedure by which participant anxiety will be managed, including the decision to terminate the interview if necessary.

The final element of the framework is *the research process*, and again the key to success is to identify any potential issues and address them clearly in the application. While health research can involve a range of processes that might be invasive, harmful or distressing (such as taking blood or tissue samples), less experienced researchers may fail to consider the ethical issues associated with more apparently 'innocent' processes. For example, in a study using interviews the researcher must be aware that the audio recording of an interview is potentially identifiable and must be transported and stored securely, while the demands of discussing a sensitive subject can be more challenging if a focus group method is being used.

So in preparing an application for REC or IRB approval it is essential to both identify and address the key ethical issues associated with the study. The framework described above aims to support the researcher to identify the range of issues involved; the challenge for the researcher is to provide clear evidence in the applica-tion that these have been addressed.

Supporting documentation

Clearly, a key aspect of successfully securing ethics approval is the quality of the submission to the committee. A common difficulty that committees face is a lack of information or indeed a lack of clarity in the documentation. This may present in the form of incomplete application or supporting documentation. The researcher should not underestimate the importance of the supporting documentation.

One factor that relates to many of the issues considered above is the responsibil-ity of the researcher to ensure that participants are fully informed as to the nature of the research and the implications of deciding to take part. In preparing an applica-tion for approval the researcher must describe the steps taken to ensure the elements of the study are clear to participants (and indeed to the REC or IRB). Unsurprisingly, the information and consent documentation are considered closely by committees. The review of REC/IRB decisions by Sansone et al. (2004) described above found that changes to consent documentation was the most common requirement and these included presentation and formatting, clarification of risks and procedures, and par-ticipants' rights. Interestingly, a study by Albala et al. (2010) examined the quality of information and consent documents submitted to an REC or IRB over the course of 25 years, and found that these documents had quadrupled in length over time and that the occurrence of discrepancies in risk levels (as reported by the application and the information sheet) had dropped over time.

Difficulties and delays can also occur if copies of research materials such as questionnaires or standardized tools are omitted. Anecdotally researchers using qualitative methods have experienced difficulties when the use of unstructured or semi-structured interviews mean that a comprehensive interview schedule cannot be included with the application. In this situation the researcher might consider provid-ing a topic guide that outlines the areas they intend to explore while recognizing that the participant may raise additional issues.

Negotiating with RECs and IRBs

The final aspect of engaging and communicating with an REC or IRB to be men-tioned is the potential to negotiate with the committee. Many academics interested in research ethics will recognize that this area is one with very few definitive right answers. As a result, researchers should consider whether there is scope to negotiate with the committee, either in response to changes or clarifications being requested or indeed in advance of a decision (typically as part of the initial application). A key concern for RECs and IRBs is the rationale behind a researcher's choice of proposed procedure, and it is worth noting that requests that are perceived as self-serving may be far less effective than those that argue that the proposed element is central to the balance of risk and benefit in the research. Furthermore, showing that the proposed element is grounded in the existing literature in the area, or indeed looking to the literature on ethics itself, can allow the researcher to present a strong rationale to pursue a course that might initially raise concerns among the members of the REC or IRB. In extreme cases researchers might pursue an appeal – for those in this situation the researcher must be pragmatic about the implications for the schedule of the research.

Conclusion

Research is a process of decision making, with researchers required to consider the different options related to the proposed course of study and identify the elements that are best suited to the proposed study. This includes the process by which ethical approval is secured from the appropriate REC or IRB. As outlined above, the ethics review processes are typically detailed and key issues can emerge in health research. In preparing an application to a REC or IRB key areas for consideration include elements of the people, process, topic and setting, and researchers should describe these issues and outline how they will be addressed as part of the application for approval. A central message of this chapter is that familiarity with the specific procedures of any committee is central to success, and time spent considering and addressing key issues as part of an application for ethics approval will prevent possibly costly delays.

Key concepts

- Research ethics: 'Principles of good conduct. In the context of research, ethics usually refers either to the protection of subjects or to honesty in reporting results' (Vogt 2005: 108).
- Ethics approval process: this refers to the procedures laid down by health and academic settings covering ethical review and approval within the organization.
- Expedited review: this refers to a shortened review process, usually limited to low-risk research.
- Voluntary informed consent: 'a communication process in which a potential [participant] decides whether to participate in the proposed research' (Sieber 2004: 493).
- Vulnerable populations: this refers to individuals who may require additional consideration in the research process. These groups typically include minors, or individuals with cognitive limitations or emotional difficulties.
- Data protection: this refers to issues regarding confidentiality and appropriate use of individuals' data in the research process.

Key readings

- H. Biggs, *Healthcare Research Ethics and Law: Regulation, Review and Responsibility.* (Abingdon: Routledge-Cavendish, 2010)
  This book provides a detailed consideration of the legislative context for research ethics, ranging from consent and confidentiality to research involving human tissue.

- T. Long, *Research Ethics in the Real World: Issues and Solutions for Health and Social Care Professionals* (Philadelphia: Elsevier Health Sciences, 2007)
  This book adopts a practical rather than a principle-based approach to research ethics, and includes debates on a number of key issues in research.
- P. Oliver, *The Student's Guide to Research Ethics* (Maidenhead: Open University Press, 2003)
  An accessible guide to the topic of research ethics, which considers issues that can arise at different phases of the research process from development to dissemination.

Examples of papers on ethics review process in health care research

The following papers provide excellent examples of issues related to ethics in health care research.

- I. Albala, M. Doyle and P.S. Appelbaum, The evolution of consent forms for research: A quarter century of changes, *IRB: Ethics & Human Research*, 32(3) (2010), 7–11
- A.M. Greaney, A. Sheehy, C. Heffernan, J. Murphy, S. Ni Mhaolrúnaigh, E. Heffernan and G. Brown, Research ethics application: A guide for the novice researcher, *British Journal of Nursing*, 21(1) (2012), 38–43
- D. Hunter, A hands-on guide on obtaining research ethics approval, *Postgraduate Medical Journal*, 87(1030) (2011), 509–13
- G. Vaughan, W. Pollock, M.J. Peek, M. Knight, D. Ellwood, C.S. Homer, L.J. Pulver, C. McLintock, M.T. Ho, E. A. Sullivan, Ethical issues: The multi-centre low-risk ethics/ governance review process and AMOSS, *Australian and New Zealand Journal of Obstetrics and Gynaecology*, 52(2) (2012), 195–203
- A.A. Vass, H.A. Minardi, R. Ward, N. Aggarwal, C. Garfield and B. Cybyk, Research into communication and consequences for effective care of people with Alzheimer's and their carers, *Dementia*, 2(1) (2003), 21–48

Useful websites

- Website of the Irish Council for Bioethics. While the Council has ceased to operate, the website contains very relevant information – www.bioethics.ie
- Website for the UK's Central Office of Research Ethics Committees – www.corec.org.uk
- A US-based research institute dedicated to bioethics – www.thehastingscenter.org/
- This site contains a range of relevant information, in particular information on the RECSAF in Ireland – www.molecularmedicineireland.ie/research_ethics
- Home page of the integrated research application system in the UK – www.myresearchproject.org.uk
- Website of the Nuffield Council on Bioethics, an independent body based in the UK that considers ethical issues in areas relevant to medicine – www.nuffieldbioethics.org

- Website of the UK Health Research Authority, which was established within the National Health Service to 'protect and promote the interests of patients and the public in health research' – www.hra.nhs.uk
- Website of the New Zealand Health and Disability Ethics Committees – www.ethics. health.govt.nz
- This website hosts the Australian National Ethics Application Form to be used when submitting applications for research with human participants – www.neaf.gov.au
- Website of the Australian Human Research Ethics Portal, which includes information on Single Ethical Review of Multi-Centre Research – http://hrep.nhmrc.gov.au/

Acknowledgements

I would like to thank Nolan O'Brien for his contribution to my thinking on the broad issue of research ethics. Nolan's PhD on decision making among research ethics committees, currently being completed with the School of Psychology at University College Dublin, has been the basis of many useful discussions on this area.

References

Albala, I., Doyle, M. and Appelbaum, P.S. (2010) The evolution of consent forms for research: A quarter century of changes, *IRB: Ethics & Human Research*, 32(3): 7–11.

Devettere, R.J. (2010) *Practical Decision Making in Health Care Ethics: Cases and Concepts*, 3rd edn. Washington, DC: Georgetown University Press.

Dyrbye, L.N., Thomas, M.R., Papp, K.K. and Durning, S.J. (2008) Clinician educators' experiences with institutional review boards: Results of a national survey, *Academic Medicine*, 83(6): 590–5.

Ferraro, F.R., Szigeti, E., Dawes, K.J and Pan, S. (1999) A survey regarding the University of North Dakota institutional review board: Data, attitudes, and perceptions, *The Journal of Psychology*, 133(3): 272–80.

Fisher, J.A. (2007) Governing human subjects research in the USA: Individualized ethics and structural inequalities, *Science and Public Policy*, 34(2): 117–26.

Gold, J.L. and Dewa, C.S. (2005) Institutional review boards and multisite studies in health services research: Is there a better way? *Health Services Research*, 40(1): 291–308.

Greaney, A.M., Sheehy, A., Heffernan, C., Murphy, J., Ni Mhaolrúnaigh, S., Heffernan, E. and Brown, G. (2012) Research ethics application: A guide for the novice researcher, *British Journal of Nursing*, 21(1): 38–43.

Hamilton, A. (2005) The development and operation of IRBs: Medical regulations and social science, *Journal of Applied Communication Research*, 33(3): 189–203.

Harbour, A. (1998) Limits of confidentiality, *Advances in Psychiatric Treatment*, 4: 66–9.

Hayes, G.J., Hayes, S.C. and Dykstra, T. (1995) A survey of university institutional review boards: Characteristics, policies, and procedures, *IRB: Ethics and Human Research*, 17(3): 1–6.

Hunter D. (2011) A hands-on guide on obtaining research ethics approval, *Postgraduate Medical Journal*, 87(1030): 509–13.

Koerner, A.F. (2005) Communication scholars' communication and relationship with their IRBs, *Journal of Applied Communication Research*, 33(3): 231–41.

Kotzer, A.M. and Milton J. (2007) An education initiative to increase staff knowledge of Institutional Review Board guidelines in the USA, *Nursing and Health Sciences*, 9(2): 103–6.

Kramer, M.W., Miller, V.D. and Commuri, S. (2009) Faculty and institutional review board communication, *Communication Education*, 58(4): 497–515.

Loh, E.D. and Meyer, R.E. (2004) Medical schools' attitudes and perceptions regarding the use of central institutional review boards, *Academic Medicine*, 79(7): 644–51.

Masterton, G. and Shah, P. (2007) How to approach a research ethics committee, *Advances in Psychiatric Treatment*, 13: 220–7.

National Commission for the Protection of Human Subjects of Biomedical and Behavioral Research (1979) *The Belmont Report: Ethical Principles and Guidelines for the Protection of Human Subjects of Research*. Federal Register, 44(76).

Parry, O. and Mauthner, N.M. (2004) Whose data are they anyway? Practical, legal and ethical issues in archiving qualitative data, *Sociology*, 38(1): 139–52.

Research Ethics Committees Review Group (2008) Review of research ethics committees and processes in Republic of Ireland. Dublin: Health Service Executive.

Rid, A. and Schmidt, H. (2010) The 2008 Declaration of Helsinki – First among equals in research ethics? *Journal of Law, Medicine & Ethics*, 38(1): 143–8.

Rosnow, R.L., Rotheram-Borus, M.J., Ceci, S.J., Blanck, P.D. and Koocher, G.P. (1993) The institutional review board as a mirror of scientific and ethical standards, *American Psychologist*, 48(7): 821–6.

Sansone, R.A., McDonald, S., Hanley, P., Sellbom, M. and Gaither, G.A. (2004) The stipulations of one institutional review board: A five year review, *Journal of Medical Ethics*, 30(3): 308–10.

Scott, C.R. (2005) Anonymity in applied communication research: Tensions between IRBs, researchers, and human subjects, *Journal of Applied Communication Research*, 33(3): 242–57.

Sharkey, S.,Jones, R., Smithson, J., Hewis, E., Emmens, T., Ford, T. and Owens, C. (2011) Ethical practice in internet research involving vulnerable people: lessons from a self-harm discussion forum study (SharpTalk), *Journal of Medical Ethics*, 37(12): 752–8.

Shuster, E. (1997) Fifty years later: The significance of the Nuremberg code, *The New England Journal of Medicine*, 337(20): 1436–40.

Sieber, J.E. (2004) Informed consent, in M.S. Lewis-Beck, A. Bryman and T. Futing Liao (eds), *The SAGE Encyclopedia of Social Science Research Methods*, vol. 2. Thousand Oaks, CA: Sage.

Smith, M., Doyle, F., McGee, H.M. and De La Harpe, D. (2004) Ethical approval for national studies in Ireland: An illustration of current challenges, *Irish Journal of Medical Science*, 173(2): 72–4.

Standard Application Form Consultation Group – Pilot Form Sub-Group (2010) *Standard Application Form for the Ethical Review of Health-Related Research Studies which are not Clinical Trials: Pilot Phase Evaluation Report*. Available at www.molecularmedicineireland.ie/uploads/files/Common_Form_Pilot_Evaluation_FINAL_DRAFT_090810.pdf [Accessed April 2013].

Vass, A.A., Minardi, H.A., Ward, R., Aggarwal, N., Garfield, C. and Cybyk, B. (2003) Research into communication and consequences for effective care of people with Alzheimer's and their carers, *Dementia*, 2(1): 21–48.

Vaughan, G., Pollock, W., Peek, M.J., Knight, M., Ellwood, D., Homer, C.S., Pulver, L.J., McLintock, C., Ho, M. T. and Sullivan, E.A. (2012) Ethical issues: The multi-centre low-risk ethics/governance review process and AMOSS, *Australian and New Zealand Journal of Obstetrics and Gynaecology*, 52(2): 195–203.

Vogt, W.P. (2005) *Dictionary of Statistics & Methodology: A Nontechnical Guide for the Social Sciences*, 3rd edn. Thousand Oaks, CA: Sage.

7   Recruiting samples from vulnerable populations

Elizabeth A. Curtis and Rhona O'Connell

Chapter topics

- Concept of vulnerability
- Regulations and guidelines on vulnerability
- Vulnerability in research
- Types of vulnerability
- Ethical issues and vulnerability
- Problems associated with using samples from vulnerable groups
- Benefits of using vulnerable groups in research
- Strategies for improving recruitment from vulnerable groups

Introduction

A vital component in planning any research study is the selection of respondents/ participants. This is particularly important since it is unlikely that everyone in a given population can participate and the success of a study will hinge on those selected. Research studies frequently require the involvement of a specific group of individuals, either with certain characteristics or from particular situations or circumstances that are considered to be vulnerable. Such individuals or groups are given special protection so that their human rights are not violated. Where potential respondents are considered to be from a vulnerable population group, it is important that specific issues – such as those contained in this chapter – are addressed, since this is likely to assist the researcher in obtaining ethical approval for the study. Research ethics committees have a key role in determining access to populations and checklists are frequently used to objectively determine the vulnerability of subjects; these vary but may include children, pregnant women, the elderly, those with mental health problems or those with learning difficulties.

The chapter does not provide the reader with material on sampling approaches. This already exists in the form of entire books on the topic (Cochran 1977; Levy and Lemeshow 2008; Daniel 2012), several chapters in research books including Chapter 6 in this book (Houser 2008; Norwood 2010; Nieswiadomy 2012; Polit and Beck 2012) and many research papers (Callaghan et al. 2010; Miller et al. 2010). Rather, the purpose of the chapter is to introduce the health care researcher to the subject of selecting samples from vulnerable populations and draw attention to the issues surrounding the recruitment and use of such samples. The chapter begins with an explanation of the term vulnerability and provides examples of groups considered by some authors and organizational bodies to be vulnerable. It then moves on to explore the concept of vulnerability, and in particular vulnerability in the context of research. Next, the chapter describes existing regulations and guidelines on vulnerability, addresses key ethical issues surrounding the use of vulnerable populations in research, and identifies some benefits and problems associated with the use of individuals from vulnerable populations. The chapter concludes by putting forward some suggestions and strategies researchers could use for improving the recruitment of samples from vulnerable populations.

What is vulnerability?

In the context of health care research, the term vulnerability is often used to describe a reduced ability to protect one's own interests, which may be manifested by a compromised capacity to give informed consent (Grady 2009). It can also refer to those with limited financial resources or where there is unequal power between disadvantaged groups and researchers (Levine et al. 2004; Grady 2009). A broad definition is provided by the United States Agency for Health Care Policy and Research (1998: 1), who define vulnerable populations as the 'groups of people made vulnerable by their financial circumstances or place of residence; health, age, or functional or developmental status; or ability to communicate effectively [and] personal characteristics, such as race, ethnicity, and sex'. Sutton et al. (2003: 106) describe vulnerable populations as 'groups of people who can be harmed, manipulated, coerced, or deceived by researchers because of their diminished competence, powerlessness, or disadvantaged status'. Some definitions are either too broad or too restrictive (Hurst 2008), yet it is consistently argued that in order to reduce the likelihood of human rights violations special justification is required when undertaking research with vulnerable participants and that special protection must be provided (Ruof 2004). Despite various international guidelines (Declaration of Helsinki, Belmont Report, Council for International Organizations of Medical Sciences (CIOMS), World Health Organization (WHO)), some authors maintain that the concept of vulnerability remains vague (Rogers 1997; Hurst 2008; Koffman et al. 2009).

While definitions of vulnerability are not always provided, lists of groups where special precautions are required are frequently encountered. In the UK, the Department of Health (DH) research guidelines state that care is needed when seeking consent from children and vulnerable adults, such as those with mental health problems or learning difficulties (DH 2005). In Ireland, guidelines from An Bord Altranais (2007: 13) identify the following as potentially vulnerable:

- patients/clients
- those who are disabled physically, intellectually, socially or emotionally
- individuals whose hearing and vision are impaired
- people who reside in institutions and residential centres
- pregnant women
- children and adolescents
- elderly people
- prisoners
- students
- people whose first language is not English

In research terms, vulnerable individuals are often considered to be at increased risk of being taken advantage of, or harmed without their consent. As will be seen later in the chapter, stronger protection is required to ensure that the rights of individuals are not compromised, particularly where participants have a limited ability to act autonomously.

The concept of vulnerability

An ongoing challenge is the lack of a clear definition of the term vulnerability. The word derives from the Latin word for wound (*vulnus*) and has a wide usage in ordinary language. It can, for example, imply 'being at risk' or 'being in touch with one's feelings' (Levine 2004: 396), but is often used to describe populations, individuals or some of their attributes.

In health care settings, 'vulnerable' is often applied to individuals at risk of adverse health-related outcomes. A vulnerable individual is, in a specific or general sense, susceptible, open to, or at an increased chance or relative risk of physiologic or psychosocial harm (Purdy 2004). A concept analysis by Purdy (2004) explored the meaning of the term vulnerability. She maintains that vulnerability is often portrayed in negative terms, which may dissuade researchers from undertaking research with vulnerable populations. Having reviewed a wide range of literature on this topic, she takes a more positive approach and maintains that the essence of this concept is openness, which can have either a positive or negative value depending on the situation of each individual. Considering the vulnerability of individuals involves weighing the advantages and disadvantages of being vulnerable, which should include an awareness of the openness of the individual and the 'prospects for change' (Purdy 2004: 27). Research involving vulnerable populations offers individuals the opportunity to benefit from the research findings and a chance to participate in something that may lead to positive change.

Furthermore, Purdy (2004) suggests that researchers are often discouraged from undertaking research in areas of disadvantage due to a presupposed difficulty in obtaining ethical approval or of accessing participants. Yet these may be the groups or individuals who are most in need of interventions or of a greater understanding of their situation. This reconceptualization of the term vulnerability, to include an *'openness to change'*, may benefit individuals or groups who are normally considered as vulnerable (Purdy 2004). Her conclusion is that vulnerability is a 'highly individualised dynamic process' of being open to circumstances with the potential to change (Purdy 2004: 25). This may seem to be an unfamiliar concept of the term vulnerability, and one not often found in research texts.

Vulnerability in research

Another challenge for researchers is that, although research guidelines classify various groups as being vulnerable, precise explanations are rarely offered as to how they are vulnerable (Grady 2009). In addition, there is little agreement with regard to the special protection required for vulnerable participants (Coleman 2009).

Vulnerability is frequently conceptualized from the perspective of whole groups of people, rather than by identifying those individuals within a group (for instance, terminally ill patients) who may have the capacity to protect their personal interests and those who cannot. Within the context of research, viewing all pregnant women, all terminally ill people, or all individuals from an ethnic minority as vulnerable has been controversial (Levine 2008). Special protection for participants who are potentially vulnerable may be more appropriately determined by: 1) their own personal circumstances; 2) the requirements of the research study itself; 3) the research environment; and 4) other factors (De Bruin 2001).

The recommendations of the National Bioethics Advisory Commission (2001) suggest six core areas of vulnerability that researchers should consider when selecting participants. One or even all of the six vulnerabilities may be present in an individual or a population group. The six vulnerabilities are:

- communication/cognition
- institutional
- deferential
- medical
- economic
- social

We will now explore each of these.

Cognitive or communicative vulnerability

This refers to individuals who are unable to understand information, contemplate and come to a decision about participating in research because of difficulties in communication or cognition. This weakens an important part of informed consent: that the participant is able to understand what the study is about, weigh up the risks and benefits, and make a decision that is free from coercion. There are several conditions that might affect a person's ability to understand or communicate, including dementia, delirium, pain, blindness, intellectual impairments, language impediments, and many psychiatric and neurologic conditions (Quest and Marco 2003). Koffman et al. (2009) reported in their study that communicative vulnerability was observed in patients who were unable to communicate as a consequence of stressful symptoms such as cancer pain.

Institutional vulnerability

Potential participants may be considered to have institutional vulnerability even if they have the cognitive ability to consent to be in a study but are under the authority of others who may have different views about whether to permit them to participate (Quest and Marco 2003). Generally, this situation centres on prisoners, but could also include those in nursing homes and health care facilities. Indeed, it has been suggested that all recipients of health care are in some way vulnerable (RCN 2011). Individuals may feel that since they are dependent on facilities for food, shelter or medical care their autonomy to decide to participate in a study is not entirely voluntary.

Institutional vulnerability can be reduced by meeting with institutional staff before beginning the study to assure them that participants will not be pressurized into agreeing to participate. Selection of participants from an institution should be fair and should not in any way be influenced by the staff in the institution (National Bioethics Advisory Commission 2001). Excluding participants with institutional vulnerability purely on grounds of potential difficulties that could arise with this participant group might be construed as 'unethical research practice' and should be avoided (Quest and Marco 2003: 1296). Koffman et al. (2009) warn that researchers should be aware of other issues when using participants from this group. Participants may be dressed differently (nightwear or hospital gowns) and this may create a relationship differential between the researcher and the participant. Also, the participant may be lying in bed at the time of recruitment or data collection (interview) and the researcher may be standing, which immediately creates a difference in height and even in perceived power. Sometimes, interviews or meetings with participants take place in busy wards with only a thin curtain to separate the participant from others, offering little privacy and protection from noise. Even when a private quiet room is available it is not always possible to move participants because of their frail condition.

Deferential vulnerability

When participants have the cognitive ability to consent to participate in a study they could still be affected by deferential vulnerability because they are subject to the authority or control of others. This control is not formal as is the case in institutional vulnerability but rather informal. This informal control can be as a consequence of ethnicity, social class, gender, and inequalities between the researcher and the participant (National Bioethics Advisory Commission 2001; Quest and Marco 2003). Where health care professionals recruit the participants directly into a study, this can be viewed as subtle coercion which may affect the relationship between the researcher/health care professional and participant. Patients or clients may feel that refusal to participate could affect their treatment or the care that they receive. It is important that, where possible, health care professionals refrain from directly selecting participants for their studies and use instead an independent recruitment process.

Medical vulnerability

This type of vulnerability refers to potential participants who are severely ill (for example those with metastatic cancer) and for whom there are no effective treatments. Individuals are usually keen to participate because they, and in some instances their medical consultants, think that the research may result in a more positive outcome than their current standard care (National Bioethics Advisory Commission 2001). In such cases, participants might find it difficult to evaluate the risks and any future benefits, and this could result in informed consent being driven by a need to find a suitable treatment. The possibility for these participants to be exploited exists because they have unrealistic views about the benefits of the research or because they have not been given honest information about the risks and potential benefits of the study. It is important to stress that the continuance of research involving potential participants who are medically vulnerable is not in question here. What is required, however, is that researchers inform potential participants about the risks and benefits as truthfully as possible (taking care not to inflate potential benefits or de-emphasize the risks), to avoid exploitation and to ensure that they fully understand the information. To reduce medical vulnerability it might be necessary for researchers to engage independent personnel to recruit participants for the study and to carry out the informed consent procedures (National Bioethics Advisory Commission 2001).

Koffman et al. (2009: 442) reported that despite informing participants who were medically vulnerable (with a poor prognosis and numerous symptoms) that they could withdraw from interview at any stage, no one did. This, together with the interview transcripts which demonstrated how compromised participants were and how much they wanted to gain relief, illustrates the point discussed above concerning participants' eagerness to become part of research studies because of their belief that it will increase their chances of finding a cure for their illness. Researchers must understand and be prepared for the effects participants' distress may have on them during data collection.

Economic vulnerability

Potential participants are considered economically vulnerable when, despite having the ability to consent, they lack adequate income, housing or health care. Paying potential participants or providing them with transportation or social services may result in them deciding to enter a study when they would not normally do so. To reduce this type of vulnerability ethics review committees should ensure that financial incentives offered are not excessive and, if appropriate, recommend that the amount of money is reduced. They may, however, find it more difficult to reduce potential benefits such as free health care or social services (National Bioethics Advisory Commission 2001). Any potential economic benefits from participating in a study could be construed as an incentive for entry and as a consequence threaten voluntary choice and increase the risk of coercion (Quest and Marco 2003).

Social vulnerability

In spite of having cognitive ability to consent, some potential participants are considered to be socially vulnerable because they belong to groups that are marginalized or undervalued in society (National Bioethics Advisory Commission 2001; Koffman et al. 2009). Generally, those who are homeless, unemployed, poor, from an ethnic or religious minority, or drug-addicted, are considered to be socially vulnerable (Quest and Marco 2003). Social vulnerability is based on the perceptions people have of individuals from undervalued groups: this can lead to discrimination and diminish the contribution these groups can make to society. Researchers planning to include participants from socially vulnerable groups must be sensitive to these perceptions and take care to include everyone in the decision-making process during the planning of the study. Koffman et al. (2009: 442) suggest that differences in ethnicity between the researcher and participants can impact on 'the veracity and accuracy of the information that participants share'. Also, ethnic differences can be intimidating to some participants (Gunaratnam 2003). Ethnic matching, which increases rapport, has been put forward as a potential solution but it is not without its problems. It presumes that ethnicity is not affected by age, gender, education and social class, and ignores the fact that similarities and differences could vary during the course of an interview. Despite these potential barriers, Koffman et al. (2009) reported data from participants from socially vulnerable groups regardless of ethnicity.

Regulations and guidelines on vulnerability

Several international bodies have guidelines for conducting ethical research and all highlight the special considerations required when undertaking studies with vulnerable populations. In the US, a national commission was set up following the revelation that research was undertaken by the US Public Health Service over a period of 40 years (1932–72) to investigate the progression of untreated syphilis in poor, rural black men in Alabama. The men were unaware that they had syphilis and thought that they were receiving free health care. This disclosure led to the National Commission (1979) and the establishment of the Office for Human Research Protections (OHRP) which subsequently developed standards in the US for ethical research. The Belmont Report highlights the principle of voluntariness and informed consent and that research involving vulnerable populations should always be appropriate and justified. It warns that inducements offered to participants may lead to undue influence being applied. Guidance is given in terms of the unjustifiable pressures which can be offered by those in authoritative positions to encourage potential participants to engage in a study. The authors maintain that it is often impossible to state precisely where justifiable persuasion ends and undue influence begins.

A key international document is the Declaration of Helsinki, which contains a set of principles to guide human experimentation. This is widely regarded as the cornerstone document for human research ethics and is updated as required. In terms of vulnerable populations, the Declaration of Helsinki (WMA 2008: 3) states that research involving a disadvantaged or vulnerable population is only justified if the research is sensitive to 'the health needs and priorities of this population or community and if there is a reasonable likelihood that this population or community stands to benefit from the results of the research'. This includes those 'who cannot give or refuse consent for themselves and those who may be vulnerable to coercion or undue influence'.

Guidance is also provided by the International Ethical Guidelines for Biomedical Research Involving Human Subjects (CIOMS 2002). This document reiterates the importance of justification for inviting vulnerable individuals to participate in research studies and that this should occur only where the research will benefit the individuals in that vulnerable class. Subjects should not be involved unless the research could not be carried out equally well with less vulnerable subjects. More recently, the Universal Declaration of Human Rights stresses the importance of autonomy for individual participants in research studies and reiterates that vulnerable individuals should be protected (UNESCO 2005). Guidance is provided for the protection required for individuals who do not have the capacity to provide informed consent.

Despite these guidelines being available to health care researchers, Leavitt (2006) questions whether medical research can ever be undertaken when the population could not be considered vulnerable. This particularly refers to experimental research where individuals, whether consenting adults or small children, participate in studies where the risks of adverse outcomes may not be fully known and that consent is inevitably limited. Individuals (or proxies) consent to studies under the assumption that there will be minimal risk to themselves (or that the potential benefit may outweigh the potential risk), or that the results of the study may be of benefit to others. It thus appears that researchers face risks associated with both inclusion and exclusion criteria. Inclusion in research, where guidelines provide inadequate protection, opens the risk of exploitation; however the exclusion of vulnerable populations may limit access to experimental treatments or beneficial interventions. Researchers are thus required to achieve a balance between protection and access.

Ethical issues surrounding the use of samples from vulnerable populations

The effective recruitment of subjects for a research study has already been identified as critical to the research process, but this activity is not always easy or straightforward. Researchers using quantitative designs in their studies must be able to recruit large representative samples in order to be able to generalize their findings to the wider population (Sutton et al. 2003). Increasingly, researchers in health care are seeking assistance from health care providers, who function as gatekeepers, to assist them with recruiting large samples or samples with specific characteristics that they wish to explore. Generally, these gatekeepers are helpful, but in some instances they do restrict individuals from vulnerable populations from participating in research (Sutton et al. 2003). However well intentioned these actions may be, these gatekeepers may actually be violating the ethical principles underpinning the conduct of research as well as obstructing the recruitment process.

The three fundamental ethical principles underpinning the conduct of research involving humans are:

- respect for person
- beneficence and non-maleficence
- justice (Tappen 2011)

Respect for persons supports the view that individuals who are autonomous can make decisions irrespective of the consequences (Norwood 2010; Polit and Beck 2012). The principle of respect for person is in two parts; the first part is concerned with treating individuals autonomously, and the term autonomous implies that they have the ability to make decisions and that these decisions should be honoured except where they are harmful to others. The second part refers to persons with 'limited ability' to make decisions and that they must be given due protection (Tappen 2011: 174).

Beneficence is an obligation to do no harm (non-maleficence) and increase potential benefits. Researchers are expected to design studies that will decrease risks and maximize benefit. Applying this principle is not always easy. For example, research involving children to test the efficacy of a drug may appear to violate the principle of non-maleficence. Such decisions are difficult for researchers and ethics review committees alike, since they have to consider how best to create a balance between participation and protection.

Justice is concerned with fair treatment and privacy. Fair treatment is about how potential participants are recruited and treated during the conduct of a study. Selection should be guided by the requirements of the study rather than on convenience or easy availability of participants. Individuals who are hospitalized are used frequently because they can be accessed easily and may feel unable to refuse (Norwood 2010). Fair treatment also implies that researchers must treat those who refuse to participate or who may withdraw from the study after they have given consent in a fair and non-discriminatory way. The right to privacy endorses the protection of participants' identity such that they are not harmed by the findings from a study. Some intrusion into the private lives of those who participate in research is to be expected, but researchers must ensure that participants' privacy is protected at all times. Procedures used to guide and uphold privacy include anonymity and confidentiality (Norwood 2010; Polit and Beck 2012).

The application of these principles to research studies is not a simple matter. Students and researchers in health care have several procedures and guidelines that they must use when designing and conducting their studies and applying for funding. For example, a student completing a research study in partial fulfilment of the requirements of a course must receive ethical approval from the university, the local research ethics committee, the hospital ethics committee (if participants are to be recruited there) and possibly a patient advisory group. In addition, the student must be mindful of relevant national or international guidelines and any *special precautions* that may apply when seeking consent from those who may be considered vulnerable. These must be considered throughout the conduct of the study.

Application of ethical principles

While most health care professionals take these principles into account when acting as gatekeepers for vulnerable people they, nevertheless, must find it difficult to decide between permitting vulnerable patients to make their own choices regarding participation and trying to protect them from perceived potential risk (Sutton et al. 2003). In such situations, the gatekeepers are functioning as patient advocates because of their concern for the patient's welfare and believe that the basis for this lies in the principle of beneficence (doing good). The refusal to allow participants to take part in the study could result in them not receiving any potential benefits the study may offer and as a consequence inhibit rather than support the principle of beneficence. Additionally, the principles of respect for persons and justice are breached when gatekeepers refuse potential participants the right to participate in a study (Sutton et al. 2003). For more information about ethical principles and communicating with ethics committees read Chapters 5 and 6 in this book.

Researchers sometimes feel that ethics review committees limit the type of research they can conduct, but ethics review committees are required not only to consider the well-being of potential respondents but also to be supportive of researchers (Tappen

2011). The principle of justice suggests that all potential subjects be treated fairly. By refusing entry into a study, gatekeepers are effectively reducing the choices of these individuals and are therefore in breach of this ethical principle (Sutton et al. 2003). Research involving people from vulnerable groups should be conducted in order to allow them the same rights and opportunities afforded those outside these groups (Gwyn and Colin 2010). Discussions about the many concerns and issues (some of which were addressed here) surrounding the inclusion of individuals from vulnerable groups in research studies will no doubt continue for some time yet. Nevertheless, it is necessary that some suggestions are put forward for resolving these issues.

Importance of using samples from vulnerable populations

If one takes the view that all research studies should be designed to protect subjects, minimize risk, and uphold the rights of individuals then it is reasonable to propose that people from vulnerable populations should be allowed to participate. Furthermore, if the views and concerns of people from vulnerable groups are not investigated, then their care and quality of life may not be enhanced (Moore and Miller 1999). Labelling individuals as vulnerable because they belong to a vulnerable group fails to distinguish between those 'individuals in the group who indeed might have special characteristics that need to be taken into account and those who do not' (Levine et al. 2004: 47). Such a stance could result in excluding large numbers of potential subjects from studies because of a group label. Exclusion on such grounds could be regarded as discriminatory and could result in the loss of a unique set of data that could be used to potentially improve the quality of the care needed by these individuals (Purdy 2004; Gwyn and Colin 2010). Populations or groups classified as vulnerable continue to increase in number and could result in everyone belonging to such a group at some point in their lives. If research involving vulnerable populations continues to be restricted it is conceivable that this will have a negative impact on the growth of new knowledge and improvement in care for these individuals who may be exluded from research for reasons of vulnerability.

Concerns and problems with recruiting samples from vulnerable populations

Where full information about a study is provided and the right to refusal discussed, opportunities to participate in health care research should not be denied to vulnerable populations. However, studies that involve samples from vulnerable groups can have many methodological challenges. One such challenge is high refusal rates.

High refusal rates

In a study involving patients with cancer pain and their caregivers, Ransom et al. (2006) reported low levels of participation. One reason put forward for this is that caregivers of patients with cancer pain are already under considerable pressure so participating in a five-week trial may not be appealing to them. One suggestion for improving participation is for researchers to recruit from a wider population, moving from single-centre to multiple-centre recruitment. This of course may provide a more representative sample. Also, the inclusion criteria must be carefully considered when planning narrowly focused studies such as those involving patients with cancer pain attending one pain clinic. It is important to consider carefully the design of the study before recruiting samples as some can be quite burdensome for individuals from vulnerable groups such as patients with cancer pain. Due consideration must also be given to the size of the sample used in intervention studies since a small sample could result in a poor uptake of the intervention (Ransom et al. 2006).

In some studies (for example, on people with acute stroke) recruiting appropriate numbers of participants can be considerably more difficult than anticipated for a number of reasons. A key factor for optimizing outcomes following a stroke is speed – speed in recognizing, admitting and rehabilitating patients (DH 2010). This speed at which patients are processed on admission to a stroke unit can affect recruitment to a study and researchers must find ways of working within such guidelines, especially since hospital stay for these patients is decreasing (Jones et al. 2010). As such, it may be difficult for the researcher to organize research activities around the clinical management of care. In some instances, patients may be too ill and fatigued to be recruited in the immediate days following admission. By the time they have improved and are thus eligible for recruitment into the study several days have elapsed and patients may have been transferred for rehabilitation to offsite facilities before consent can be obtained (Jones et al. 2010).

Another factor that might impact on recruitment to a study concerns a definitive diagnosis. If diagnosis of a stroke by means of a CT (computerized tomography) scan is identified as part of the inclusion criteria then this may hamper recruitment because early CT scans are usually used to rule out cerebral haemorrhage rather than diagnose a stroke. Therefore, it is important that inclusion criteria for studies of this kind are developed using a well-validated clinical diagnosis framework or strategy (Parsons et al. 2009).

Timing of data collection

The timing of data collection, which may include the completion of detailed assessments of patients at different phases of a study, could present challenges for the researcher. A patient's condition may deteriorate or the patient may be discharged back to a referring hospital or home before the completion of data collection. It is important therefore that the researcher anticipates these likely scenarios when designing studies involving patients (Jones et al. 2010). It is necessary to bear in mind also the complexity of the data-collection tool when planning a study as patients may find them too long and complex, and this could have an impact on recruitment. Enrolment into a study can be affected even when a study has few or no known risks. Potential participants may decline entry because they believe that coping with the demands of their illness and the requirements of a study simultaneously will be too difficult. For example, research using participants in palliative care continues to cause concern because of its potential to increase distress in this cohort and also because there may be no immediate benefit from the research (Barnett 2001). Participants who are terminally ill may find interviews very tiring and emotionally difficult so researchers may wish to consider short interviews over a number of days if this is feasible. Similarly, participants who are at the early stage of their illness may have a positive outlook but this may not be the same for those who are in the terminal stages of their illness. Therefore, strategies must be put in place for dealing with participants who become emotionally upset. In her study, Barnett (2001) found that terminally ill patients lost their independence as a result of their illness and consenting to participate in a research study could help restore their independence. Difficult though these situations might be, researchers and gatekeepers cannot take a paternalistic approach when recruiting potential participants for studies that will investigate issues that are relevant to them (Barnett 2001).

Women who are pregnant or in labour

Women who are pregnant or in labour are another group that are often considered vulnerable in terms of obtaining consent, and as such may be disadvantaged. The fear of obtaining an 'informed refusal' may deter researchers from approaching pregnant women (Reid et al. 2011: 491). 'The primacy of competent pregnant women's autonomy is supported in both ethics and law and it is considered unacceptable both ethically and medically to routinely exclude pregnant women from clinical trials' (Reid et al. 2011: 491). Where studies of women in labour are proposed, staged recruitment is suggested, which involves providing information antenatally and obtaining informed consent when the woman is in labour. Provided the ability to obtain informed consent was present prior to labour, women retain their capacity to express explicit, voluntary and revocable consent during labour (CIOMS 2002; Kottow 2004).

Informed consent from children

It is also good practice to seek informed consent from children. The extent to which this will be feasible will vary with age, but information can be provided in written or pictorial format as appropriate (Neill 2005). Where a child does not have sufficient understanding of what is involved their assent should still be sought. Children should be made aware that, where information concerning risks to themselves or others emerges, confidentiality cannot be guaranteed. Where a child objects to being a research participant, this should be respected. In all cases, parental consent will also be required.

Strategies for improving the recruitment of samples from vulnerable populations

Successful recruitment of potential subjects is critical to the success of every research study. Yet, accruing suitable individuals including those from vulnerable populations can be quite difficult (Sutton et al. 2003). Below are some suggestions for addressing the recruitment of participants from vulnerable populations.

Cultivating a culturally safe space for research

Cultural safety is concerned with respecting the worldviews of the people being investigated (research subjects/participants), recognizing the range of differences that may exist and incorporating these into the research design protocol. This demands commitment from the researcher to respect the rights of participants and to work closely with them to develop a better understanding of the culture of the vulnerable population (Wilson and Neville 2009). This can occur only if the researcher respects the views and experiences of the participants, listens to them and observes what takes place before they communicate their views. Engaging in self-reflection will allow the researcher to examine their own worldviews and how these may impact on the research process, and provide insights into how they may affect the relationships with those being researched.

Collaboration

The importance of collaboration has been identified as essential to the recruitment of participants from vulnerable groups (Sutton et al. 2003). Collaboration with health care providers, potential participants and community members were reported as invaluable to recruiting participants with human immunodeficiency virus (HIV) and acquired immune deficiency syndrome (AIDS) (Regan-Kubinski and Sharts-Hopko 1997). Collaboration was critical in reducing mistrust felt by the clinicians regarding the reasons for the research and in increasing the researchers' awareness of the expertise of the clinicians and also the barriers to participation by potential participants. Collaboration between the researcher and staff in the clinical environment is essential for maintaining the integrity of data collected, particularly in randomized controlled trials (RCTs). It has been suggested that 'without data integrity (valid, sufficient, and high quality data), the results of RCTs would be uninterpretable' (Moody and McMillan 2002: 130). Data should be collected using a well-designed protocol developed jointly by the researcher and clinical staff. Despite this strong support for collaboration, researchers must always be aware of the influence or effect that clinical staff, family members and friends have on potential participants' decision to participate in a study (Gorelick et al. 1998).

Collaboration is essential when recruiting potential participants from vulnerable groups into studies. Patel et al. (2003) identified three key areas for consideration: establishing collaboration, methods of collaboration, and maintaining collaboration.

Establishing collaboration

Successful recruitment of potential participants from health care agencies hinges on early contact with administrative and clinical staff from key recruitment centres such as hospitals. Determining the level of administration support, the views of clinical staff, and patient statistics (e.g. volume, turnover) at these initial meetings is vital to the recruitment strategy. Worthy of note is that some health care professionals request that administrative staff do not encourage any enquiries about research studies (Patel et al. 2003) which can compound the problem of participant recruitment. Therefore, identifying health care professionals who encourage and support research at an early stage of the research process is recommended as it will reduce unnecessary visits to sites and delays in commencing the study. Early collaboration with health care professionals is useful for other reasons too. It provides sufficient time for staff to familiarize themselves with the study and understand what is expected from them, plan effectively for facilitating data collection, and establish what the data will be used for. All health care professionals as well as other staff (medical records personnel, ward clerks) who might be expected to assist with data retrieval and the data-collection process must feel comfortable with the researcher, accept his or her credentials, and be convinced of the potential value of the research before endorsing the study (Patel et al. 2003).

Methods of collaboration

Promoting the study before it commences is essential to successful collaboration. Strategies that could be used to assist with this process include presentations in key recruitment centres, pre-arranged meetings with relevant health care professionals or clinical staff, and forums (Patel et al. 2003). During this stage of collaboration, the researcher must discuss and agree procedures for sampling, inclusion and exclusion criteria, participant information sheets, ethical protocol for guiding the study, and consent with clinical staff. For clinical trials, the role of the medical consultant or physician must be established and procedures and regulations for dealing with an acute emergency (for instance, if the patient's condition deteriorates) outlined and if possible rehearsed. Mutual respect and trust among all those involved is critical to the success of this stage of collaboration and essential groundwork for a successful research project (Patel et al. 2003; Sutton et al. 2003).

Maintaining collaboration

Having established collaboration, it is necessary that the researcher maintains regular contact with the research site to promote the study and recruit participants. Ways in which this can be achieved include attending ward rounds in hospitals, attending staff meetings, and giving a presentation or lecture. In other words, researchers need to demonstrate enthusiasm and participate in some of the activities taking place in the recruitment centres (Patel et al. 2003; Sutton et al. 2003). Sending thank you notes or emails in appreciation of the assistance received from health care professionals may be time-consuming but is a necessary part of maintaining collaboration. Health professionals are busy people so any appreciation for their time is sure to boost relationships and therefore cooperation. Finally, providing regular feedback on how the study is progressing, giving updates on the medical condition of participants/patients, and sharing tentative results with health care professionals are activities that are often overlooked by researchers. These activities must be addressed properly and in a timely manner by the researchers or they could have a negative impact on any future collaborations and recruitment in centres such as hospitals (Patel et al. 2003).

Education

Education is necessary for the successful recruitment of potential participants from vulnerable groups. Researchers, health care professionals, and others who may be involved in research projects must all receive correct information and education about the study prior to its commencement and during its implementation. Clarity about the aim of the study, the ethical principles guiding the study and informing decision making, recruitment procedures for selecting potential participants, planned procedures/treatment and activities for data collection, the data-analysis procedures, and activities for the dissemination of findings must be communicated to all individuals involved (Sutton et al. 2003). Communicating the need for research and its impact on evidence-based practice must remain ongoing, open and honest since it makes a significant contribution to the education process. Integral to the education process is the need to identify and debate the ethical issues surrounding human rights. When the procedures and principles used to protect the rights of potential participants are understood by all involved this promotes trust not only in the research process but also the researcher. Where public trust in medical research is threatened, this could undermine research endeavours and reduce participation. Hall et al. (2006) reported that race, education, health status, prior participation and willingness to participate were significantly associated with researcher trust. Therefore, all possible interventions to improve trust among the general public and potential participants must be considered and utilized.

Education is especially important in clinical trials. Researchers must ensure that participants from vulnerable groups fully understand the randomization process since some may incorrectly assume that participation in a trial will deny them treatment for their illness. Therefore, an important part of education is to explain that participants will receive the care and treatment they have been prescribed even though they are allocated to the control group for the study (Sutton et al. 2003).

Recruiting an ethicist

In some research projects (for example, RCTs), it may be necessary for the researcher to invite an ethicist to contribute to discussions on ethics and human rights and clarify any issues that may arise before the study commences. This type of collaboration can help to allay fears and enhance the significance of the role of ethics in the research process (Sutton et al. 2003). Furthermore, members of the research team, health care professionals and potential participants must understand the regulations and procedures that have been put in place to protect the confidentiality and safety of research participants. To facilitate this process, education sessions on ethics may be necessary and the principal investigator must ensure that all research staff involved are familiar with the procedures and regulations guiding the study and that they adhere to them at all times. Depending on the nature of the study, some institutional review boards (IRBs) and ethics committees can request that members of a research team labelled as key personnel undertake education in the protection of human subjects before the study begins (National Institutes of Health 2000; Sutton et al. 2003).

The role of research ethics committees in protecting vulnerable populations

Research ethics committees have an important role in the protection of the public and to ensure that research studies are conducted ethically. This will include that the study has a robust design, that there is care and protection of research participants and that the study is justified. Protection of participants will include the principles of confidentiality and anonymity, informed consent, and awareness of potential risks to individuals and methods of addressing these issues. Where risks are identified, there is a requirement to undertake the study with the smallest number of participants that will provide statistically sound results.

Regulations about vulnerability can vary from country to country and in many instances vulnerability is defined using a list of categories. Moreover, ethics committees within the same country can have different views about vulnerability (Hurst 2008). These anomalies will, hopefully, decrease in time but for the present they can result in frustration and misunderstanding for researchers.

With regard to research involving people from vulnerable groups, ethics committee reviewers will be particularly concerned with how potential participants were sourced and recruited. Recruitment must be free from coercion while at the same time taking care not to exclude individuals from certain groups (Smith 2008). The reviewers will examine the reasons for excluding such groups because although usually warranted, this is not always the case. They will also examine all documents submitted to ensure that adequate information about the study and its potential benefits and risks have been communicated. For more information about communicating with research ethics committees read Chapter 6.

Conclusion

There are many areas in health care research which are poorly researched due to the presupposed difficulties of undertaking studies with vulnerable population groups. Researchers are often deterred due to anticipated difficulties in acquiring ethical approval, difficulties in accessing samples or difficulties in obtaining informed consent. Research ethics committees highlight that special precautions are required when studies involve individuals from vulnerable groups, yet it is not always clear what is required other than that ethical principles are maintained. For those interested in researching hard-to-access populations, it is worth persevering, finding out what special precautions are required, taking time to approach and seek approval from gatekeepers and, most importantly, exploring options for ensuring that the potential participants remain autonomous, with the right to provide consent, to decline to participate, or to withdraw from a study at any stage as required. All researchers are grateful to the individuals who consent to participate in their studies, and as such they must be valued and treated well at each stage, including, where appropriate, being respectfully informed of results. Addressing these issues will involve time and resources, which may be difficult for individual researchers to surmount without the support of the relevant health care professionals who endorse the proposal. The benefit of undertaking research with vulnerable populations is that these are the individuals who are most in need of good-quality studies to address their needs. This chapter has explored the issues and challenges in undertaking research with people who are considered vulnerable and has provided a range of strategies that may be useful to researchers.

Key concepts

- The concept of vulnerability remains vague, with many definitions of the term either too broad or too restrictive.
- Several international guidelines highlight the special considerations required for undertaking research with vulnerable populations.
- Researchers should consider six core areas of vulnerability when selecting subjects/participants from vulnerable populations. These areas of vulnerability include cognitive, institutional, deferential, medical, economic and social.
- The three fundamental principles underpinning research involving humans are respect for person, beneficence and non-maleficence, and justice.
- Studies that involve individuals from vulnerable populations can have many methodological challenges, including refusal rates, recruiting sufficient numbers, timing of data collection, and obtaining informed consent.
- It is important to include individuals from vulnerable populations in research because to exclude them could result in the loss of a unique set of data that could be used to improve the quality of care required by such individuals.

Key readings on sampling vulnerable populations

- M. De Chesney and B. Anderson (eds), *Caring for the Vulnerable: Perspectives in Nursing Theory, Practice and Research*, 3rd edn (Burlington, MA: Jones & Bartlett Learning, 2012) *This book provides examples of studies undertaken with vulnerable populations. It includes guidance on undertaking research with vulnerable populations including developing research proposals in preparation for review by ethics committees.*
- F. Delor and M. Hubert, Revisiting the concept of 'vulnerability', *Social Science and Medicine*, 50(11) (2000), 1557–70 *This paper addresses the concept of vulnerability in the context of research on HIV/AIDS as well as research in other fields such as mental health and famine.*
- J. Faugier and M. Sargeant, Sampling hard to reach populations, *Journal of Advanced Nursing*, 26(4) (1997), 790–7 *Studies using samples from populations such as homeless people, prostitutes and drug addicts can give rise to several methodological issues or questions that are not encountered when using samples from other populations. The authors of this paper explore the benefits and drawbacks to using such samples.*
- G.A. Jacobson, Vulnerable research participants: Anyone may qualify, *Nursing Science Quarterly*, 18(4) (2005), 359–63 *This paper outlines the roles, responsibilities and processes of institutional review boards and concludes by calling for nurses to become active members of institutional review boards.*

- F. J. Leavitt, Is any medical research population not vulnerable?, *Cambridge Quarterly of Healthcare Ethics*, 15(1) (2006), 81–8
  This paper provides an interesting classification of vulnerable populations and argues that all research populations are potentially vulnerable and therefore require protection. It further discusses the issue of whether medical researchers and their sponsors should be the ones providing protection for participants from vulnerable populations.
- L.W. Moore and M. Miller, Initiating research with doubly vulnerable populations, *Journal of Advanced Nursing*, 30(5) (1999), 1034–40
  Research studies using participants from vulnerable populations can offer invaluable information about the concerns and needs of these individuals. But using such populations can present many challenges for the health care researcher. This paper discusses two challenges often encountered by nurse researchers – pre-investigation issues and gaining access to vulnerable populations – and outlines strategies for dealing with them.

Examples of studies involving samples from vulnerable populations

- R. Chapman, J. Wardrop, P. Freeman, T. Zappia, R. Watkins and L. Shields, A descriptive study of the experiences of lesbian, gay and transgender parents accessing health services for their children, *Journal of Clinical Nursing*, 21(7–8) (2012), 1128–35
- C. Cook, Email interviewing: Generating data with a vulnerable population, *Journal of Advanced Nursing*, 68(6) (2012), 1330–9
- J. Koffman, I.J. Higginson, S. Hall, J. Riley, P. McCrone and B. Gomes, Bereaved relatives' views about participating in cancer research, *Palliative Medicine*, 26(4) (2011), 379–83
- D.G. Moore, J.J.T. Turner, A.C. Parrott, J.E. Goodwin, S.E. Fulton, M.O. Min, H.C. Fox, F.M.B. Braddick, A. Toplis, E.L. Axelsson, S. Lynch, H. Ribeiro, C.J. Frostick and L.T. Singer, During pregnancy, recreational drug-using women stop taking ecstasy (MDMA) and reduce alcohol consumption but continue to smoke tobacco and cannabis, *Journal of Psychopharmacology*, 24(9) (2010), 1403–10
- S. Pickens, J. Burnett, A.D. Naik, H.M. Holmes and C.B. Dyer, Is pain a significant factor in elder self-neglect?, *Journal of Elder Abuse & Neglect*, 18(4) (2006), 51–61
- M.Y. Veenstra, P.N. Walsh, H.M.J. van Schrojenstein Lantman-de Valk, M.J. Haveman, C. Linehan, M.P. Kerr, G. Weber, L. Salvador-Carulla, A. Carmen-Cara, B. Azema, S. Buono, A. Germanavicius, J. Tossebro, T. Maatta, G. van Hove and D. Moravec, Sampling and ethical issues in a multicentre study on health of people with intellectual disabilities, *Journal of Clinical Epidemiology*, 63(10) (2010), 1091–100
- L.C. Wilson and A. Scarpa, Level of participatory distress experienced by women in a study of childhood abuse, *Ethics & Behaviour*, 22(2) (2011), 131–41

Useful websites

- British Society of Criminology: Code of ethics – provides information on the requirements for conducting ethical research in the field of criminology – http://www.britsoccrim.org/codeofethics.htm
- General Medical Council: Consent to research: Research involving vulnerable adults – provides guidance to the medical profession on the ethical issues for undertaking research with vulnerable adults – http://www.gmc-uk.org/guidance/ethical_guidance/6471.asp
- National Centre for Guidance in Education: Research code of ethics – provides information on the values and principles to be considered when undertaking research in education – http://www.ncge.ie/resources_publications.htm
- NSPCC: Ethical issues in research with children – provides links to resources for undertaking ethical research with children – http://www.nspcc.org.uk/Inform/research/reading_lists/ethical_issues_in_research_with_children_wda55732.html
- Health Research Authority UK – provides information for conducting ethical research in the UK which protects and promotes the interests of patients and the public – http://www.hra.nhs.uk/hra/
- NIHR Research Governance: HR Good Practice Resource Pack: The Research Passport: Vetting and barring scheme guidance – provides information and resources for researchers in the UK who do not have contractual arrangements with the NHS but who may wish to carry out research which requires access to NHS facilities – http://www.nihr.ac.uk/systems/Pages/systems_research_passports.aspx/
- Research Ethics Canada – provides links to various Canadian sources of information on conducting ethical research – http://www.researchethics.ca/canada.htm
- National Health and Medical Research Council Australia – provides links to various Australian resources of information on conducting ethical research and human health – http://www.nhmrc.gov.au/health-ethics/human-research-ethics
- Health and Disability Ethics Committees (HDEC) New Zealand: Guidance on Ethical Research Review – provides links to various resources for conducting ethical research in New Zealand – http://www.ethicscommittees.health.govt.nz/moh.nsf/indexcm/ethics-resources-guidanceethicalresearch

References

An Bord Altranais (2007) *Guidance to Nurses and Midwives Regarding Ethical Conduct of Nursing and Midwifery Research*. Dublin: An Bord Altranais.

Barnett, M. (2001) Interviewing terminally ill people: Is it fair to take their time? *Palliative Medicine*, 15(2): 157–8.

Callaghan, P., Khalil, E. and Morres, I. (2010) A prospective evaluation of the transtheoretical model of change applied to exercise in young people, *International Journal of Nursing Studies*, 47(1): 3–12.

Cochran, W.G. (1977) *Sampling Techniques*, 3rd edn. New York: John Wiley and Sons.

Coleman, C.H. (2009) Vulnerability as a regulatory category in human subject research, *Journal of Law, Medicine & Ethics*, 37(1): 12–18.

Council for International Organizations of Medical Sciences (CIOMS) (2002) *International Ethical Guidelines for Biomedical Research Involving Human Subjects*. Geneva: CIOMS.

Daniel, J. (2012) *Sampling Essentials: Practical Guidelines for Making Sampling Choices*. London: Sage.

DeBruin, D. (2001) Reflections on vulnerability, *Bioethics Examiner*, 5(2): 1–4.

Department of Health (2005) *Research Governance Framework for Health and Social Care*, 2nd edn. London: DH. Available at http://www.dh.gov.uk/en/Publicationsandstatistics/Publications/PublicationsPolicyAndGuidance/DH_4108962 [Accessed March 2013].

Department of Health (2010) *Progress in Improving Stroke Care*. London: National Audit Office.

Gorelick, P.B., Harris, Y., Burnett, B. and Bonecutter, F.J. (1998) The recruitment triangle: Reasons why African Americans enrol, refuse to enrol, or voluntarily withdraw from a clinical trial: An interim report from the African American Antiplatelet Stroke Prevention Study (AAASPS), *Journal of the National Medical Association*, 90(3): 141–5.

Grady, C. (2009) Vulnerability in research: Individuals with limited financial and/or social resources, *Journal of Law, Medicine and Ethics*, 37(1): 19–27.

Gunaratnam, Y. (2003) *Researching Race and Ethnicity: Methods, Knowledge and Power*. London: Sage.

Gwyn, P.G. and Colin, J.M. (2010) Research with the doubly vulnerable population of individuals who abuse alcohol, *Journal of Psychosocial Nursing*, 48(2): 38–42.

Hall, M.K., Camacho, F., Lawlor, J.S., DePuy, V., Sugarman, J. and Weinfurt, K. (2006) Measuring trust in medical researchers, *Medical Care*, 44(11): 1048–53.

Houser, J. (2008) *Nursing Research: Reading, Using, and Creating Evidence*. Boston, MA: Jones and Bartlett.

Hurst, S.A. (2008) Vulnerability in research and health care: Describing the elephant in the room?, *Bioethics*, 22(4): 191–202.

Jones, S.E., Hamilton, S., Perry, L., O'Malley, C. and Halton, C. (2010) Developing workable research methods: Lessons from a pilot study with vulnerable participants and complex assessments, *Journal of Research in Nursing*, 16(4): 307–18.

Koffman, J., Morgan, M. and Edmonds, P. (2009) Vulnerability in palliative care research: Findings from a qualitative study of Black Caribbean and White British patients with advanced cancer, *Journal of Medical Ethics*, 35(7): 440–4.

Kottow, M. (2004) The battering of informed consent, *Journal of Medical Ethics*, 30(6): 565–9.

Leavitt, F.J. (2006) Is any research population not vulnerable?, *Cambridge Quarterly of Healthcare Ethics*, 15(7): 81–8.

Levine, C. (2004) The concept of vulnerability in disaster research, *Journal of Traumatic Stress*, 17(5): 395–402.

Levine, C. (2008) Research involving economically disadvantaged participants, in E. Emanuel, C. Grady, R. Crouch, R. Lie, F. Miller and D. Wendler (eds) *The Oxford Textbook of Clinical Research Ethics*. New York: Oxford University Press, pp. 431–6.

Levine, C., Faden, R., Grady, C., Hammerschmidt, D., Eckenwiler, L. and Sugarman, J. (2004) The limitations of 'vulnerability' as a protection for human research participants, *The American Journal of Bioethics*, 4(3): 44–9.

Levy, P.S. and Lemeshow, S. (2008) *Sampling of Population: Methods and Applications*, 4th edn. New Jersey: John Wiley and Sons.

Miller, P.G., Johnston, J., Dunn, M., Fry, C.L. and Degenhardt, L. (2010) Comparing probability and non-probability sampling methods in ecstasy research: Implications for the internet as a research tool, *Substance Use and Misuse*, 45(3): 437–50.

Moody, L.E. and McMillan, S. (2002) Maintaining data integrity in randomised clinical trials, *Nursing Research*, 51(2): 129–33.

Moore, L.W. and Miller, M. (1999) Initiating research with doubly vulnerable populations, *Journal of Advanced Nursing*, 30(5): 1034–40.

National Bioethics Advisory Commission (2001) *Ethical Policy Issues in Research Involving Human Participants*, i: *Report and Recommendations of the National Bioethics Advisory Commission*. Washington, DC: US Government Printing Office.

National Commission for the Protection of Human Subjects of Biomedical and Behavioral Research (1979) *The Belmont Report: Ethical Principles and Guidelines for the Protection of Human Subjects of Research*. Washington, DC: US Government Printing Office. Available at http://www.hhs.gov/ohrp/humansubjects/guidance/belmont.html [Accessed 21 November 2012].

National Institutes of Health (2000) *Required Education in the Protection of Human Research Participants*. Available at http://grants2.nih.gov/grants/guide/notice-files/NOT-OD-00-039.html [Accessed March 2013].

Neill, S.J. (2005) Research with children: A critical review of the guidelines, *Journal of Child Health Care*, 9(1): 46–58.

Nieswiadomy, R.M. (2012) *Foundations of Nursing Research*, 6th edn. Boston, MA: Pearson Education.

Norwood, S.L. (2010) *Research Essentials: Foundations for Evidence-Based Practice*. New Jersey: Pearson Education.

Parsons, M., Miteff, F., Bateman, G., Spratt, N., Loiselle, A. and Attia, J. (2009) Acute ischemic stroke: Imaging-guided tenecteplase treatment in an extended time window, *Neurology*, 72(10): 915–21.

Patel, M.X., Doku, V. and Tennakoon, L. (2003) Challenges in recruitment of research participants, *Advances in Psychiatric Treatment*, 9(3): 229–38.

Polit, D.F. and Beck, C.T. (2012) *Nursing Research: Generating and Assessing Evidence for Nursing Practice*, 9th edn. Philadelphia: Wolters Kluwer/Lippincott Williams & Wilkins.

Purdy, I.B. (2004) Vulnerable: A concept analysis, *Nursing Forum*, 39(4): 25–33.

Quest, T. and Marco, C.A. (2003) Ethics seminars: Vulnerable populations in emergency medicine research, *ACAD Emergency Medicine*, 10(11): 1294–8.

Ransom, S., Azzarello, L.M. and McMillan, S.C. (2006) Methodological issues in the recruitment of cancer pain patients and their caregivers, *Research in Nursing & Health*, 29(3): 190–8.

RCN (2011) *Informed Consent in Health and Social Care Research: RCN Guidance for Nurses*, 2nd edn. London: RCN.

Regan-Kubinski, M.J. and Sharts-Hopko, N.C. (1997) Accessing HIV-infected research subjects: The need for collaboration, *Journal of the Association of Nurses in AIDS Care*, 8(2): 83–6.

Reid, R., Susic, D., Pathirana, S., Tracy, S. and Welsh, A.W. (2011) The ethics of obtaining consent in labour for research, *Australian and New Zealand Journal of Obstetrics and Gynaecology*, 51(6): 485–92.

Rogers, A.C. (1997) Vulnerability, health and health care, *Journal of Advanced Nursing*, 26(1): 65–72.

Ruof, M.C. (2004) Vulnerability, vulnerable populations, and policy, *Kennedy Institute of Ethics Journal*, 14(4): 411–25.

Smith, I.J. (2008) How ethical is ethical research? Recruiting marginalised, vulnerable groups into health services research, *Journal of Advanced Nursing*, 62(2): 248–57.

Sutton, L.B., Erlen, J.A., Glad, L.M. and Siminoff, L.A. (2003) Recruiting vulnerable populations for research: Revisiting the ethical issues, *Journal of Professional Nursing*, 19(2): 106–12.

Tappen, R.M. (2011) *Advanced Nursing Research: From Theory to Practice*. Sudbury, MA: Jones and Bartlett.

UNESCO (2005) *Universal Declaration on Bioethics and Human Rights. Paris*: UNESCO. Available at: http://www.unesco.org/new/en/social-and-human-sciences/themes/bioethics/bioethics-and-human-rights/ [Accessed March 2013].

United States Agency for Health Care Policy and Research (AHCPR) (1998) *Final Report of the President's Advisory Commission on Consumer Protection and Quality in the Health Care Industry*, cited by the Agency for Healthcare Research and Quality. Available at http://archive.ahrq.gov/news/press/vulnpr.htm [Accessed March 2013].

Wilson, D. and Neville, S. (2009) Culturally safe research with vulnerable populations, *Contemporary Nurse*, 33(1): 69–79.

World Medical Association (2008) *Declaration of Helsinki: Ethical Principles for Medical Research Involving Human Subjects*. Available at http://www.wma.net/en/30publications/10policies/b3/ [Accessed March 2013].

PART 3

Quantitative research designs

8 Designing and conducting quantitative research studies

Elaine Pierce

Introduction

In health and social care, as in other spheres, quantitative research refers to the collection and interpretation of statistics, while qualitative research focuses on the significance of observed experiences. Both are used for interpretation and analysis. Quantitative research is systematic and empirical, utilizing various methodological approaches and techniques. Theories and hypotheses are proposed and developed, with measurement underpinning it all. In general the research question for quantitative research tends to be more specific and narrow, whereas for qualitative research it may be broader. All the processes involved in quantitative research can be said to fall within four phases:

- conceptual
- planning
- operational
- dissemination

Common approaches encompassed under the banner of the quantitative paradigm include: the classic or true experiment, quasi-experiments, and randomized controlled trials. Other designs, such as surveys, interviews and questionnaires, can be either quantitative or qualitative. The design is made up of characteristics and specifics (the ingredients) such as variables, reliability, validity and statistics. Illustrated in Figure 8.1 are some examples of designs for what will be described as the quantitative menu for health and social care, while Figure 8.2 shows examples of the ingredients. Topics that make up the ingredients and the menu will be discussed in more detail later in the chapter.

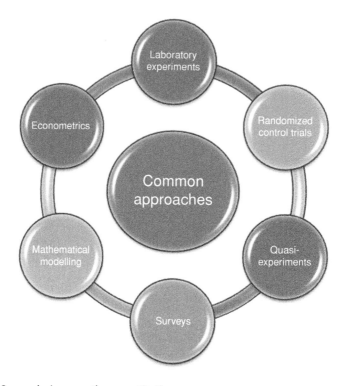

Figure 8.1 Some designs on the quantitative menu.

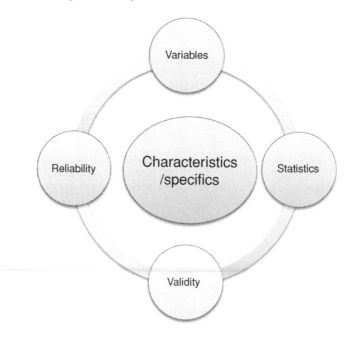

Figure 8.2 Some examples of design ingredients for the quantitative menu.

Quantitative research designs aim to produce findings that are:

- objective
- reliable
- valid
- reproducible

Replication could be undertaken by anyone, including the original researcher, and could be conducted anywhere as long as the exact same protocols are followed and the same conditions of the original experiment are met. In quantitative studies, the numbers making up the study population can range from tens to hundreds, to thousands or millions. Hence, for the smaller population, for basic statistics, for example, a calculator can be utilized, whereas bigger numbers require more advanced statistical procedures and packages. There may be a need to build mathematical models for complex theories, and in some cases to engage a statistician as part of the research team. As with qualitative research, there are a number of methodological approaches that can be used when conducting quantitative research.

Quantitative research methodologies are widely employed in not only scientific research, but also other types of research conducted by health and social care investigators and scientists in the fields of mathematics, education and so on. Quantitative research incorporates causality, variables and a well-defined pre-structure (Bryman 1992), as will become apparent throughout this chapter.

Positivism

Positivism was detailed in Chapter 1. Below is a brief description of how quantitative research is grounded in philosophy and has its origins in positivism. According to Krauss (2005), epistemology (from Greek, meaning 'knowledge philosophy or how we acquire it') is closely aligned with ontology (the philosophy and study of reality) and methodology (identification of specific practices to acquire knowledge). Thus in the positivist paradigm the research is independent of the investigator; knowledge is acquired and confirmed through direct observation and/or measurement of phenomena; and detailed examination of the phenomenon/phenomena will reveal the facts (Krauss 2005). In broad terms, this sums up what quantitative research entails.

Many authors (Qureshi 1992; Straub et al. 2004; Gray 2009) cite Karl Popper's *'scientific'* theory and *'myth'* as being instrumental in positivism. The theory is based on the falsification principle, which states that scientific theories cannot be proved right, but they can be shown to be wrong. Post-positivism, on the other hand, tends to have a more realistic outlook. It is based on there being a real world irrespective of our perception, referred to as critical realism. Science should try to understand the real world, and there should be awareness that measurements and observations are not perfect and so require multiple corroboration or triangulation (Straub et al. 2004).

One can envisage science as endeavouring to capture the truth about the world and the universe and understanding it sufficiently to predict and control it (Krauss 2005). The universe is a single determinate operating and governed by the rules of cause and effect. According to Hoefer (2010), causal determinism – that is, cause and effect – implies that, against the backdrop of the laws of nature, each event is unavoidable, having been determined by a preceding occurrence, condition, cause or event. The relationship between cause and effect is experienced in daily activities (Cota 2006), for example, you set the alarm clock (cause) to wake up (effect) at a certain time. Science can therefore be regarded as mechanical, because of the major role positivism plays within it and because it may also influence and control scientific methodologies. Positivism is one of the many instruments at the disposal of the researcher.

Deductive and inductive approaches

Knowledge can be obtained through the processes of both deduction and induction. In general, research obtained by deduction relates to the testing of established theory – deductive research. Induction refers to research where theories are developed or generated from, for example, observation – inductive research. In other words, using deduction involves generating an idea (to test established theory) and progressing through the research process to obtain data, whereas with induction you start by looking at the data and then progress through the research process to obtain the idea (generate theory) (Figure 8.3).

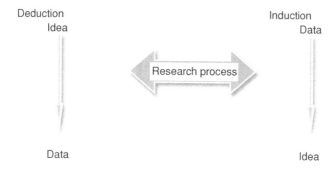

Figure 8.3 The deductive and inductive approaches.

Figure 8.3 is a simplified version of the deductive and inductive approaches, which omits the detail between the idea and the data and vice versa. According to Gray (2009), the process of deduction involves a number of phases. A literature search needs to be undertaken, in order to choose the theoretical concepts and theories most relevant to the research, followed by the development of the hypothesis. The research is conducted according to the chosen method and the data compared with the theory to ascertain if the latter has been established. Depending on the outcomes, the hypothesis is accepted or rejected. On the other hand, the inductive process does not confirm or falsify a theory; instead, it attempts to discover patterns, consistencies and meanings from the research (Gray 2009).

In the main, the deductive or hypothetico-deductive approaches refer to quantitative research, because of the testing of a hypothesis, and the inductive approach refers to qualitative research. For example, the randomized controlled trial uses the hypothetico-deductive approach. However, not all quantitative research involves the testing of a hypothesis (for example, descriptive surveys), whereas some qualitative researchers such as ethnographers may accept the hypothetico-deductive method (Hammersley 1992). Both quantitative and qualitative methodologies are needed and there may be elements of deduction and induction in all research; therefore research should not be seen as purely quantitative or qualitative (Hammersley 1992). However, hypothesis-testing research and research primarily concerned with generating theoretical ideas are easily distinguishable (Hammersley 1992).

Empirical data

Of importance in science and scientific method is that the evidence is empirical. Positivism is based on scientific theory supported by empirical data. Empirical data are derived from experiment and/or the senses (observation, smell, hearing, taste and touch). Straub et al. (2004) cite Karl Popper to the effect that Einstein's theory of relativity is a first-class example of a scientific theory that would have been rejected had it not been tested and supported by empirical data. A number of authors quote Popper's notion of falsifiability, as opposed to verifiability, as being a key component of science: that is, findings are not verified but supported or corroborated by evidence every time they are tested (Qureshi 1992; Straub et al. 2004; Gray 2009).

Science demands that assumptions are supported by empirical evidence and that this evidence has been obtained by following a methodical process in order to minimize or control errors that may arise (Ruane 2005). If evidence is not obtained systematically it should be considered less favourably and regarded as less trustworthy. If it is to be regarded as scientific and reliable, the evidence obtained must be capable of being tested and replicated in other studies (Ruane 2005).

To pursue the quest for accurate scientific knowledge with minimal or no error there are methodological processes or standards to adhere to. According to Ruane (2005) they include criteria for:

- sampling
- measurement validity
- internal validity
- external validity

The above methodological standards are integral to research methods and their adoption offers assurance that the evidence provided is reproducible, reliable and less likely to contain errors (Table 8.1) (see Chapter 10). Researchers should ensure that:

- the study sample is representative in order for it to be generalizable
- the outcome can be accurately and confidently assessed and interpreted
- data have been systematically observed, collected, measured and/or manipulated (Table 8.1)

Table 8.1 Standards integral to research methods

Methodological process	Explanation	Example
Sampling	The sample is made up of the participants in a research study. This group is identified as being representative of the population being studied and participants are selected from the sampling frame.	If in your research study, for a representative sample, you were to interview all the nurses at your hospital, the list of nurses would be your sampling frame. However, they will not all be included in the sample, as some may decline to be interviewed and others may start and then opt out.
Measurement validity	Relates specifically to whether operationalization and the scoring of cases sufficiently captures the idea or concept the researcher is aiming to measure (Adcock and Collier 2001).	Operationalization refers to the transformation of your idea, concept or construct into a functioning and operating reality (Trochim 2006). In the example above, your idea is to use the nurses as your sampling frame. Recruiting your sample from this frame is putting it into action and making it a reality.
Internal validity	Refers to accuracy of the research findings and determines whether the research has achieved what it set out to measure so that the outcome may be considered valid and trustworthy (see Chapter 10).	Doing a pilot study prior to commencing the research has substantial benefits. Subjects used in the pilot should not be used in the actual study, because the effect or their responses may be affected by their awareness of what to expect, making the research findings less reliable.
External validity	Refers to the generalizability of the research and asks whether or not the results can be safely generalized and/or extended to other settings, areas, populations or groups.	A health and safety study on a single neonatal ward could not be generalized to all children's wards and departments in a hospital or to all hospitals in the country.

Why a quantitative research design?

The research design encompasses the overall plan of data collection, utilization, measurement and analysis. If the design is ill-conceived, the likelihood of obtaining solutions to the research question is jeopardized. Quantitative research designs include, among others:

- experimental
- quasi-experimental

- analytical (for example, surveys (Chapter 10))
- developmental (cross-sectional study)
- factorial
- designs employing mixed methods, such as action research

The most common design types are covered in more detail in other chapters in this book. The above designs all have commonalities in their methodologies and because they fall under the quantitative banner their methods and approaches are all highly structured. According to Gray (2009), they tend to seek the truth in order to provide the evidence as opposed to seeking perspectives which provide qualitative data. Gray (2009) states that classification can be made according to purpose, for example exploratory, descriptive and explanatory studies.

There are numerous influences, factors and combinations of factors which will influence the choice of a design. The quantitative researcher will be influenced by the knowledge they have acquired of research philosophies and paradigms and their interpretation of how the theory should be utilized and implemented. By choosing a quantitative research design, the theoretical route the researcher chooses to follow is likely to be the deductive approach (see deductive and inductive discussion above). The design is also dependent on the nature of the research question. For example, are they setting out to make a new discovery, such as a new drug to cure a disease? Are they exploring associations between variables such as in an analytical survey? Are they exploring effects of different drugs on a particular disease? Are they reproducing an experiment under the same conditions? Regardless of what philosophy, paradigm, approach, design or method is adopted, the researcher should be able to justify it in relation to the research question or questions.

How strong or how weak the internal validity of a research study is may depend on the research design. Hence the purpose of the design, and the use of techniques to improve it, is to minimize experimental error and maximize the possibility of the research producing reliable and valid results (Burns 2000). Any well-designed quantitative study – for example, a clinical trial – will provide strong internal validity.

Variables

As an investigator, you will be examining characteristics or values within your research which have impact, and can be changed and/or measured. Variables, also referred to as fields, are these characteristics or values. You will be assessing, for example, how well they are distributed within your population and what you can infer from the relationships, associations and correlations between them. Although quantitative research enables such relationships, associations and correlations between variables to be ascertained, it may be more difficult to explore the reasons underlying them. The latter is probably more suited to a qualitative study. In your dataset you will also have a case (also referred to as a record), which is a collection of information about one participant or observation in your research. If you are analysing your findings quantitatively, then your research variables have to be isolated, defined and measured (Hohmann 2006).

The nature of the research will determine the type of variables, their number and how they are to be analysed (Hohmann 2006). To do this you will need clear operational definitions, so that it is explicit what is being measured. To illustrate the above terms, an example from a research study conducted by Pierce and McLaren (2012) is in Box 8.1.

Box 8.1   An example of research to illustrate terms used to describe variables

The aim of this research study (Pierce and McLaren 2012) was to assess to what extent neurological patients were dependent on the staff caring for them. For the purposes of the study there had to be a clear definition of *dependent*; the neurological diagnoses of the patients who were to be included in the sample and the relevant participating staff in the multidisciplinary team had to be specified. All the information that was collected on each patient – how dependent they were on staff, their diagnosis and the different staff who cared for them – constitutes the case or record. The headings that were the same for each case or record (for example, degree of dependency, diagnosis and so on) are the variables. In this study the dataset is multivariate – that is, it contains information on many variables (one variable is referred to as univariate and two, bivariate). The information that changes for each variable is the value or the entry. For example, in patient 1's case/record the value/entry under dependency (variable) is *very dependent* and the diagnosis (variable) *traumatic brain injury*. For patient 2, the entries may be *moderately dependent and multiple sclerosis*; for patient 3 *independent* and *subarachnoid haemorrhage*; and so on.

Through operational definitions you and others will better understand what you are measuring; you will be able to exert control. For example, if you are investigating groups, you will be able to ensure that the variable categories remain constant between the groups; or you may be able to manipulate the independent variables.

Earlier in this chapter causal determinism was mentioned and the example of the alarm clock and waking up was given to illustrate the concept of cause and effect. The cause (alarm clock) can be described as the independent variable and the effect (wake up) as the dependent variable. Gray (2009) points out that independent variables may not always directly affect dependent variables: that is, cause and effect does not always necessarily follow. The effect may come indirectly from an intermediary known as an intervening variable. Using the previous example, although the alarm clock (cause) has been set to wake up the person sleeping (effect), they may be disturbed by a loud noise or movement (intervening variable). If the experiment is to ensure the participant sleeps a set number of hours, in order to collect relevant and accurate data relating to the effectiveness of the alarm, then any extraneous variables need to be controlled. This would imply that extraneous variables can indeed be controlled. Control can be exerted by, among others, elimination and randomization, and the study should be designed so that intervening variables have no impact on the data collection and analyses at all. Once again using the alarm clock example, this time including the intervening variables, to prevent disturbance by extraneous factors the participant may be asked to sleep alone in a soundproof room.

Experimental research

Experimental research can be defined as truly scientific if it displays certain characteristics. These characteristics are as follows (Gray 2009):

- By its very nature it is quantitative.
- The methodology is well defined.
- The methodology is reproducible.
- There is generation of a hypothesis.
- The variables are controlled and/or manipulated.
- There is accurate measurement and quantification of the data.
- The findings can be generalized to other similar populations.

These characteristics incorporate a number of important factors which together constitute and underpin a true or classic experiment (Gray 2009):

- deduction
- manipulation
- randomization
- control and control group(s) or conditions

Deduction: Experimental research can be assumed to be generally deductive,
because it tends to utilize hypotheses which the experiment sets out to confirm
or refute. Refer also to the section on deductive and inductive approaches discussed earlier in this chapter.

Manipulation: For effect in experiments, it is necessary to manipulate and therefore control the independent variables (Gray 2009). For example, in an experiment on behaviour, the environment may be systematically manipulated and
the effects of this manipulation observed. What is observed, or the effect, is the
dependent variable and the manipulation of the area of the environment is the
independent variable (Burns 2000).

Randomization: This is the process whereby participants have an equal chance of
being selected or assigned to an experimental or control group (Burns 2000). Random selection refers to how you select your sample from a population and random
assignment to how you randomly assign the sample to, for example, a control or
treatment group (Research Methods Knowledge Base 2006). We have seen under
the heading of variables that randomization is one way of controlling extraneous variables, and for it to be achieved there needs to be equality and/or equi-
librium in terms of variables in experimental groups. Randomization in its true
sense may not always be achievable in practice (Gray 2009). For instance, the
research method may specify a random selection of the first 100 patients to walk
through the outpatient department door. However, it also specifies for equality, and for it to be representative the sample should consist of 50 men and
50 women. This would mean that the first 100 patients walking through the
door, although randomly selected, may not meet the criteria (there may be say 65
women and 35 men). To be both random and equal, the first 50 women and the
first 50 men to walk through the door would have to be selected. Randomization

strengthens control over any threats there may be to internal validity and it can be said to remove bias (Gray 2009). Other forms of randomization include the use of tables of random numbers and computer-generated random numbers.

Control and control group(s) or conditions: Control can be achieved by manipulation, randomization, use of experimental controls and use of control groups. The latter is where participants are randomly assigned to either an experimental or a control group or the experiment is conducted under controlled conditions. The experimental group receives the intervention or treatment and the control group does not. The theory behind this is that all independent variables are controlled. Extraneous variables too need to be controlled.

Experimental research differs from quasi-experiments and non-experiments in that sample selection is random (Gray 2009). Another difference is that variables can be manipulated, although this also takes place in quasi-experiments (see Chapter 11).

Randomized controlled trials

In a randomized controlled trial (RCT) there is control and comparison. The researchers study perhaps two groups of individuals (experimental group and control group), who receive the intervention randomly for the purpose of measurement and comparison (see Randomization above). The control can be: usual practice (for comparison with a new or different practice yielding better results); a placebo; or no intervention at all. The RCT is a simple, effective and powerful tool in clinical research (MedicineNet.com 2004).

Characteristics of an RCT

- It is quantitative.
- It uses the hypothetico-deductive approach.
- The sample is usually large and heterogeneous.
- It is necessary to perform a power calculation initially to determine the sample size to increase the chances of statistical significance and also to prevent type 2 statistical error. (Type 2 statistical error occurs when the null hypothesis is accepted, when it should be rejected, and usually occurs as a result of the sample size being small).
- There is random assignation to control and intervention groups. Data on both groups are collected at a specified time.
- The RCT may be 'single blind' or 'double blind'. 'Single blind' means the participants are unaware of the nature of the treatment or intervention they are receiving; for example, in the case of medication they do not know whether they are receiving the real thing or a placebo. If it is a 'double-blind' study, then neither the researcher(s) nor the participants are aware of who is receiving the intervention or the treatment.

According to Greenhalgh (1997), the main advantages of the RCT are that it:

- allows for rigorous evaluation of a single variable
- can be prospective

- may eliminate bias when comparing two or more identical groups
- allows for meta-analysis

The main disadvantage is that it is expensive and time-consuming. This has knock-on effects and may lead to improper or inaccurate randomization of all eligible participants. For example, a multinational company that provides the funding may be allowed to dictate the research agenda (Greenhalgh 1997).

Statistics and the role of the statistician

Quantitative research by its nature implies that the information obtained will be quantifiable. Therefore data will be presented numerically and analysis will be aided by statistical tests, whether basic or advanced, in the hope that the findings will be unbiased and generalizable. For the positivist, the role of statistics is to falsify or reject the null hypothesis (Robson 2011).

There is a frightening array and variety of statistical tests available to the quantitative researcher. Most novice and some seasoned researchers find statistics daunting, and for some it is the reason why they shy away from quantitative research. Although you will need an understanding, you do not require in-depth knowledge of statistical methods and should not be deterred, because help is available in the form of the statistician for those who feel they are statistically challenged. As the terms imply, descriptive statistics is used to describe or summarize the sample, whereas inferential statistics is used to make inferences about the sample which can be extended to other studies (Gray 2009). Chapters 9 and 16 to 19 give more detailed and thorough descriptions and explanations of statistics.

Once a decision has been made to follow the quantitative research pathway, it is important to consult the statistician as early as possible in the research process (Pierce 2003) (see Figure 8.4 below). In my experience, the statistician can advise and make recommendations on the research design, data collection, data analysis and useful statistical packages. Some statisticians extend their services to reading and commenting on research proposals, funding applications, abstracts of oral and poster presentations, as well as the actual presentations of completed research and manuscripts for publication before they are submitted.

The quantitative researcher or investigator

Traditionalists who are staunch pursuers of quantitative research regard themselves as either positivists or post-positivists. Neither of these approaches stands alone: they were both developed and stem from various theories and theorists. Although the theorists had different views and standpoints, there were also commonalities in their theories (Gray 2009; Robson 2011). Researchers should regard positivism as another element to consider (Straub et al. 2004) as they embark on their research journey.

While the researcher may be considered to be independent of the research, the subject and/or the participant (Krauss 2005), it is important to also acknowledge that their background, knowledge, experience and values may influence their work. Quantitative researchers should positively commit to being objective and constantly aware of possible biases (Krauss 2005). In my experience this may at times prove to be extremely difficult for the researcher, especially if she or he has two roles. For example, the researcher may be a health professional undertaking a research project in part fulfilment of a degree, such as an MSc, professional doctorate or PhD, which they are doing part time while working full time at the organization where they are undertaking their research. Switching from one role to the other can also result in the researcher experiencing dilemmas and conflict. This is especially problematic and stressful in cases where in their role as researcher they may be observing a patient's safety being compromised or malpractice, whether major or minor, and they have to make a decision as to what to do next.

The researcher should therefore ensure that they have had adequate and relevant training and additionally, in the case of those who undertake research while being a student, appropriate supervision. The training should be directed at acquiring knowledge and skills that encompass paradigms, philosophies, designs, statistics, ethics, research governance, proposal and report writing, as well as funding applications. This will enable them to deal with, among others, dilemmas as in the examples stated above. It is also imperative that the researcher finds out who is able to assist them and avails themselves of the necessary support, whether at their work or their educational institute. The author of this chapter recommends that a pilot study should always be conducted (Table 8.1). If the researcher finds that the results of their study are not consistent, this should not be regarded as a failure, but could be used as an opportunity for a new line of enquiry. The original study could then be regarded as a pilot study (Gray 2009).

The quantitative research process

This process encompasses planning and conducting the research study (Figure 8.4). The manner in which the thoughts and ideas about the research are put into operation and become a reality will decide the success of the study (Gray 2009).

1 **Research idea:** Ideas for research can come from a variety of sources. In the work setting there are often problems which require solutions or questions which arise from thinking differently or 'out of the box'. These questions may be triggered by an incident in the clinical setting or perhaps by a student, a relative or even the self-questioning of clinical practices. Other sources may arise from reading the literature or from equipment, treatments, medication, surveys, questionnaires or pilot studies.

2 **Literature search:** Once the researcher has an idea that he or she thinks may be a viable one for a quantitative research study, an extensive literature search (Hohmann 2006) needs to be conducted around it. This will help to: clarify the idea and improve understanding around it; improve

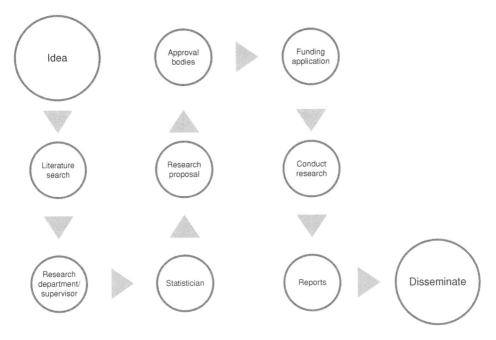

Figure 8.4 Steps in the quantitative research process.

the researcher's knowledge and skills on theories and the research process; and through learning from others it may even give the researcher further ideas to either improve or modify aspects of the entire process. A literature search will create an awareness of who the experts are in the field of the study, which can be useful if the necessity arises for external review of the study or for seeking further information and advice. It is important to stress that the literature search is not a one-off exercise: it should be ongoing throughout the whole process, as outlined in Figure 8.4.

3 **Consult with a research department/supervisor:** Now that there is better understanding of the idea and the way forward, the next stage is to consult with more experienced staff who can advise and direct the researcher on the research process journey. If the researcher is employed in an organization where there is a department able to assist, then this department should be approached to discuss the research idea, find out who else to consult and seek advice on any protocols, policies and procedures in relation to conducting research (Pierce 2003). Additionally, if the researcher is a student conducting research in part fulfilment of a degree, they should consult with their supervisor and elicit the same information as they would from the research department.

4 **Consult with a statistician:** As already stated under the heading 'Statistics and the role of the statistician', this individual can be an extremely useful partner to have on board and should be consulted at an early stage.

5 **Write a research proposal:** There is often a set way to do this or a template obtainable from the research centre of the organization (Pierce 2003). If not, there is a wide array of examples which can be downloaded from the internet. The headings may differ slightly from one template to another, but the basic information required remains the same. The proposal is a detailed document requiring all the information about the study (the why, how and where), such as:
   • its rationale and background
   • literature search
   • research question(s)
   • hypothesis
   • aim(s)
   • objectives
   • design
   • method
   • implementation
   • protocols
   • personnel involved
   • ethics
   • finances
   • sponsors
   • time frames
   • dissemination
   • contact details of the lead researcher and others significant in the research team

6 **Seek approval from relevant approval bodies:** Having sought the necessary information from either the research department (Pierce 2003) and/or the supervisor, the researcher should now be aware of where the research proposal should be submitted and what the documents required for ethical approval are. The ethics application, the format and the information required may be somewhat different from that of the research proposal. The research approval bodies generally have a wide remit to ensure that the entire process meets the requirements for research, that it conforms with governance and parliamentary acts: among others, data protection, human rights, human tissue, animal rights, and health and safety (Pierce 2007). Members of ethical approval bodies, on the other hand, also assess the above, but with greater emphasis on ethical aspects (Stanley and McLaren 2007). It may be non-obligatory or mandatory for the researcher to attend when the approval committee meets to examine a research proposal or ethics application and decide on an outcome. The researcher may be required to deliver a presentation and answer questions. In such cases it is advisable for novice researchers

to be accompanied by a more experienced researcher and for a student to be accompanied by their research supervisor.

7   **Consider funding applications:** Serious thought should be given to the resources, whether human, equipment or other, and the time frame for conducting the study, to ensure adequate funding. In my experience most funding bodies have their own application forms which should be completed by the researcher. Again these may vary in length, format and information required, but the essential information relating to the research remains common to all. If attendance is mandatory at a funding board assessment the same guidelines as for attendance at approval boards above apply.

8   **Conduct research:** Throughout the process, the researcher should remain an active agent. The lead researcher has overall responsibility for the content and delivery of the research and for any individuals involved. She or he also has a duty to ensure that protocols are followed and the research is conducted within the rules of governance (Pierce 2007) and ethics (Stanley and McLaren 2007).

9   **Write reports:** Submission of regular update reports on the progress of the research is mandatory for most approval and funding bodies. In my experience the researcher is generally informed by the relevant body when to submit the report. For most bodies submission of a report occurs annually, but this is dependent on the duration of the study. If the funding body has a template or specific report form, this should be completed and submitted. All bodies will require a final report. This should contain similar information to that of the original application, except that now the study is completed, additional inclusions will be: the results of the study; acceptance or rejection of the hypothesis; and the conclusions that have been arrived at. It should also be specified where and how the results will be disseminated.

10 **Dissemination of the research findings:** In my view, failure to disseminate results in one form or another should be regarded as unethical, especially if the research was funded from the public purse or by a charity. Dissemination can be active or passive. Active dissemination includes: informal verbal reports to colleagues and participants; more formal oral presentations to, for example, stakeholders or others or at conferences. Passive dissemination includes: written reports, such as the final reports to sponsors and funders; flyers, leaflets and poster presentations. It is imperative that participants are informed of the outcome of the study. This not only will bode well for any future research, but also serves to inform and thank the participants and is regarded as good research practice. Please note it is equally important to disseminate negative results as it is positive ones. The reasons are that others can learn from the mistakes made, negative findings may trigger new lines of enquiry, or it can serve as a pilot for a new research study.

Combining quantitative and qualitative research

Quantitative and qualitative approaches can both be used in the same research or single research study, and this practice is becoming increasingly popular as health care researchers are becoming more conversant with their philosophies, paradigms, designs and methodologies (see Chapter 10). This was not always the case: there were many advocates of quantitative research who argued that the scientific approach was crucial if a research project was to be regarded as legitimate, reliable and valid, and if the findings were to be adopted by others. They were sceptical as to the value of qualitative research. The advocates of qualitative research argued that it was a better method for eliciting and understanding behaviours and problems than through the use of statistics and numbers (Robson 2011). It has now been recognized that both are important and that they can be underpinned by and conducted from the utilization of a number of research philosophies and/or paradigms (Robson 2011).

According to Kroll and Neri (2009), there are numerous terms used for the combined approach, which can be confusing, but it is essential to focus on the aim(s) of the research and to relate everything else to that, including the most appropriate design. Some researchers may adopt their own name or term, although two terms commonly appearing in the literature are mixed-methods research and multi-method research. Quantitative and qualitative approaches each have strengths and weaknesses, depending on the type of research design conducted. A strength of adopting a mixed-methods design approach is the resultant balance between the qualitative flexibility of the research and its exploratory nature and that of the fixed elements encompassed in many quantitative approaches, such as the theoretical grounding and hypothesis testing (Kroll and Neri 2009). Weaknesses may include a poor or ill thought out rationale and a lack of expertise for the approach.

There are arguments for and against using a mixed-methods approach. For example, those in favour argue that embracing both quantitative and qualitative methods results in a body of knowledge that is:

- more holistic
- improved
- more extensive

Those against postulate that:

- neither can inform the other
- the quantitative approach deals with objective factual knowledge
- the qualitative approach deals with subjective interpretation of experience (Slevin 2010)

The weighting for each of the quantitative and qualitative elements within a single research project can and does vary from study to study. Whatever the weighting, a combination of the two methodologies does not necessarily imply that the research is of a sufficiently high standard and quality. The researcher(s) should be conversant with both quantitative and qualitative methodologies and designs if they are to implement mixed methods in their study. Each has different emphases, as well as contrasting strengths and weaknesses. It is the researcher's responsibility to make an informed choice as to what would best suit their research, as well as to be able to clearly justify the approach used.

Conclusion

The quantitative traditionalist can mainly be regarded as being a positivist or a post-positivist. Researchers should consider positivism, among other theories, as they embark on the road to conducting research. They will need at some stage during the process to engage with the theoretical aspects, which in quantitative research usually occurs beforehand – the deductive approach.

The accuracy of measurement and quantification is integral to quantitative research. Unless there is empirical evidence which can be established and replicated, it cannot be deemed to be science or scientific. Hence the aim, research question(s), or objectives of the study relating to it and the research design should be clarified very early in the research process. The sample should be representative of the population studied and the data analysed statistically. The statistician is a useful adjunct to the research team and should be consulted once the researcher has decided on journeying down the quantitative research road. Additionally, the research protocol should be sufficiently detailed and robust for the study to be replicated.

It can be assumed that the utilization of mixed methods not only involves a combination of different quantitative and qualitative approaches, but also includes differing philosophical underpinnings, theories, data collection and modes of analysis. Mixed methods can be a useful design option for the researcher.

The researcher should avail themselves of the knowledge and skills necessary for conducting quantitative research. They should know where to obtain additional information, assistance and resources. The quantitative researcher should commit to being objective and try to eliminate biases from their research. Adherence to the principles and standards of quantitative research should result in studies that are truly scientific and capable of being replicated.

Key concepts
- If the researcher wants their research to be grounded in a philosophy originating in positivism, systematic and empirical, they should consider the quantitative research method.
- Quantitative research is generally deductive or hypothetico-deductive.
- A quantitative research design includes the overall plan of data collection, utilization, measurement and analysis; therefore, the researcher should positively commit to being objective and aware of possible biases.
- Some of the common quantitative research designs for consideration are: experimental research, where the experiment is set out to confirm or refute the hypothesis; and randomized controlled trials where there is control and comparison.

- Quantitative research implies that the information obtained is quantifiable, hence the researcher should, early in the research process, think about statistical tests that will aid their analyses, and consult a statistician.
- Adherence to the quantitative research process and the manner in which the thoughts and ideas of the research are put into operation and become a reality will decide the success of the study.

Key readings on designing and conducting quantitative research

- D. Hartung and D. Touchette, Overview of clinical research design, *American Journal of Health-System Pharmacy*, 66(4) (2009), 398–408
  This article outlines the concepts and terminology of clinical research design (described as either observational or experimental research in human subjects) for the clinical researcher.
- C.M. Hicks, *Research Methods for Clinical Therapists: Applied Project Design and Analysis* (London: Churchill Livingstone Elsevier, 2009)
  This book focuses on design and analysis of experimental research and is suitable for students as well as clinicians in health care. Research concepts and statistics are explained using examples from different clinical settings.
- D.G. Tincello, The joys and pitfalls of organising a research study, *Journal of the Association of Chartered Physiotherapists in Women's Health*, 94 (2004), 19–25
  This is a practical framework covering all the relevant stages of development and design of research, from idea through to the approval stage.

Examples of quantitative studies in health care research

- S. Ameringer, R. Serlin and S. Ward, Simpson's Paradox and experimental research, *Nursing Research*, 58(2) (2009), 123–7
  This is an illustration of the importance of rigour in study design. It uses an example of an experimental study as a reminder of potential threats to internal validity that can lead to a paradox.
- A. Lash, D. Plonczynski and A. Sehdev, Trends in hypothesis testing and related variables in nursing research: A retrospective exploratory study, *Nurse Researcher*, 18(3) (2011), 38–44
  The relevance of hypothesis testing to quantitative research has been described in the above chapter. This is a comparative study of the influences and inclusion of variables on hypothesis testing. The authors conclude that there has been a decrease in the use of hypothesis testing in the last decades of the twentieth century.
- M. Murtonen, Learning of quantitative research methods: University students' views, motivation, and difficulties in learning. PhD dissertation, Finland: University of Turku (2005). Available at http://users.utu.fi/marimur/Murtonen%20dissertation%20without%20articles.pdf [Accessed 22 June 2012]

The aim of the research was to examine difficulties experienced by students studying quantitative research at the university. The results showed that factors such as quantitative method courses, research orientations and motivational factors are related to and do affect content learning and importance of research skills in students' future work.

- J.E. Squires, C.A. Estabrooks, P. Gustavsson and L. Wallin, Individual determinants of research utilization by nurses: A systematic review update, *Implementation Science*, 6 (2011), 1. Available at http://www.implementationscience.com/content/6/1/1 [Accessed 18 June 2012]

  It is important not only to conduct quantitative research, but also to utilize it. Included in this review were randomized controlled trials, clinical trials and observational study designs in order to examine characteristics influencing nurses' utilization of research.

Useful websites

- SpringerLink – allows open access and free downloads of book chapters, journal articles, protocols and e-reference entries – http://www.springerlink.com
- Royal College of Nursing (RCN) International Nursing Research Conference – annual showcase conference of the RCN's research society – http://www.rcn.org.uk
- Iowa State University e-library – scientific research resources that are free to access from anywhere in the world. No affiliations or subscriptions are required to access the full texts – http://instr.iastate.libguides.com/freescientific

References

Adcock, R. and Collier, D. (2001) Measurement validity: A shared standard for qualitative and quantitative research, *The American Political Science Review*, 95(3): 529–46.

Bryman, A. (1992) Quantitative and qualitative research: Further reflections on their integration, in J. Brannen (ed.) *Mixing Methods: Qualitative and Quantitative Research*. Farnham: Ashgate Publishing, pp. 57–81.

Burns, R.B. (2000) *Introduction to Research*. London: Sage.

Cota, C. (2006) #3743: Cause and Effect SDAIE Lesson. Available at http://teachers.net/lessons/posts/3743.html [Accessed 5 March 2012].

Gray, D.E. (2009) *Doing Research in the Real World*, 2nd edn. London: Sage.

Greenhalgh, T. (1997) How to read a paper: Getting your bearings (deciding what the paper is about), *British Medical Journal*, 315(7102): 243–6.

Hammersley, M. (1992) Deconstructing the qualitative–quantitative divide, in J. Brannen (ed.) *Mixing Methods: Qualitative and Quantitative Research*. England: Ashgate Publishing, pp. 39–56.

Hohmann, U. (2006) Quantitative methods in education research. Available at http://www.edu.plymouth.ac.uk/resined/Quantitative/quanthme.htm [Accessed 12 June 2012].

Hoefer, C. (2010) Causal Determinism, in E.N. Zalta (ed.) *The Stanford Encyclopedia of Philosophy (Spring 2010 edn)*. Stanford, CA: Metaphysics Research Lab, Stanford University. Available at http://plato.stanford.edu/archives/spr2010/entries/determinism-causal/ [Accessed 5 March 2012].

Krauss, S.E. (2005) Research paradigms and meaning making: a primer, *The Qualitative Report*, 10(4): 758–70. Available at http://www.nova.edu/ssss/QR/QR10-4/krauss.pdf [Accessed 31 January 2012].

Kroll, T. and Neri, M. (2009) Designs for mixed methods research, in S. Andrew and E. Halcombe (eds) *Mixed Methods Research for Nursing and the Health Sciences*. Oxford: Wiley-Blackwell, pp. 31–49.

MedicineNet.com (2004) Definition of randomized control trial. Available at http://www.med terms.com/script/main/art.asp?articlekey=39532 [Accessed 13 April 2012].

Pierce, E. (2003) Research notes: How research and development offices and centers can assist you, *Nursing Standard*, 17(33): 21.

Pierce, E. (2007) Ethics: Research governance for health and social care, in A. Leathard and S. McLaren (eds) *Ethics: Contemporary Challenges in Health and Social Care*. Bristol: The Policy Press, pp. 53–68.

Pierce, E. and McLaren, S. (2012) Development of an assessment tool for the Multidisciplinary Evaluation of Severe Neurodependency (MEND): Preliminary findings, *Scandinavian Journal of Caring Sciences*, doi: 10.1111/scs.12018.

Qureshi, H. (1992) Integrating methods in applied research in social policy: A case study, in J. Brannen (ed.) *Mixing Methods: Qualitative and Quantitative Research*. England: Ashgate Publishing, pp. 101–26.

Research Methods Knowledge Base (2006) Random Selection and Assignment. Available at http://www.socialresearchmethods.net/kb/random.htm [Accessed 24 May 2012].

Robson, C. (2011) *Real World Research*. Chichester: John Wiley and Sons.

Ruane, J.M. (2005) *Essentials of Research Methods: A Guide to Social Science Research*. Oxford: Blackwell Publishing.

Slevin, O. (2010) Approaches to healthcare research, in P. Roberts and H. Priest (eds) *Healthcare Research: A Textbook for Students and Practitioners*. Chichester: Wiley-Blackwell, pp. 11–38.

Stanley, R. and McLaren, S. (2007) Ethical issues in health and social care research, in A. Leathard and S. McLaren (eds) *Ethics: Contemporary Challenges in Health and Social Care*. Bristol: The Policy Press, pp. 35–52.

Straub, D., Gefen, D. and Boudreau, M.-C. (2004) The ISWorld Quantitative, Positivist Research Methods Website, ed. D. Galletta. Available at http://dstraub.cis.gsu.edu:88/quant/ [Accessed 5 March 2012].

Trochim, W. (2006) Research Methods Knowledge Base: Measurement Validity Types. Available at http://www.socialresearchmethods.net/kb/measval.php [Accessed 29 March 2012].

9 Sampling issues in health care research

Gloria Crispino

Chapter topics

- From research hypotheses to sampling
- Population and samples
- Sample designs
- Sampling strategies
- Sample size calculation

Introduction

A typical conversation between a health researcher (HR) and a statistician (ST) regarding sample size calculation may go like this:

HR: 'Hi, I am submitting a grant proposal, the deadline is tomorrow. I have completed the application, I just need to know how many patients I need for the study. It shouldn't take more than a few minutes of your time.'

ST: *silence* . . .

HR: *with some hesitation* – 'I want to do a study on patients with Alzheimer's, male, over 55. There are 3,000 cases in this county. I thought a sample size of 30–50 patients would be OK.'

ST: *more silence* . . .

Eventually, ST answers . . . with a question: 'What are you trying to measure exactly?'

HR replies with information on how to prove that treatment X works better than treatment Y.

ST: 'What do you mean by "better"?'

And a long conversation (much longer than 'a few minutes') starts with the statistician 'peeling off' the many layers of the study proposal in search of the original, *primary question* to which a *primary* outcome measure is attached and on which the entire study rests. This 'peeling off' process, or for a more technical word, *'inductive'* process, is the thread that guides the structure of this chapter, with typical questions and useful answers, hints on how to make the statistician's life easier and, more importantly, how not to waste the patients' time. It is also important to understand that it is unethical for a statistician to support a study that has no clear methods for sampling and sample size calculations. The aim of this chapter is to help the researcher to develop clear, simple and effective sampling strategies and to address the most common issues that arise during the sampling process.

The first section of the chapter introduces a three-step process to flow from the research question to the study design to the statistical analysis plan, and in doing so shows how to gather the correct information to compute a sample size. The second section of the chapter offers some points for discussion on the meaning and reasoning behind sampling, inferential statistics and the issue of small versus large sample sizes. The third section introduces the most common issues for sampling strategies and how these issues are addressed. The fourth section describes in statistical terms the most common methods for sample size calculation, and the fifth draws together some final conclusions.

A note: throughout the chapter the terms 'participant', 'patient' and/or 'individual' are used interchangeably to describe the human cases of the study.

Research hypotheses and sampling: the link

Sample size calculations and sampling strategies are strictly linked to the research hypothesis and the study design (see Chapter 4 for a further discussion of these topics). Such a statement might sound obvious to most researchers, but finding this link is often not obvious and it requires extensive knowledge of the study protocol, the patient population and what data are to be collected.

Before a study is carried out, three main steps are taken in order to *set up the study*. They describe the *'flow'* from the research idea to the study design, and the statistical analysis that leads to the delivery of the study results. In these three steps, the statistical issues behind sample size and sampling are raised and resolved (Figure 9.1).

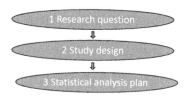

Figure 9.1 Flow chart of the three main steps of a research study.

In very generic terms, the steps are:

1 Research question: a research question is stated in relation to an issue that needs to be investigated. The answer to the research question will provide evidence on that issue.
2 Study design: a study is designed to answer the research question. The design of the study defines the research hypothesis, what data will be collected, what variables will be measured and how many subjects will be required.
3 Statistical analysis plan: a plan is drafted to introduce the statistical methods that will be used to describe and process the data.

Details of steps 1 to 3 are collated in the **study protocol**. Once they are finalized and regulatory and ethical requirements have been satisfied, the study is carried out according to such a protocol, the data are analysed and conclusions are drawn about the original research question.

Performing steps 1 to 3 can take anything from a couple of months to one year or, in some cases, longer. Often the final version of the protocol is released many months after the first draft was circulated, with many revisions in between. This lengthy process is due to the fact that it takes time to design the appropriate study, to understand the technicalities behind collecting specific measurements and to appreciate the profile of the patient population.

Sample size calculations, sampling strategies and statistical planning are an integral part of this three-step process. It is highly recommended to involve a statistician in the process as early as possible – the earlier, the better.

The main issues when attempting a sample size calculation are what type of information is required, where to find it and how to use it. Identifying the key components for a correct calculation often requires a multidisciplinary approach in which the researcher extracts information from multiple sources: for example clinical data, current practices and pilot studies.

Below are two examples on how to flow from the research question to the statistical plan and in doing so how to gather the correct information to compute a sample size.

Example 1 The key performance indicator study (Wakai et al. 2011)

In the health sector, key performance indicators (KPIs) are used to measure the quality of care. They are used broadly for many health services, but they are reliable only if the information gathered to build the KPIs is available, accurate and consistent.

This study wishes to address the feasibility of collecting 'good' data for a set of KPIs that measures the quality of emergency departments in Ireland. The three-step process described in Figure 9.1 has been implemented as follows.

1 *Research question: the primary question of the study is 'Can we measure KPIs with accuracy, reliability and consistency?'*

Such a primary question is very valid, but also very broad. There is a wide variety of KPIs that could be used in emergency departments, some related to the process management, others to the structure or the outcomes of the service. Therefore, the original question needs to be narrowed down by a series of related questions: 'Which KPIs do we wish to measure?' is a good one. 'What do you mean by accuracy?' is another very good question to ask at this stage of the process, or 'Do you think it is more important to measure accuracy or consistency or reliability?' The answers to these questions initiate the process of developing the study design, and start to **quantify the study**.

It would be very common at this stage for the process to go 'off at a tangent' and 'to drown' in the vast amount of approaches that could be taken. All aspects become important, including the scientific aspect of the study, the clinical implications of the results and the link to current working practices. These are all 'high-level' points of discussion that should be addressed during this phase. The aim is to 'nail' one approach, to stay focused on the primary research question and to move on to the study design.

2 Study design

After the initial attempt to define a primary research question, an in-depth analysis of the KPIs suitable for emergency departments is undertaken. At this stage of the process a large amount of information is submitted for consideration. Details are gathered about everything: the medical condition, staffing levels, working practices and so on. The databases currently available are considered, and practical issues such as resources, time and logistics are discussed, together with issues on subgroups of the patient population and treatment effects.

A first draft of the study design would include **a selection of endpoints** (that is, the occurrence of a specific event), chosen to describe the KPIs, the emergency department and the patients. In general, it is good practice to limit the number of primary endpoints to a minimum, but it is often the case that researchers get very 'attached' to their choices and it requires a broad and multidisciplinary approach to identify the primary ones and to 'declass' others as secondary endpoints.

For this study, the primary analysis focuses on process KPIs, which include endpoints such as 'time to analgesia', 'time to antibiotics in sepsis', 'time from ED arrival to first electrocardiogram in suspected cardiac chest pain'. The primary endpoints are chosen from among these constructs.

The study design should also include initial estimates of the sample size and sampling strategies, but not enough information is available at this point. A sample size calculation can be performed when a **primary variable** has been identified. The study design needs to be unfolded further; the role of the endpoints and how the data will be collected must be clarified, so that the link can be made between the research question, the primary endpoints and the primary variable.

The critical leap is made when the question 'Where do we find the information about process KPIs?' is answered. The answer is: KPIs are built from data collected in the **patient records**. Thus, the study design starts to take shape around the **data required** to build process KPIs and the source of such data – patient records. The original research question ('Can we measure KPIs with accuracy, reliability and consistency?') is transformed into a question about patient records, and the quality of the KPI is really about the accuracy, reliability and consistency of the data collected in such records. This leap is the most important step for this study process: the design of the study now focuses on **datasets** and **variables** which describe a set of KPIs and can be found in the patient records.

3 Statistical analysis plan

Once the study has been quantified, the statistical methodology can be described. This is the last step to take and it leads to the computation of the sample size.

The choice of the statistical methodology depends on the choice of the primary variable, which depends on the research question. In this study, there are two distinct questions:

Q1 – Can we measure KPIs?
Q2 – Can we measure KPIs with accuracy, reliability and consistency?

With regard to Q1, 'Can we measure KPIs?' should be interpreted as: 'Are data available to measure KPIs?' A note of caution: it is not a good idea at this stage of the process to pose 'closed questions' – questions that only require a 'yes' or 'no' answer. Imagine the conversation:

HR1: Are data available to measure process KPIs?
HR2: Yes!
End of the study!

It is useful to expand the question in a more quantifiable way. A good angle from which to look at the 'can we measure' question is by addressing it as: 'How many data items in the patient records are there to build a KPI?' The study now is about **counting** the data items in the patient records, and the *primary variable* of the study is the *number of data items* available in the patient records for a set of KPIs.

The statistical method used to count the data items – that is, to measure availability – can now be chosen. For this study the following method was selected: 'A binary (dichotomous) scoring method will be used in this project to assess the availability and completeness of dataset items in the ED records. The scoring method will involve recording a score of 1 if a dataset item is present in an individual patient ED record and a score of 0 if a dataset item is absent. The availability in the ED records of the dataset items relevant to each of the timeliness KPIs will be assessed based on the following calculation: mean and median score of the number of relevant dataset items available per KPI per participating emergency department. Furthermore, a composite score of 8 dataset items to assess medical record completeness will be used and the overall mean of the dataset items will be measured.'

This statement quantifies in full Q1 – Can we measure KPIs? – and provides details on how to collect the data. It might not be obvious yet, but from a statistical point of view, the computation of a sample size for this study is very close. Once Q2 is unfolded, the job is done.

With regard to Q2, it can be argued that all three aspects – accuracy, reliability and consistency – may define quality, and that they are all important. This is a very reasonable argument, but the dilemma – the statistical dilemma – is which one should be chosen to measure the availability of the relevant data items? Each one would have a different statistical method and it would require a different sample size.

For this particular study, accuracy became the most important way to measure availability. Obviously, many points can be brought forward to argue both for and against this choice; all arguments would be valid but irrelevant once the choice has been made. So, let's move on and define accuracy.

The rationale for defining accuracy is stated clearly in the protocol as follows: 'The desired accuracy of the availability, measured as a mean number of items, is a confidence interval of ±0.25.'

The sentence above is neat, but it took quite a deal of inductive thinking process to finalize it. The milestones of this thinking process are:

1   The researcher wishes to provide a score for the availability of a set of data items relevant to a set of chosen KPIs: an average availability score.

2   It is reasonable to anticipate that the average availability score would vary depend-
      ing on the department, time of year, and choice of data items.
3   The question to be answered is: 'What level of accuracy do you wish to provide for
      the average score?'
4   The answer is: a confidence interval of ±0.25.

This is it! The study is about counting the number of data items in the patient records
and computing an average availability score that has an accuracy of ±0.25. The study
design for the primary variable is complete and a **sample size calculation** can be
computed.

   The sample size required to estimate the mean to within ±0.25 uses Formula 7 (see
Example 5 below). The sample size is 96. Therefore, it is required to collect 96 unique
patient records in order to show an average availability score with an accuracy of
±0.25.

Example 2   The ICS study (Crispino-O'Connell 2010)

Studies have shown that physical activity after diagnosis and treatment of breast cancer
reduces the risk of recurrence and improves survival. The Irish Cancer Society launched
a pilot physical activity programme; the aim of this programme was to introduce breast
cancer survivors to a structured physical activity programme and to evaluate how effectively such a programme could be implemented on a national scale.

   An evaluation study has been carried out to measure the success of the programme
(Crispino-O'Connell 2010). The protocol of the evaluation study was developed following the three-step process in Figure 9.1.

**1 *Research question: while there is already scientific knowledge of the benefits of
physical exercise, the main question for this pilot programme is 'Does it work?'***

The research question is valid, but it is too broad. More precisely, what do we mean
by 'does it work'? A vast selection of derived questions can unfold, such as: 1) Does it
reduce the risk of recurrence? 2) Does it improve the fitness level of the participants?
3) Is it realistic to expect cancer survivors to engage in a 15-week fitness programme?
4) Are they happier/healthier individuals at the end of the programme? Each one of these
questions requires a unique study design with its own unique variables and sample size.

   For this study, it was decided to narrow down the investigation to three aspects:
recruitment, retention and outcome. The outcome was physical fitness at the end of
the programme. Therefore, it was decided that the **primary outcome** of the training
would be to enhance the physical fitness of the participants.

2 *Study design*

The study is now quantifiable and it is about **measuring the fitness level** of the participants. The research question can now be defined as follows: 'What is the change in
fitness level before, during and after the programme?'

An incredibly vast amount of information is available at this stage of the process, with, for example, fitness, training programmes and survival curves. The study design needs to take into consideration all the aspects of the study, so a lengthy process of including and disregarding information is initiated until final decisions are made on what data will be collected to measure the primary outcome – fitness level – and the associated secondary outcomes.

3 Statistical analysis plan

The last decision to take is to define 'fitness' – that is, what are the data that can validly measure the construct 'fitness'? Once that is defined, a statistical method can be chosen to analyse such data and a sample size calculation can be computed. For this type of study, the key to a successful training programme is adaptation to a given stress load. The stress load is defined by the time, volume and intensity of the workout, that increases over time. The overall fitness level of each participant is assessed by four indicators: 1) fitness test – a one-mile walking time trial; 2) improvement in oxygen consumption (VO_2); 3) metabolic equivalent of tasks (METs) hours per week; and 4) body fat analysis. The four indicators are measured at baseline, and then at weeks 5, 10 and 15. The programme is designed to allow the participants to achieve a minimum of nine METs/hr/wk on completion of the programme, which is the minimum weekly requirement shown for lowering the risk of a reoccurrence of breast cancer. Figure 9.2 shows the data-acquisition process.

Baselines and follow–up results

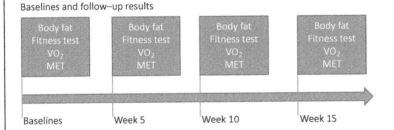

Figure 9.2   Flow chart of baseline and follow-up results.

The statistical dilemma is now: 'Which indicator is the primary outcome measure?' It was agreed that METs would be the **primary outcome measure**. In fact, a lengthy discussion took place within the team to make this the final choice. To help the decision process a metaphor was used: 'If there was a fire in your lab and you could save only one indicator, which one would you choose?' It might sound drastic, but it is interesting to know that it took the principal investigator less than a second to make up their mind.

Following this process there is now a primary variable – METs – on which to compute a sample size. In particular, what sample size is required to estimate to within 10 per cent the proportion of participants who would reach nine METs at the end of the programme?

The level of precision, in this case 10 per cent, is a clinical choice not a statistical one, and it depends on the medical condition, the intervention and the practicalities of the study. Using Formula 7 (see Example 5 below), a sample size of 62 women would be required to estimate this value. For this particular study, the sample size was fixed to 50–60 participants due to logistical limitations; however the sample size calculation shows that there were enough participants to get a meaningful answer with regard to fitness level at the end of the programme.

The leap from sample to population: why sample?

Before we proceed, we need to ask: why do we sample in the first place? How can a small sample tell us something valuable about an entire population of individuals? Should we not just ask everybody in the population?

Let's think about it: even if we ask everybody today, the population will probably change tomorrow anyway; someone will die, someone will get better. So, why is the answer from a particular study applicable to a whole population over time?

In the language of research we would ask the following question: what inference do we hope to make from the study – what conclusions can we draw from our study that may be valid for a larger population?

It is often said that it is impossible to make a decision in the field of science and that statistics gives 'an educated guess'. The statistical reasoning behind inference has a vast literature, going back to the definition of probability (Fisher 1956, Moore 1985 and van Belle et al. 2004 are some examples).

Let's use an example: a study is run to compare the effect of one type of painkiller (X) with another (Y), in terms of side effects during the first three days in intensive care with patients following cardiac surgery. Every year approximately 1,000 patients present to the local hospital with such a condition. It may be possible to enrol all of the patients in the study – to make it more robust. The point is there is no need to. A sample from that population, which is representative in terms of key characteristics such as age, gender, medical history and so on, is expected to provide robust evidence of the effects of X and Y. In other words, it is expected that the patients that are not enrolled in the study or the patients presenting to the hospital after the study has been completed would have an equivalent profile to that of the patients that participated in the study. Therefore, the conclusions drawn by the study are 'transferable' to the overall population of patients carrying this condition.

At this stage, the health researcher (HR) may have some doubts and would start a conversation with the statistician (ST), that goes more or less like this:

HR: 'Are you sure?'
ST: 'Sure enough.'
HR: 'What do you mean?'
ST: 'If the study design is correct and if the protocol has been implemented appropriately with a limited number of deviations, we can state that there is evidence (or

strong evidence or very strong evidence, depending on the results) that, on average, patients treated with X suffer fewer side effects than patients treated with Y. Then, if possible, the conclusions derived from the study can be used to create simulation models and to predict what side effects an individual patient with certain characteristics would suffer. There is always a chance that we might be wrong, but that chance as measured within the study is small, let's say less than 5 per cent.

The chance of being wrong is defined as type 1 error and it is described in more detail in the section 'Comparing means (two groups)' below. (Further details on hypothesis testing are provided in Chapter 4.)

The inferential process described above does not make a decision about X and Y; it provides evidence (robust, if the study is carried out appropriately) that can be used to make a decision. Whether the sample size is small or large, the key issue is the framework of the overall study, its strength in terms of the quality of the data, the clarity of the design and the execution of the protocol. In many cases, studies fail to provide robust evidence not because of their sample size calculation, but because of the challenges in completing the study according to the protocol. This is not an educated guess, it is hard work.

There are also situations where sample size is limited due to the inherent characteristics of the condition under investigation. Rare types of cancer and biomarker studies are typical examples. For these cases, studies with low power, $\beta = 0.5$ or 0.6, and low significance levels, $\alpha = 0.1$, have been run.

Of course, there is a counterargument. More precisely, there are many cases in which 'size matters'. When designing a study, there are inherent statistical uncertainties that are difficult to remove. Chance always plays a role, even though it can be minimized by an effective study design. Bias may occur if proper randomization and sampling strategies are not introduced. Chance and bias mislead the conclusions of any study. A large sample size, in terms of thousands of patients, is capable of limiting the impact of those factors.

Below are two examples: mega-trials, and large observational studies.

Example 1   Mega-trials

Clinical trials often only show a moderate effect of treatment. If the sample size is not large enough, this effect may not be detected at all or it may appear as trivial, although moderate or even small effects over a large population of patients and over a long period of time may bring life-changing improvements capable of reducing morbidity and improving mortality. In order to capture such changes, very large trials – mega-trials – enrolling tens of thousands of participants, are run. Interesting examples can be found in breast cancer research (see, for example, the Early Breast Cancer Trialists' Collaborative Group 1988) or cardiovascular diseases (see, for example, the International Studies of Infarct Survival 1986, 1988, 1992, 1995).

Example 2 Large observational studies

Observational studies are carried out to identify factors that cause disease and death. Risk factors have been established for some of the most common diseases and are widely accepted in the scientific community, such as smoking for lung cancer or hypertension and cholesterol levels for cardiovascular diseases. Although the effect of those factors may vary from one population to another and over time, their relevance may change in different socio-economic contexts or when comparing subjects from developed and developing countries. They may also impact subgroups of the population differently and become age-, gender- or ethnic origin-specific.

Therefore there is a real need for large observational studies, with hundreds of thousands of participants, in which to study extensively the causes of mortality and how those causes change when the settings change.

Sampling strategies: how to sample from a population and deal with issues of recruitment, retention and follow-up

The three-step process described in Figure 9.1 is used to set up the study. After that, the success of the study relies on the ability to resolve all the practical issues of recruiting, following up and retaining the participants. The sample size calculation gives an estimate of the number of participants needed to compute with enough confidence an estimate or to detect a difference in treatment effect, i.e. 95 per cent confidence when $\alpha = 0.05$. Sampling strategies depend on the population of interest, the pattern of the condition studied and the context in which treatments and services are provided. An in-depth knowledge of these key concepts is required in order to develop effective strategies.

The recruitment process can be lengthy. It takes time to recruit participants into a study, whether it is a short pilot study or a large clinical trial, whether it administers a brief questionnaire or a complex medical procedure. Often the resources needed to 'stay on schedule' are underestimated, in terms of personnel, logistics, sites and the profile of the population. Some of the most common issues are outlined in Box 9.1.

Box 9.1 Issues in the recruitment and retention of participants in a research study

- The rate at which individuals use a facility is not constant. For example, if a study were recruiting children with asthma from a paediatric hospital, seasonal effects would affect the frequency and the number of cases per month.
- The individual's response to entering a study or not is unpredictable and, even when an individual agrees to participate, it may take time and 'a change of heart' when it comes to understanding and signing the consent form.
- There are hard-to-reach populations that would make the recruitment process challenging. When conducting a study in a middle-class, well-educated subgroup

of the population residing in settled homes, recruitment should be achievable. In contrast, a study of heroin drug users, such as the ROSIE study (Comiskey et al. 2003), where many of the participants are homeless and others are trafficking drugs and sex, poses great challenges and raises obstacles that are inherent in the socio-economic context and beyond the technicalities of the study.

- There are regulatory requirements, particularly in the clinical research area, where regulatory bodies expect that a proportion of the participants will be recruited in the country where the drug, service or device will be used. The logistics of recruiting in some of these countries may be challenging.

Once recruitment to the study is in process, retention becomes the next priority. Individuals drop out of a study for many reasons: they die, they move to another part of the country, their medical condition changes – for better or worse – or they do not see the need to be part of the study any more. These are usually considered external forces that cannot be managed, but there are other reasons why an individual would withdraw from a study, and the impact of such decisions can be reduced by an appropriate study design (see Box 9.2).

Box 9.2   Strategies that can help the retention of participants in a research study

- The medical procedure used may be invasive, painful and lengthy; therefore a patient may decide not to return for a follow-up visit. Consideration should be given during the study design phase to alternative procedures that could provide the same level of information and be less invasive.
- The questionnaire administered may be too long and complex. For example, the primary set of questions may be hidden somewhere after question 53 and it is approached only after 30 minutes of investigation – not a good strategy. For the ROSIE study (Comiskey et al. 2003), the questionnaire, in many cases, was administered to heroin drug users in a methadone clinic while they were waiting for their medication. It was clearly not an ideal situation, therefore the field researchers were trained to gather the primary information first and then attempt to collect further details if possible. Careful considerations must be given to the design of a questionnaire, especially for hard-to-reach populations (see Chapters 14 and 15 for further discussion on questionnaire design).

If extra resources are not added to compensate for the cases lost to follow-up, the consequences are an incomplete dataset and a smaller sample. An incomplete dataset may be biased because those who withdraw are often the ones the study requires the most – they are often sicker and more vulnerable; they are the ones for whom the effect of treatment or service may be most beneficial. A smaller sample may not be robust enough: that is, there may not be enough measurements to detect a difference in treatment, or the p-value may not show the pre-specified significance. These obstacles may be overcome, at least partially, by inflating the sample size calculation, with 10–20 per cent more cases and with an in-depth knowledge of the context from which the participants are recruited.

Randomization and other sampling strategies

Finally, a note on randomization and other sampling strategies. A fully randomized study is indisputably a robust framework for high-quality results. This is because most of the statistical analyses that would be carried out for the study assume that the data are random. Randomization reduces bias and therefore strengthens the results, but not all studies can or should be designed as fully randomized, double-blind clinical trials. A tight, double-blind trial creates a constrained environment that may have very little applicability to the intended population. There is a trade-off between the rigour of the study design and the logistic and representativeness of the context in which the study is carried out. This trade-off must be evaluated as early as possible in the study and justifications for the sampling strategies must be included in the protocol.

Alternative sampling strategies, such as stratified sampling or quota sampling, are commonly used. Stratified sampling implies stratifying the population into relevant subgroups and then drawing a random sample from each group. When stratifying a population, the researcher attempts to increase the representativeness of the population. For example, if a drug has a different effect on over-55 males and females, it is advisable to create blocks – that is strata – of different age groups and gender that are randomized within each block. Quota sampling is a type of non-random sample design. This approach is usually designed on a 'first-come-first-served' basis. As long as the sample size is reached, it is somewhat irrelevant how the data have been collected. Quota sampling has limitations in terms of representativeness as the participants may not be representative of the population under investigation.

Methods for sample size calculations

As shown above, once a research question is quantified and the appropriate study has been designed, with primary and secondary outcome measures, sample size calculations become a straightforward exercise.

The choice of the primary outcome measure dictates the sample size calculation and therefore the sample size. It is often the case that a series of sample size calculations is performed to make the researcher aware of the differences in terms of number of patients, the size of the treatment effect detected and the certainty of the results. Considering the complexity of most health studies in terms of clinical, medical and statistical outputs, it would be wise to streamline the design as much as possible and 'translate' a research question into an easily quantifiable outcome. Most regulatory bodies, and myself as the author of this chapter, would advise using one of the following approaches: 1) **comparing** means or proportions, or 2) **estimating** means or proportions. These are the two most commonly used approaches for study design – and for good reasons. They focus on one, unique primary outcome, either **measured** on a continuous scale – a mean, such as the average height, weight, MET etc. – or **counted** from a population set – a proportion, such as the percentage of patients who survive, the percentage of women who show a side effect, and so on.

In the following section, these two approaches are explained in statistical terms.

Other methods, such as comparing correlation coefficients and estimating variances, are also commonly used, but are beyond the scope of this chapter. Literature on these methods can be found in Cohen 1988, van Belle et al. 2004, Munro 2004 and Julious 2009.

Comparing means or proportions

When a study is based on the comparison of means or proportion, the research question is usually stated in one of the following formats:

- Is the average value of X in group 1 different from the average value of X in group 2?
- Is the proportion of individuals who show improvement after treatment in group 1 different from that in group 2?
- Has the average value of X changed after treatment in the patient population?

The concept is that the study aims to investigate the **difference between groups** (two or more groups) or **change over time** (one group) in terms of the effect of 'treatment', where treatment may mean a health care intervention, a service provided or any other aspect of care. Such effect is represented by a primary variable expressed as an average or a proportion.

In statistical terms, the research question is translated into a null (H_0) and an alternative (H_1) hypothesis (see Chapter 4 for a further discussion on hypothesis testing). Hypothesis testing is a broad subject of inferential statistics, with many detailed examples available in the literature. Here, we wish to use the concept of null and alternative hypotheses to explain sample size calculations. The choice of a null hypothesis determines what statistical test is to be carried out – for example, a t-test, two-way ANOVA, repeated measures ANOVA. Depending on the type of statistical test, a specific formula for sample size is derived.

Comparing means (two groups)

A standard format for H_0 and H_1 when comparing the means of two groups is as follows:

$$\begin{cases} H_0 : \mu_1 - \mu_2 = 0 \\ H_1 : \mu_1 - \mu_2 \neq 0 \end{cases} \qquad \text{(Formula 1)}$$

where μ_1 = average value for group 1 and μ_2 = average value for group 2.

Formula 1 can be considered the statistical interpretation of the following research question: 'Is the average value of X in group 1 different from the average value of X in group 2?

The null hypothesis states that 'group 1 is equivalent to group 2'. The alternative hypothesis states that they are different. If the study is trying to show that the treatment effect for group 1 is different from that for group 2, then it is expected that the data would consist of 'unlikely' measurements if H_0 is true. Therefore we would reject the null hypothesis in favour of the alternative one.

Formula 1 implies a two-tailed study, in which the direction of the difference of the treatment effect is not specified. A one-tailed system would have an alternative hypothesis:

$$H_1 : \mu_1 - \mu_2 < 0 \ \text{ or } \ H_1 : \mu_1 - \mu_2 > 0$$

To compute a sample size for Formula 1, the following information is required:

- size of the effect of treatment to be detected – a clinical question, not a statistical one
- variability of the data – estimates for variance or standard deviation
- level of certainty required to detect the treatment effect, also defined as the power $1 - \beta$
- the chance you are willing to accept 'being wrong', also defined as the significance level α

Let us look at each of these points in more detail.

Size of the effect of treatment: $\mu_1 = \mu_2$. Estimating the magnitude of the effect to be detected is mainly a clinical issue, not a statistical one. Researchers are usually unaware of the impact that different effect sizes have on the sample size calculation. It is often the case that many calculations are attempted in order to appreciate the magnitude of this impact and its direction. A very small difference in treatment effects requires a large sample size, while a large effect can be detected with a small sample. The challenge is to identify a meaningful difference that is relevant from a clinical point of view. Cohen (1988) has written extensively about the subject and a review of his approach is recommended.

Variability of the data: σ^2, the variance. The more variability in the data, the more difficult it will be to detect any difference in the effect of treatment. Larger variability requires larger sample sizes. An estimate of the variance is usually derived from previous pilot studies or previously published data.

The significance level: α, the probability of a type 1 error. This is the chance you are willing to take for 'being wrong', when the conclusions of the study are that there is a significant difference between groups. Significance level may be interpreted as follows: for $\alpha = 0.05$, there is 95 per cent confidence that the results of the study are true, for $\alpha = 0.01$, there is 99 per cent confidence that the results of the study are true, and so on. The probability of type 1 error implies that there is always a level of error when inferring conclusions from data. The researcher, with the help of the statistician, must quantify the significance of this level. In most cases, the choice of α is derived from previous studies, standard practices or regulatory requirements, but it is important to understand why a choice must be made in the first place. Let's use an example. A quality audit was carried out in a small pharmaceutical company when oversize tablets were discovered in a batch. The tablets were used to treat depression and the oversize tablets appeared to contain twice the amount of active ingredient required. The side effects, if those tablets were swallowed, included cardiac arrest and death. The company did not have specific guidelines on how to handle the sampling strategy or how to compute the sample size in order to audit the suspect batches, but they were adamant that they 'could not be wrong' in their conclusions due to the potential consequences of 'making such a mistake'. Eventually, a list of α levels and related sample sizes was produced, ranging from $\alpha = 0.05$ to $\alpha = 0.001$, but the level of uncertainty was considered too high in all cases and it was decided that all tablets from all suspect batches (100 per cent inspection) had to be audited. Guidelines are provided by the main regulatory bodies to address the level of significance and choices are made based on many considerations, including patient safety, established practices and practicalities.

Level of certainty: $1 - \beta$, the power of the study. β is the probability of a type 2 error, that is the probability of accepting that there is no difference between groups – accepting H_0 – when it is not true. The value of β is usually set between 0.1 and 0.2, giving a power of 90 per cent or 80 per cent. Higher values may be required. The higher the power required, the larger the size of the sample. In some circumstances lower powers, as low as 0.5 or 0.6, have been accepted when the number of participants in a study is limited by external factors such as rare diseases.

Once the information is gathered, a computer package can be used to compute the sample size. An example is outlined below with a standard formula for the comparison of two means. The formula is derived from the two-sample t-test, the statistical test used to accept or reject the null hypothesis when comparing two means. It assumes that the data are normally distributed, or approximately normally distributed, or that they can be transformed into normally distributed data. It also assumes that the data are independent – statistically independent – and that the variance in each group is equivalent. Each of these assumptions must be satisfied with a certain degree of accuracy, otherwise the t-test and the sample size calculation are meaningless.

Example 3

A study similar to the one discussed in Example 2 has been designed to investigate the effect of resistance training on the level of fitness. In this case, two independent groups are enrolled. Group 1 receives only cardiovascular training, group 2 receives cardiovascular and resistance training. As it is not known in which direction the fitness level – measured using metabolic equivalent of tasks (METs) – would go due to the different training programme, the study is designed as a two-group comparison and is two-tailed.

Information required:

- size of treatment effect: a clinically relevant difference between the two groups is estimated to be 4 METs, thus $\mu_1 - \mu_2 = 4$

- variability of the data: σ^2. From previous studies published in the literature, $\sigma = 6$
- significance level: $\alpha = 0.05$
- level of certainty: $1 - \beta = 0.0$

The sample size formula for comparing means of two groups is:

$$n = \frac{2\left(z_{1-\frac{\alpha}{2}} + z_{1-\beta}\right)^2}{\Delta^2} \qquad \text{(Formula 2)}$$

where n is the number of participants required in each group, $z_{1-\frac{\alpha}{2}}$, and $z_{1-\beta}$ are derived from the normal distribution tables, and $\Delta = \frac{|\mu_1 - \mu_2|}{\sigma}$. Substituting the values in Formula 2 as follows:

$$\Delta = \frac{4}{6} = 0.67$$

and

$$n = \frac{2\left(z_{1-0.025} + z_{1-0.2}\right)^2}{0.67^2} = \frac{2(1.96 + 0.842)^2}{0.45} = 35$$

We obtain $n = 35$. Therefore, 35 women are required in each group, in order to detect a significant difference of 4 METs between the group that undertakes cardiovascular and resistance training and the group that undertakes cardiovascular training only.

A one-tailed study would use Formula 2, but with $z_{1-\alpha}$.

Comparing means for one group

A derived application from Formula 1 is the case when one group, instead of two, is investigated in a paired or related experiment. The research question in this case would be 'Is the average value of X different from a hypothesized value?' or 'Has the average value of X changed after treatment?' These are defined as 'paired comparison' studies, in which one group is compared to itself, or each individual serves as his or her own control. Paired studies have higher statistical power due to the fact that the standard deviation is expected to be smaller when a change occurs within one group of individuals. Formula 1 would be adapted as follows:

Comparing means (one group):

$$\begin{cases} H_0 : \mu - \mu_0 = 0 \\ H_1 : \mu - \mu_0 \neq 0 \end{cases} \qquad \text{(Formula 3)}$$

The formula for sample size calculation becomes:

$$n = \frac{\left(z_{1-\frac{\alpha}{2}} + z_{1-\beta}\right)^2}{\Delta^2} \qquad \text{(Formula 4)}$$

where n is one-half the size estimated for the two groups, everything else remaining equal.

Comparing proportions

When comparing proportions, the study compares the percentage of individuals that show a particular characteristic in each group and evaluates if the difference is significant. The null and alternative hypotheses may be stated as follows (for two groups):

$$\begin{cases} H_0 : \pi_1 - \pi_2 = 0 \\ H_1 : \pi_1 - \pi_2 \neq 0 \end{cases}$$

(Formula 5)

where π_1 = proportion in group 1 and π_2 = proportion in group 2.

The null hypothesis states that the proportion of individuals (with a specific characteristic) in group 1 is equivalent to the proportion in group 2. The alternative hypothesis states that these proportions are different. Formula 5 represents a two-tailed study, where the direction of the difference between group 1 and group 2 is unknown. As for Formula 1, the alternative hypothesis can be adapted to a one-tailed study as follows:

$$H_1 : \pi_1 - \pi_2 < 0 \ \text{ or } \ H_1 : \pi_1 - \pi_2 > 0$$

Formula 5 may be considered the statistical interpretation of the following research question: 'Is the proportion of individuals who show improvement after treatment in group 1 different from that in group 2? Or, for example, 'Is the percentage of males (group 1) with a certain condition different from the percentage of females (group 2) with the same condition?'

To compute a sample size for Formula 5, the following information is required:

- π_1 and π_2 = the proportions in group 1 and in group 2 (under the alternative hypothesis)
- level of certainty required to detect the treatment effect, the power $1 - \beta$
- the chance you are willing to accept of 'being wrong', the significance level α

Considerations about the power and the significance level have been provided for Formula 1 and are equivalent for this case.

Estimates for π_1 and π_2 are usually derived from previous studies or published data. The difference between the two groups, expressed as $\pi_1 - \pi_2$, is the size of the effect of treatment and quantifying it carries the same challenges as the quantification of $\mu_1 - \mu_2$ discussed for Formula 1.

The variability of the data is included in the formula, implicitly within π_1 and π_2.

Once the information is gathered, a computer package can be used to compute the sample size. The following is an example with a standard formula for the comparison of two proportions.

Example 4

A study aims to measure the effect of a probiotic drink in gestational diabetics and its ability to reduce the number of pregnant women who require insulin to manage their glucose levels. Participants are randomized into either the treatment group (probiotic drink) or placebo group (placebo drink) and followed until the end of their pregnancy.

The primary variable is the percentage of women who require insulin. It is expected that the probiotic drink can reduce the number of women who need insulin by 20 per cent. A sample size can be computed to estimate the number of participants needed to observe such a difference.

Sample size formula for comparing proportions of two groups (two-tailed):

$$n = \frac{\left(z_{1-\frac{\alpha}{2}}\sqrt{2\bar{\pi}(1-\bar{\pi})} + z_{1-\beta}\sqrt{(\pi_1(1-\pi_1) + (1-\pi_2))}\right)^2}{(\pi_1 - \pi_2)^2} \qquad \text{(Formula 6)}$$

where $\bar{\pi} = (\pi_1 + \pi_2)/2$.

Information required:

- π_1 and π_2 = the proportions of women who require insulin in the treatment group (π_1) and the proportion of women who require insulin in the placebo group (π_2). It is estimated that $\pi_1 = 0.25$ and, under the alternative hypothesis, $\pi_2 = 0.45$
- the power $1 - \beta = 0.8$
- the significance level $\alpha = 0.05$

Substituting the values in Formula 6, the sample size n is 88. It is required to enrol and retain 88 women in each group in order to detect a change of 20 per cent.

Formula 6 assumes equal sample sizes for the two groups. It also assumes equal variances or that the variance can be replaced by the average variance $\bar{\pi}$. A one-tailed study would use Formula 6, but with $z_{1-\alpha}$.

Estimating means and proportions

When a study is designed to estimate a mean or a proportion, the result is a confidence interval (CI), with confidence levels usually between 95 per cent and 99 per cent. In generic terms, the conclusions of the study would state that the average value or proportion lies within a certain interval with a certain level of confidence.

These types of studies compute point estimates for a specific parameter, irrespective of any hypothesized value. They are often used in pilot research or new fields of research. They may be conducted when very little knowledge is available on any hypothesized value and the comparison between groups may be premature. The aim of these studies is to derive an estimate for a clinically relevant parameter (the primary variable) with the highest level of precision that is practically achievable. The sample size calculations become an iterative process where the trade-off between the precision of the answer and the logistics of recruiting and retaining the required sample size is resolved – or at least attempted to be resolved.

Estimating a mean value

When estimating a mean, the research question may be stated as follows: 'Can we detect an average value for X, i.e. the availability score in the KPI study, within an interval of ± δ?'

To compute the sample size calculation, the following information is required:

- the chance you are willing to accept of 'being wrong', the significance level α
- variability of the data
- size of the interval

Considerations about the significance level have been provided for Formula 5 and are equivalent for this case.

Variability of the data. Variability has the same effect on estimation studies as it does on comparison studies – the bigger the variance, the larger the sample size. Large variations in the data negatively affect the precision of the estimate as they require larger confidence intervals. To gain greater precision, that is, to obtain a narrower confidence interval, larger sample sizes are required.

Size of the interval: ± δ. The size of the interval plays the same role as the size of the treatment effect in the comparison case. The smaller the size of the interval, the larger the sample size. A clinical and practical decision, not a statistical one, is reached after many attempts have shown the effect of different interval widths on the sample size.

As for all previous examples, once the information is gathered a computer package can be used to compute the sample size. Below, an example is provided – the KPI study from earlier in the chapter – with a standard formula for estimating a confidence interval for the mean.

Example 5

The KPI study aims to estimate the number of data items available in the patient records as an average availability score with a confidence interval of ±0.25.
Information required:

- the significance level $\alpha = 0.05$, i.e. a 95 per cent CI
- variability of the data, σ: based on results from a pilot study, the average number of data items reported is expected to be 4.04, with a standard deviation of 1.25
- size of the interval, ± δ: the accuracy required is a confidence interval for the mean of ±0.25 or total interval width of 0.5

Sample size formula for estimating the mean of a population:

$$n = 4\left(\frac{z_{1-\frac{\alpha}{2}} * \sigma}{\delta}\right)^2 \qquad \text{(Formula 7)}$$

where δ is the *total* width of the interval, σ is the standard deviation, and $z_{1-\frac{\alpha}{2}}$ is given by the standardized normal distribution tables.

Substituting the value for $\sigma = 1.25$, $\delta = 0.5$ and $z_{1-\frac{\alpha}{2}} = 1.96$, the sample size n is 96.

The formula assumes the data are normally distributed or that they may be normalized. It does not require a value for the power.

Estimating a proportion

In this type of study, the research question may be stated as follows: 'Can we detect the proportion of patients with a specific medical condition/treatment effect, with a precision of 1 per cent?'

In this case, the following information is required:

- p = a preliminary estimate of the proportion itself
- δ = the precision of the interval, i.e. ±10 per cent, 5 per cent, 3 per cent etc.?
- the chance you are willing to accept of 'being wrong' – the significance level α

As before, considerations about the significance level have been provided in the section 'Comparing means (two groups)' above, and are equivalent for this case.

A preliminary estimate of the proportion p is usually derived from pilot studies or from previously published research.

The precision of the interval is often set between ±1 per cent and 10 per cent. As for many of the examples before, it is often the case that a series of sample size calculations is performed to make the researcher aware of the increasing effect that higher precision has on sample sizes. Issues of practicality, and in some cases regulatory requirements, would dictate the choice of δ.

Once again, when the information is gathered computer software is used to estimate the sample size. Below are two examples that use a standard formula for estimating a proportion.

Example 6

Population-based studies are carried out to compare the outcome of stroke in many regions. For example one of the parameters investigated in studies of this kind is the proportion of individuals over 85 years of age who experienced a stroke for the first time. It is hypothesized that the percentage of strokes in this age group is approximately 15 per cent. In order to detect this estimate with a precision of ±10 per cent a sample size calculation would be computed as follows.

Sample size formula for estimating a proportion from one population:

$$n = 4\frac{z_{1-\frac{\alpha}{2}}^{2} * p * (1-p)}{\delta^{2}}$$

(Formula 8)

Information required:

- p = a preliminary value has been estimated at 15 per cent
- the precision of the interval is set at ±10 per cent, the total width δ is 0.2
- the significance level α is set at 0.05, i.e. a 95 per cent CI

Substituting the values in Formula 8, the sample size n is 49.

Example 7

The study from Example 2 is also a case of estimating a proportion from one population. To answer the question of how large a sample size is required to estimate the proportion of women who would reach 9 METs with a precision of ±10 per cent, Formula 8 would be applied as follows.
   Information required:

- p = a preliminary value has been estimated at 80 per cent
- the precision of the interval is set at ±10 per cent, the total width δ is 0.2
- the significance level α is set at 0.05, i.e. a 95 per cent CI

Substituting the values in Formula 8, the sample size n is 62.

Conclusion

As shown in this chapter, the importance of a well-designed study cannot be stressed enough. If the flow from the research question to the statistical analysis is clear and well defined, the sample size calculation is a straightforward exercise of choosing the correct mathematical formula.

   Whether the sample is large or small, sampling is the tool for inferential statistics. It has its limitations, but it is capable of providing reliable and robust answers, if fitted with the appropriate design. Once again, the stress is on the overall framework of the study, its implications and the practicalities to implement it accurately.

   As mentioned in the introduction, it is statistically unethical to support a study that has no clear design and no justifications for the sample size. The general advice is to 'keep it simple'; clear comparisons and easily measurable parameters reduce the effect of noise and provide robust tools for evidence-based research.

Key concepts
- The difficulty in identifying the path from the research hypotheses to the primary and secondary outcomes of a study is the greatest obstacle to effective sampling.

- Unclear study designs and the lack of data affect sample size calculations, impact on the robustness of the sampling strategies and subsequently weaken the final results. Instead, simplicity and clarity of design strengthen the study and increase the quality of the results.
- Small samples versus large samples: while larger samples may give more robust answers, it is often impractical and logistically too difficult to obtain large samples of data. Also, incomplete datasets, invasive procedures and lengthy questionnaires may affect the quality of the data collected, in some cases making the study statistically unethical. Sample size calculations and sampling strategies should be used to minimize the effort of collecting data, for the benefit of the study and the participants.
- Sampling strategies depend on the population of interest, the pattern of the condition studied and the context in which treatments and/or services are provided. An in-depth knowledge of these key concepts is required in order to develop effective strategies.
- The main issues when attempting a sample size calculation are what type of information is required, where to find it and how to use it. Identifying the key components for a correct calculation often requires a multidisciplinary approach in which the researcher extracts information from multiple sources – clinical data, current practices, pilot studies etc.
- Comparing groups and estimating values are the most common strategies for study design. The researcher must learn how to 'translate' such designs into a mathematical formula for a sample size calculation. A step-by-step framework can be used to facilitate this process.

Key readings in sampling issues

- G. van Belle, P.J. Heagerty, L.D. Fisher and T.S. Lumley (2004) Biostatistics: *A Methodology For the Health Sciences*, Wiley Series in Probability and Statistics. New York: John Wiley and Sons
  This book provides a broad and in-depth overview of the statistical methods for the health sciences, including sampling, with examples from clinical, epidemiological and health services research.
- S.A. Julious (2009) *Sample Size for Clinical Trials*. London: Chapman and Hall/CRC
  A comprehensive reference book, it covers the majority of study designs for clinical trials. It uses thorough processes and useful tables, many of which are applicable beyond clinical trials and can be a useful reference for many health research studies.
- Shein-Chung Chow and Jen-Pei Liu (2003) *Design and Analysis of Clinical Trials: Concepts and Methodologies*, Wiley Series in Probability and Statistics. New York: John Wiley and Sons
  This book provides a comprehensive account of the clinical trial process, including sampling issues. It also provides detailed information of the regulatory process with ethical and quality issues applicable to all health research studies.

- B.H. Munro (2004) *Statistical Methods for Health Care Research*. Philadelphia: Lippincott Williams & Wilkins
  A good reference book to understand the foundations of statistics applied to nursing and health care research, including sample size calculation and sampling strategies.
- W.L. Carlson and B. Thorne (1997) *Applied Statistical Methods for Business, Economics and the Social Sciences*. New Jersey: Prentice Hall
  A good teaching book that provides a variety of examples and applications of statistics in economics and social sciences.

Examples of the use of sampling issues in health care research
- R.A. Crosby, L.F. Salazar, R.J. Di Clemente and D.L. Lang, Balancing rigour against the inherent limitations of investigating hard-to-reach populations, *Health Education Research*, 25(1) (Feb 2010), 1–5
- M. Manson, Methodological and ethical challenges in investigating the safety of medication administration, *Nurse Res.*, 18(4) (2011), 28–32
- S. Fernandes-Taylor, J.K. Hyun, R.N. Reiden and A.H.S. Harris, Common statistical and research design problems in manuscripts submitted to high-impact medical journals, *BMC Research Notes*, 4 (2011), 304

References

Cohen, J. (1988) *Statistical Power Analysis for the Behavioral Sciences*, 2nd edn. Hillsdale, NJ: Lawrence Erlbaum Associates.

Comiskey, C.M., Crispino, G. and Cassidy, T. (2003) *ROSIE, Research Outcome Study in Ireland Evaluating drug treatment effectiveness: Project Objectives Document (Protocol and study design)*. Dublin: NACD.

Crispino-O'Connell, G. (2010) *The Implementation of a Pilot Physical Activity Programme for Breast Cancer Patients after Surgery: Evaluation Study Protocol*. Dublin: Irish Cancer Society (ICS). Extracts have been reproduced with the permission of the ICS.

Early Breast Cancer Trialists' Collaborative Group (1988) Effects of adjuvant tamoxifen and of cytotoxic therapy on mortality in early breast cancer: An overview of 61 randomized trials among 28,896 women, *New England Journal Medicine*, 319(26): 1681–91.

Fisher, R.A. (1956) *Statistical Methods and Scientific Inference*. London: Oliver & Boyd.

Julious, S.A. (2009) *Sample Size for Clinical Trials*. London: Chapman and Hall/CRC.

Kelly, P.J., Crispino-O'Connell, G., Giles, M., Sheenan, O. et al. (2012). Incidence, event rates, and early outcome of stroke in Dublin, Ireland: The North Dublin Population Stroke Study, *Stroke*, 43(8): 2042–7.

Moore, D.S. (1985) *Statistics: Concepts and Controversies*, 2nd edn. New York: W.H. Freeman.

Munro, B.H. (2004) *Statistical Methods for Health Care Research*. Philadelphia: Lippincott Williams & Wilkins.

The First International Study of Infarct Survival Collaborative Group (1986) Randomised trial of intravenous atenolol among 16,027 cases of suspected acute myocardial infarction: ISIS-1. *Lancet*, ii: 57–66.

The Second International Study of Infarct Survival Collaborative Group (1988) Randomised trial of intravenous streptokinase, oral aspirin, both, or neither among 17,187 cases of suspected acute myocardial infarction: ISIS-2. *Lancet*, ii: 349–60.

The Third International Study of Infarct Survival Collaborative Group (1992) A randomised trial of streptokinase vs tissue plasminogen activator vs anistreplase and of aspirin plus heparin vs aspirin alone among 41,299 cases of suspected acute myocardial infarction: ISIS-3. *Lancet*, 339: 753–70.

The Fourth International Study of Infarct Survival Collaborative Group (1995) A randomised factorial trial assessing early oral captopril, oral mononitrate, and intravenous magnesium sulphate in 58,050 patients with suspected acute myocardial infarction: ISIS-4. *Lancet*, 345: 669–85.

van Belle, G., Heagerty, P.J., Fisher, L.D. and Lumley, T.S. (2004) *Biostatistics: A Methodology For the Health Sciences*, Wiley Series in Probability and Statistics. New York: John Wiley and Sons.

Wakai, A., O'Sullivan, R., Crispino-O'Connell, G., et al. (2011) *Feasibility Analysis of Key Performance Indicators for Emergency Departments in Ireland*, Study Protocol. Dublin: The National Children's Research Centre. Extracts have been reproduced with the permission of the principal authors.

10   Planning and conducting surveys

Susan McLaren

Chapter topics

- Survey approaches
- Sampling strategies
- Methodological diversity

- Validity and reliability
- Sources of error
- Response styles

Introduction

Contemporary definitions of survey design tend to emphasize common features in relation to populations of interest, purposes of investigation and the testing of relationships between variables. For example, Sapsford (2007: 2) defined a survey as a 'collection of quantified data from a population for purposes of description or to identify covariance between variables which may point towards causal relationships or predictive patterns of influence'. In contrast, the definition by Whittaker (2009: 61) also associated survey design with a quantitative research approach, but emphasized the type of attributes measured in the population of interest: 'surveys are used to study large groups or populations usually using a standardized quantitative approach to identify beliefs, attitudes, behaviors and other characteristics'.

Traditionally, survey designs have indeed been used for both quantitative, descriptive and correlational studies, that is, used either to describe and classify phenomena or to test links between variables of interest. In scope, this text is devoted to quantitative methods, but it is important to appreciate from the outset of this chapter that although the use of questionnaires (quantitative) has tended to become synonymous with survey design, other methods can be used. Contemporary survey approaches can employ the use of single or multiple quantitative or qualitative methods or a rich combination of both quantitative and qualitative approaches. In quantitative research, combining methods can be used to enhance the validity of findings or, in qualitative research, to obtain an in-depth understanding through exploration of different perspectives.

Considerable debate exists regarding the merits or otherwise of combining qualitative and quantitative methods in a single design: in health care research a strong argument has been made for the use of mixed methods justified on the basis of the complexity of phenomena studied. In a recent critical methodological review of combining quantitative and qualitative approaches, Ostlund et al. (2011) concluded that using triangulation as a methodological metaphor could facilitate integration of findings from both perspectives and enable researchers to clarify theoretical propositions. The reader who is interested in developing a mixed-methods survey design is advised to consider the arguments put forward by Morgan (2007) and Sale et al. (2002), the nature of their research question(s) and the research context in which their study would be conducted, as a preliminary to decision making. Further essential reading on the use of mixed methods can be found in the following sources.

- Cresswell and Plano Clark (2007) address the design and conduct of mixed-methods research, including frameworks for converging, connecting and embedding datasets.
- Brannen (2008) reviews the practice of mixed-methods research from various viewpoints, including choice of methods related to research questions and their epistemological framing.
- Bergman (2008) provides an insightful text on mixed-methods research addressing theoretical foundations and applications.

Evolution of survey design – historical perspective

Survey design has a long and fascinating history: analysis of documentary evidence in historical records can provide invaluable insights into social and economic circumstances prevalent during a particular period of time, many sources including information on health and mortality. While the findings of such surveys are of great interest, the enthusiastic researcher of today can find much in the finer detail of historical accounts that is exciting in terms of evolving ideas on survey design, approaches to sampling, the range and type of methods employed and attempts which were taken to address the rigour and reliability of findings. Notable examples of early surveys include the following (see also Twitchett et al. 1986; Scheidel 2009).

- The census (Latin *censere*; to estimate): decennial surveys of the total population on one night, describing households and residents (age, gender, occupation, place of birth, marital status and relationship to the head of household) have been conducted since 1801, although survival of complete records is of later date (see http://nationalarchives.gov.uk and http://www.nationalarchives.ie).
- The Domesday Book (1085–86): commissioned by William the Conqueror in 1085, this descriptive land survey, probably intended to inform taxation and asset management, has been conserved in the National Archives at Kew (http://www.nationalarchives.gov.uk; http://www.domesdaybook.co.uk).
- John Graunt (1620–74): Graunt conducted a retrospective survey based on an analysis of London Bills of Mortality. Findings included a classification of death rates according to causes and a life table presenting mortality in terms of survivorship, which made an invaluable contribution to the development of epidemiology.
- The Manchester Statistical Society (established 1883): this organization (learned society) with a focus on improving social conditions was the first in the UK to investigate these problems and collect statistical data about them (http://www.manstatsoc.org).

- Charles Booth (1840–1916): with co-investigators, Booth conducted the survey 'An Inquiry into the Life and Labour of the People in London' (1886–1903). Outputs included street maps of London showing areas of poverty and wealth. Findings provided invaluable insights into working lives in the context of social and economic conditions prevalent at the time (http://booth.lse.ac.uk/static/a/2.html).

Contemporary survey design

A number of features have evolved to mark contemporary survey design:

- collection of information from the total population or a subsample of the population of interest
- cross-sectional and longitudinal approaches
- diversity in use of methods
- standardization and methodological rigour
- a measurement focus on events, attributes, behaviours, beliefs, feelings, preferences and attitudes

With regard to the collection of data at a single point in time (cross-sectional) or at intervals (longitudinal), either of these approaches can be prospective and/or retrospective in nature – that is, investigate phenomena by collecting information on current/future events, or by collecting information on past events, respectively. Retrospective studies can be challenging, given the potential for bias due to fallible or selective memory recall where participants are questioned about past events. Another problem which can arise where documentary analysis is a method of choice, is that such documents may be incomplete and difficult to access after the passage of time.

Cross-sectional surveys

The cross-sectional survey describes a phenomenon of interest and its associations in the population; typically the phenomenon is described in relation to gender, age, ethnicity and other population characteristics. For this reason, cross-sectional surveys are used extensively to measure the prevalence of a phenomenon: for example, the prevalence of smoking in young people; the prevalence of malnutrition in the elderly, or the prevalence of type 2 diabetes mellitus in ethnic groups. Survey participants can be questioned about current (prospective) and/or past (retrospective) attitudes, beliefs, feelings, behaviours, events. Measuring phenomena at one point in time precludes any indications of cause and effect relationships between variables, however the cross-sectional survey possesses the advantages of providing information which can inform the development and testing of hypotheses in experimental studies and offers economies in terms of time and resource utilization. The serial cross-sectional study is sometimes utilized in situations where a longitudinal study is rejected due to the impact of sample attrition, and information about change is needed (Haw and Gruer 2007; DH 2011) – see below. Exemplars of cross-sectional surveys which embody the different design features noted above, utilize an interesting range of methods and were conducted in health and social care settings include the following.

- Prevalence and risk factors for experiencing phantom vibrations (a form of sensory hallucination) in medical staff using mobile phones (Rothberg et al. 2010).
- Prevalence of abuse of people with dementia by family carers (Cooper et al. 2009).
- UK National Diet and Nutrition Survey (DH 2011): a cross-sectional rolling survey to assess diet, nutrient intake and nutritional status of the general population living in private households.
- Cross-sectional surveys conducted before and after the introduction of legislation in Scotland to determine changes in adult non-smokers' exposure to second-hand smoke in public and private places (Haw and Gruer 2007).

Longitudinal surveys

This analytic survey approach using multiple timed data-collection points can suggest the direction of cause and effect associations. Three prospective variants can be distinguished: 1) the panel study in which the same sample drawn from the population of interest is followed up; 2) the trend study, in which different samples are recruited and followed up at each time period; and 3) the prospective cohort study, a variant in which a sample with a common characteristic (e.g. year of birth: see below) is followed over time. In a review of the value of prospective cohort studies, Watts (2011) cites sources listing their advantages as follows.

- ready determination of sequence and timing
- absence of retrospective recall introducing memory bias
- allowing estimation of effect size and opportunities to examine expected and unexpected outcomes

In contrast, disadvantages were perceived to be as follows.

- the need for large sample sizes, particularly where outcomes were uncommon
- the long time frame over which studies need to be conducted
- the 'cohort effect', which is a consequence of shared life experiences, attributed to the impact of time and context on attitudes, beliefs, preferences etc.

Trend studies 2), by recruiting a new representative random sample at each time point, have the advantage of allowing changes in the population of interest to be identified and can be used to determine incidence rates of diseases.

More generally, problems which can arise in prospective longitudinal surveys include the following.

- Sample ageing and sample attrition due to geographic relocation, refusals to continue participation, morbidity and mortality. Rates of attrition can also be affected by the length of time between data-collection points and also by demands placed on participants.

- Long-term funding is needed, which can be costly, and the management of a complex dataset, which involves maintenance of up-to-date databases to follow up participants, can be very time-consuming.
- Over time a number of extraneous variables can exert an impact on findings (for instance, environmental factors).
- Panel studies are vulnerable to the Hawthorne effect, whereby conditioning of panel members over time can result in learned responses to questionnaires.
- Expectations about the findings of prospective longitudinal studies have to be realistic, given that early stage results may not offer value for money and greater benefits are yielded in mature years of the survey.

Harpham et al. (2003), noting the above issue about expectations in panel studies and their expansion in developing countries to investigate transitory and persistent states (such as poverty and unemployment), has explored how challenges can be addressed in resource-constrained environments. Watson and Wooden (2009) also provide an in-depth discussion of challenges associated with longitudinal surveys. Exemplars of different types of longitudinal survey utilizing a diversity of methods are summarized below.

- **British Household Panel Study:** ongoing since 1991, a multipurpose panel study following a representative sample of households over a period of years; involves interviews with every adult member of sampled households (wave 1: 5,500 households and 10,300 participants drawn from 250 areas). Findings have illuminated the impact of a cultural divide on wages and job satisfaction and the consequences of financial capability on income and psychological well-being.
- **French GAZEL Occupational Cohort Study:** prospective cohort study investigating the effect of retirement on chronic conditions and fatigue in 11,246 men and 2,858 women, seven years before and seven years after retirement (Westerlund et al. 2010). Findings concluded that retirement did not alter the risk of major chronic disease but decreased mental and physical fatigue, notably in people with chronic conditions.
- **Medical Research Council National Survey of Health and Development:** a prospective cohort survey investigating the impact of health and ageing on a socially stratified sample of 5,562 babies born to married parents in a single week in March 1946 in England, Scotland and Wales (MRC 2009). Findings so far have informed UK health and social care policy for over 60 years, notably by illuminating the impact of events in early years on adult life.
- **Regional UK Trend Study:** population-based time trends and socio-economic variation in the use of radiotherapy and radical surgery for prostate cancer: a study based in a cancer registry surveyed 35,171 patients over 51 years diagnosed with prostate cancer between 1995 and 2006. Findings showed a significant rise in the use of radical surgery, while radiotherapy use remained constant: both treatments were used most commonly in least deprived patients (Lyratzopoulos et al. 2010).

Planning a survey – key development questions

In the early stages of proposal development considerable thought needs to be given to a number of key questions which if not carefully considered at the outset can lead to problems in obtaining ethical approval or in the later stages of design implementation.

Survey purpose: what is the purpose of the survey? Is it to test a hypothesis, or to test causal models, to estimate the prevalence of a characteristic or a belief, or to follow up groups over time to determine changes in attributes, characteristics, behaviours? Clarity about purpose has relevance to a number of design decisions, for example sampling frameworks, sampling and determination of time needed to complete the study in relation to resources available (Czaja and Blair 2005).

Quality issues: how will requirements for quality and rigour be addressed? Has appropriate time been allowed for the design and pretesting of instruments (reliability and validity), pilot studies, training of interviewers, development of a protocol for data collection and verification, debriefing of participants?

Legal issues: if previously published and validated questionnaires are to be used, what copyright issues may arise and how will author permission be sought? How will the requirements for data protection and security be ensured?

Ethical issues: what are the ethical issues which may arise related to project design and implementation? How will the informed consent of participants be obtained, and their anonymity and confidentiality ensured? Will debriefing of participants be necessary? How will feedback be provided as agreed with participants?

Data-collection mode: how will the data be collected? Web-based surveys, postal survey, face-to-face interviews or mixed mode? How will choice of data-collection mode impact on time and project costs?

Access to study population: are there gatekeepers who may restrict access to the study sample? How will access be negotiated through gatekeepers? Will the study sample be accessible using the chosen mode of data collection?

Minimizing bias: how can bias due to low unit and item response rates (questionnaires, structured interviews), sampling approaches and sample attrition be minimized?

Sampling – probability and non-probability sampling

Sampling is the process whereby subjects of the survey are selected from a defined population according to specific criteria. The rationale for sampling, selecting a representative subset of the population, is that the researcher wishes to make inferences (generalize) about the population of interest and that it can be impractical and costly to survey the total population. Effective sampling is predicated on the sampling frame, which determines how well a sample represents the population, and probability methods, wherein each individual (or other unit of analysis) has a known, non-zero chance of selection based on a random procedure (see below):

- Simple random sampling: selection at random from a numbered list using either a table of random numbers or computer program to generate random numbers.

- Stratified random sampling: selection at random from homogeneous sub-groups in the population based on predetermined key characteristics.
- Cluster (or multistage) sampling: sequential selection of random samples from larger to smaller units using either of the above approaches.

With non-probability sampling, which encompasses convenience, quota, snowball and purposive approaches, the probabilities of selection may not be known and statistical inferences cannot generally be supported. However, their use can be helpful as a basis for preliminary quantitative research focused on developing hypotheses, defining response categories for questionnaire construction and identifying hard-to-find populations.

Defining populations, constructing sampling frameworks

The population of interest is the group to whom generalization is intended: essentially this is informed by the research question, aims and objectives. It is important to identify clearly the units of analysis (individuals, households, groups, organizations etc.) together with their boundaries. For individuals, boundaries encompass those relating to study area, study setting, demographic characteristics, inclusion and exclusion criteria. Having defined the population of interest, it is then necessary to identify a sampling framework: essentially, this is the 'lists or other resources that contain the elements of a defined population' (Czaja and Blair 2005). Dependent on survey purpose and method, these can encompass organizational directories (listing email and contact telephone numbers); regional telephone directories; databases listing contact details for membership of organizations or interest groups, individuals attending specialist health clinics or receiving specific services on the basis of medical diagnosis. A number of problems can arise with the listings that comprise sampling frameworks: these relate to the inclusion of erroneous or outdated information, missing data and also re-entry data; furthermore, the list may include information on individuals or units ineligible for inclusion. Issues of non-coverage may present other problems in terms of exclusion of members of the defined population; some may not be accessible via email or do not possess a landline telephone. At the outset of pilot work, researchers should evaluate these issues, the likelihood of their impact on results and take any pre-emptive actions which may be necessary: sources of error are discussed later in this chapter.

Sample size

Determination of sample size is influenced by study design and purpose: is the purpose to establish a population value and/or test hypotheses? If it is intended to generalize results to the population from which the sample was drawn, then the following information is required (Price et al. 2005):

- population size (N); the extent of variation of the variable investigated; the smallest subsample for which sample size estimates are needed
- the extent of acceptable sampling error

A number of published tables are available citing sample sizes at various levels of error (for example, 1 per cent, 3 per cent, 5 per cent, 7 per cent) at 95 per cent confidence intervals (Barnett (1974), Salant and Dillman (1994) and Price et al. (2005) draw attention to the software packages also available).

When testing a hypothesis, it is important to determine a sample size which minimizes type 1 and type 2 statistical errors when drawing conclusions from the data. These errors are defined as follows:

- Type 1 error: incorrect rejection of a null hypothesis when it is true.
- Type 2 error: incorrect acceptance of a null hypothesis when it is false.

The probability of making a type 1 error is reduced when setting the significance level (p-value, also known as the alpha level) at 0.05 or less. The probability of making a type 2 error (beta) is reduced by setting statistical power (1 − beta) at 0.8 or higher: in effect this means that 80 per cent of the time a false null hypothesis will be correctly rejected – that is, there is a 20 per cent risk of committing a type 2 error. Based on the considerations above, sample size is determined a priori by conducting a power analysis based on the following, of which only the first three factors are known:

- the level of significance (alpha): conventionally specified at 0.05 or less
- the population effect (gamma): the magnitude of the effect of the independent variable on the dependent variable in the population
- statistical power (1 − beta): conventionally specified at 0.8 or higher
- sample size (n)

Effect size can be approximated on the basis of published evidence (appraisal of precedent research literature), pilot studies, or the utilization of the general effect sizes published by Cohen (1988). When relationships between variables are relatively small, then larger sample sizes are needed to detect the effect at statistically significant levels, and vice versa. It should be noted that the determination of gamma differs according to level of measurement and use of statistical test. Attention of survey researchers is drawn to the fact that a questionnaire may contain different levels of measurement (Bartlett et al. 2001). In the conduct of power analysis, researchers are not required to do the calculations by hand: software packages are available (for example, G-Power). For a more detailed discussion see Price et al. (2005) and Polit and Beck (2006). Attention is drawn to the impact that low response rates can have on effective sample size: oversampling to allow for this can be based on stepped sampling techniques, pilot studies or using response rates from previously published research. Not all researchers agree with some of these approaches (Bartlett et al. 2001).

Survey methods

As is evident from the examples cited earlier in this chapter, surveys can utilize a range of methods: in this chapter some of the most common approaches, notably questionnaires administered by post, telephone, face-to-face structured interviews, email and websites are reviewed in relation to their relative advantages and disadvantages. For further discussion on this in relation to 'error' and 'response rates' see later sections of this chapter.

Postal questionnaires

Postal questionnaires are one of the most commonly used approaches: advantages are that a large volume of data can be collected over a large geographical area in situations where other approaches would be unwieldy, interviewer bias is avoided, respondent convenience is ensured and anonymity is safeguarded (Curtis and Redmond 2009). Furthermore, structured questionnaires are easy to code and analyse using computer packages such as SPSS. Structure and predetermined responses are easy to evaluate with regard to reliability (see below). Set against these advantages are the challenges of possible low response rates and lack of researcher supervision, which means that no control is exerted over who answers the questions and no information can be obtained from probes, prompts and observations of body language indicative of frustration, confusion and anxiety. Researchers should ascertain the accuracy of mailed addresses when sampling frameworks are developed. Although postal questionnaires are relatively less costly, this may not be the case in large-scale surveys, hence Weitzel (1990) has emphasized the benefits of utilizing third class bulk and business reply mail to reduce costs. Poor levels of literacy and the presence of disability can preclude the use of postal questionnaires in these groups, although attendance to font size and visual presentation can enable completion in some instances of disability.

Telephone interviews

Increased numbers of households with telephones has resulted in the telephone interview becoming one of the most widely used survey methods. Advantages include the wide access offered to general populations using random-digit dialling, relatively low costs (fewer staff needed although it is labour intensive) and versatility in terms of interviewer locations, which can be remote. Other advantages are that the interviewer can build rapport with the respondent, offer clarification of any misunderstanding and supervise the order of questions, and use computer-assisted telephone recording techniques (CATI). Some researchers have suggested that telephone interviews can increase comfort of both interviewers and respondents, who are less affected by each other's presence (Smith 2005) and that this method offers interviewer safety, inasmuch as travel to risky settings is avoided. Limitations are that the omission of populations without a telephone can lead to problems of non-coverage, the interviewer cannot observe body language, the respondent's environment may not be conducive in terms of noise or privacy and the method may be unsuitable for use with some sensitive topics. In a review of the use of telephone interviewing in clinical nursing research, Musselwhite et al. (2007) concluded that supportive training for interviewers, standardized operating procedures and effective communication were vital and have made further recommendations which can benefit researchers using this method.

Face-to-face structured interviews

This approach involves the use of a structured, standardized questionnaire which is administered in person by the researcher in the respondent's own home or in a predetermined setting which is convenient for both. In contrast to other interview approaches, the researcher does not deviate from the question format and sequence laid out in the questionnaire, although predetermined, non-directive prompts may be used. This approach has the advantages of allowing the interviewer to build up rapport and confidence with the respondent and enables clarification of anything that is misunderstood – observing body language of respondents can be helpful here. The advent of computerized assisted personal interviewing (CAPI) enables researchers to code and enter responses directly – a substantial time- and cost-saving measure. Structured interviews can be a useful alternative to other methods for obtaining information from disabled or otherwise frail respondents and those whose reading and writing skills would preclude the use of a postal questionnaire. Disadvantages are that it can be more time-consuming, is not suitable for gathering information on sensitive topics and is more costly than other modes of data collection: costs incurred include travel costs, and employing and training interviewers. Issues of researcher safety are a paramount consideration in the conduct of fieldwork interviews (see guidelines: Social Research Association 2003).

Internet – email and websites

Innovations introduced by the expansion of the internet over the last 20 years have been exploited in survey design by either sending the survey questionnaire within the body or attachment of an email, or by providing hyperlink or browser access to a dedicated website. Potential advantages of such survey approaches are that they can access local, national and international populations, elicit rapid responses, reduce costs and facilitate respondent convenience (time can be taken over answers and respondents can interrupt and re-enter a website). Furthermore, Stewart (2003) and Huntington et al. (2009) have emphasized the added convenience to researchers of rapid data handling and analysis due to direct feeding into analysis software and rapid follow-up of non-respondents via email.

Schonlau et al. (2002) point out that making initial contact with respondents by post or phone is costly and that savings can be made by using email instead. However this requires access to a reliable address system or database. In weighing up benefits versus costs of electronic surveys it is important to bear in mind the costs of setting up and maintaining websites, which can be substantial. Other disadvantages of using the internet include problems of non-coverage (the survey is limited to internet users) and lack of interviewer involvement (see other methods above). Password protection and use of personal PIN numbers to authenticate participants, together with data encryption, are vital to ensure that the privacy and anonymity of respondents is ensured and risks of unwanted observers accessing data is eliminated. Research ethics committees and some professional bodies offer guidance on the conduct of internet research, for example, the British Psychological Association (2007).

Experiences of using the internet to establish a web-based longitudinal survey of the nursing and midwifery workforce in three countries has been reported by Huntington et al. (2009), illustrating many of the benefits and challenges of conducting web-based survey research. Challenges included website development costs, needs for fast broadband connections and the need for computer literacy in the nursing and midwifery population. Offsetting these were the benefits of being able to establish international e-cohorts of respondents, who could continue participation as long as they could access the internet (a benefit in the investigation of workforce migration) and the enhanced recruitment and retention which could result from use of an interactive website: factors such as this are discussed later in this chapter under the heading, 'Sources of error and bias'.

Pilot studies

Beyond commenting on testing of methods, comparatively few surveys report details of this vital early stage in survey development, yet the conduct of pilot fieldwork is intrinsic to success, as discussed in relation to response rates later in this chapter.

The rationale for conducting pilot studies is variably reported in the literature to include the following (Robinson et al. 1998; Baird 2000; van Teijlingen et al. 2000):

- development of a rigorous survey protocol and evaluation of its workability
- development and pretesting of questionnaires and other instruments to establish validity, reliability, practical utility, issues affecting participant response
- identification of any logistical problems which could mar data collection
- training of researchers in specific research techniques and processes
- establishing the adequacy of the sampling framework, determination of sample size and potential response rates
- evaluating data-analysis techniques to ensure they are non-problematic
- determination of the resources needed for the main study
- establishing communication networks with key stakeholders
- providing feedback to funding bodies related to feasibility issues

Validity and reliability

Establishing validity and reliability in relation to method is intrinsic to quality design and implementation. Survey research can utilize questionnaires which are designed *de novo* but will require validity and reliability to be established, or those which have already been published and possess demonstrable reliability and validity: in the case of the latter, researchers should establish copyright issues and request author permission before use. Questionnaires may also include valid and reliable instruments which have been used to measure health status, quality of life or other outcome variables: if these are to be used, then researchers should establish the mode of administration for which they have been validated, to assess suitability for inclusion in a questionnaire. Alongside the content of this chapter, readers may find the publications of De Vellis (2003) and Streiher and Norman (2008) on scale development and measurement invaluable reading, as well as the specialist text on questionnaire design, evaluation and analysis by Saris and Gallhofer (2007). Apart from the use of questionnaires, it is recognized that surveys may use a diverse range of quantitative methods which include indicators of disease, biological and psychosocial measures: readers of this chapter are referred to specialist texts for approaches used to establish validity, reliability, sensitivity and specificity of such methods.

Validity

Validity generally refers to the extent to which the questionnaire measures the dimension of interest, i.e. what it is intended to measure. Different dimensions of **internal validity** (Chapter 8) can be distinguished in the literature: of these, content, criterion-related and construct validity are briefly considered here.

- Content validity is determined by the extent to which the questions are representative of what is known about the specific topic. Approaches to establish content validity can include preliminary interviews and/or focus groups with a subsample drawn from the population of interest, thematic analysis subsequently informing questionnaire content. The use of an expert panel to review questionnaire content and structure offers another independent view to establishing content validity.
- Criterion-related validity: here, the relationship between scores on the questionnaire and their correlation with an independent criterion are tested. An example would be to correlate scores on a self-report questionnaire designed to assess dietary patterns with measurements recorded in food diaries or weighed food intakes.
- Construct validity: depending on the survey purpose and content of the questionnaire, researchers may wish to establish construct validity, that is, the attributes which underlie a series of scaled measurements: the key question which is answered here is what construct is really being measured? A number of approaches can be used to determine construct validity: these include factor analysis, which identifies clusters of related variables (see Brown 2006).

Distinct from internal validity is **external validity** (Chapter 8) which refers to the generalizability of research findings to the wider population of interest. Rigour in the construction of a sampling framework, use of probability sampling, ensuring sample size is adequate to overcome type 2 statistical error and appropriate use of inferential statistics are vital considerations here. Threats to the validity of survey research findings can also arise due to other sources of error and bias, including unit and item non-response and interviewer bias, which are addressed later in this chapter.

Reliability

Reliability is concerned with consistency in use: essentially, this is the consistency, stability and dependability with which it measures an attribute.

- Stability: this can be established by measuring test–retest reliability. The scaled questionnaire is distributed at two different time points to a subsample of the population of interest and the magnitude, direction and statistical significance of correlation coefficients between the two sets of scores are determined for each question. Positive correlation coefficients >0.7 are generally accepted as evidence of reliability: poor correlations may indicate problems with question wording. However, researchers should also ascertain whether anything has happened in the time period between administering the questionnaires to change a respondent's view: this can be done by incorporating an additional open question on the second questionnaire. It is also necessary to determine, as part of pilot fieldwork, what the optimal time period is between administering the questionnaires to attenuate memory bias: opinions vary, but intervals of around two to three weeks have been cited (Bohannon et al. 2004).

- Internal consistency: a questionnaire may be considered to be internally consistent to the extent that all the questions are measuring the same characteristic. The extent to which internal consistency has been achieved can be determined by measurement of Cronbach's coefficient alpha (Cronbach 1951). Values of coefficient alpha >0.7 are generally accepted as evidence of homogeneity. For a discussion of other approaches to internal consistency see De Vellis (2003) and Saris and Gallhofer (2007).

- Practical utility: rigorous pretesting of pilot questionnaires on a representative subsample of the population is also vital to ensure wording lacks ambiguity, and the format and order of questions has clarity and continuity. Cognitive interviewing may also be helpful in identifying questions that respondents are likely to find problematic and/or sensitive (Drennan 2002; Willis 2005). Questionnaire length in relation to time for completion should not exceed circa 20 minutes or problems with low response rates can occur.

Sources of error and bias

Conducting a survey can be challenging: error and bias can arise in relation to problems relating to sampling and recruitment, attrition, response rates, respondents' characteristics and behaviours. This is not an exhaustive error checklist: readers will find more detailed information in specialist survey texts (Schonlau et al. 2002; Czaja and Blair 2005; Fowler 2009) which are recommended further reading at the end of this chapter.

Missing data

Sampling frameworks should ensure that subgroups in a population are represented in the sample data accurately reflecting their representation in the population from which the sample was drawn. If under-representation occurs, weighting of questionnaire responses can be performed to adjust for different probabilities of selection. Statistical weighting procedures can also be used to adjust for non-response and non-coverage. Further details of these weighting methods are described in the guidelines for household surveys published by the United Nations Statistics Division (2005).

One of the major challenges which can arise in longitudinal studies (panel and prospective cohort) is sample attrition over time, causes of which were discussed earlier in this chapter. The impact of attrition can be serious in terms of loss of representativeness of the sample ('healthy survivor effect') and the potential for statistical error. Strategies to minimize sample attrition and maintain participant commitment include initial personal meetings with researchers at the outset of the study, the maintenance of frequent contact with participants (feedback on progress), setting in place arrangements for notification of change of address (prepaid postcards) and ensuring that intervals between successive periods of data collection are not too lengthy. In highly mobile populations (developing countries) rigorous tracking procedures are necessary to reduce substantial attrition in panel studies (Hill 2004). Attention to the strategies summarized below, which minimize unit and item non-response, are also vital. Where possible, details of drop-outs (demographic details, reason for attrition) should be documented for inclusion in analyses and results. In terms of making statistical comparisons at successive time points, unless sample attrition is very small, these should be made between participants who took part at each stage of data collection. This can have the effect of introducing bias due to the 'healthy survivor' effect; thus, analyses should also be completed on drop-outs to ascertain whether any differences exist between them and the remaining sample – this can help to modify bias. (See also Robinson and Marsland 1994; British Household Panel Study 2011.)

Unit and item non-response

Response rate is the number of eligible sample members who complete a questionnaire (postal or electronic) or structured interview (telephone or face to face) divided by the total number of eligible sample members, expressed as a percentage. Although researchers aspire and strive to obtain answers from all the sample units, together with answers to every item on a questionnaire or structured interview, the reality is that some of the sample will not return the questionnaire (unit non-response) or refuse to take part in an interview. Of those who do return questionnaires or take part in structured interviews, a proportion may decide not to answer every question (item non-response). Missing data at either of these levels can exert serious effects on data quality, for example by introducing bias (for respondents may differ from non-respondents) and raising the possibility of statistical error though reduction of effective sample size and power in the analysis stage. How can such problems be attenuated and what corrective measures are available? Furthermore, what is an acceptable response rate (RR)? Opinions vary, but Kelley et al. (2003) suggest that this is 75 per cent for interviews and 65 per cent for self-completion questionnaires. In contrast, Fowler (2009) cites a standard of >80 per cent based on specific government requirements in the USA, where an RR below this level requires a non-response analysis. Where unit non-response is high, attempting to assess the direction and magnitude of bias in the sample by contacting and characterizing the non-respondents, for example in relation to demographic characteristics, can be helpful in assisting interpretation. However, it may not be possible to do this for a number of reasons: for example, time, resources and ethical issues can be constraining.

Unit non-response – questionnaires

Strategies most frequently cited to improve unit response rates are to send two to three re-mailings (electronic or postal) of questionnaires to non-respondents, and to ensure rigorous pretesting prior to distribution through pilot fieldwork (obtaining feedback on content, structure and utility from participant focus groups, expert panel review). Cognitive interviewing can also benefit both unit (and item) non-response by identifying problematic questions in pretesting with a sample of respondents; this approach appears to be most helpful in pretesting questions which can be complex, sensitive and intrusive (Drennan 2002; Willis 2005).

A Cochrane Review (Edwards et al. 2008), conducted to identify strategies to increase responses to postal and electronic questionnaires, has generated findings which have important implications for questionnaire design, recruitment strategies, resources and funding. With regard to **postal** questionnaires, findings were that strategies likely either to increase or reduce the odds of response at different levels included:

- Increased response: monetary incentives, use of recorded delivery, envelope teasers and a greater level of topic interest, use of prenotification, follow-up contact, shorter questionnaires, unconditional incentives, obligations to respond and university sponsorship, use of stamped addressed envelopes and assurances on confidentiality.
- Reduced response: inclusion of sensitive topics.

In relation to **electronic** questionnaires Edwards et al. (2008) also found that the following were likely either to increase or reduce odds of response:

- Increased response: a picture included with an email, use of non-monetary incentives, shorter questionnaires, interesting topic, using a white background, the offer of notification of survey results, textual formatting of response categories.
- Reduced response: use of the term 'survey', gender of email signatory (male).

The influence of survey mode (postal, email or website) is also relevant to the issue of non-response. A meta-analysis of comparative studies by Shih and Fan (2008) found that response rates for paper questionnaires resulted in a 10 per cent higher response rate than web-based questionnaires. In contrast, other investigations have suggested equivalence between the two modes of approach. Ritter et al. (2004), Dillman (2007) and Balter et al. (2005) found in comparing web-based and mailed questionnaires that interactivity in web-based research could increase retention and completion.

In recent years the mixed-mode survey has become popular, in which two or more modes are used to collect a single dataset with the intention of increasing response rates. This can be approached in different ways, for example distributing a first wave of mailed questionnaires followed up by web mode for non-respondents, or allowing respondents a choice with regard to mode. However, concerns have arisen with regard to a possible 'mode effect' occurring where responses and content of returned questionnaires differs between modes: this creates problems where data need to be combined into a single dataset, for it is vital to know that respondents provide the same answers irrespective of mode used (Borkan 2010). An experimental crossover study by Borkan (2010) utilizing questionnaires found that web surveys had lower unit response rates than mail surveys and that web survey respondents were significantly younger; however, item non-response was not affected by survey mode. In contrast, Guise et al. (2010) found that while mixed-mode design increased overall unit response rates, significant differences were present between responses to emailed, paper and web-based questionnaires. Implications are that researchers need to consider the potential for the 'mode effect' in the planning stages of survey design.

Item non-response – questionnaires

Approaches to reduce questionnaire item non-response include the conduct of rigorous pretesting of pilot questionnaires on a representative subsample of the population, to ensure wording lacks ambiguity, and the format and order of questions has clarity and continuity. Cognitive interviewing may also improve item response (see Drennan 2002). It is also vital to ensure during pretesting that instructions on questionnaire completion which include clarity relating to any 'skip details' for individual questions are clear and unambiguous. At the data-analysis stage, Fowler (2009) has suggested that if item non-response is <5 per cent, then the potential for this to impact negatively is small, so this could require no further action by the researcher. However, if the level of non-response on items is much higher, then decisions could be either to omit respondents' questionnaires, or to attempt to estimate what answers they would have given: this is usually done by substituting the average answer for the missing value. This has the advantage of keeping all the respondents in an analysis, reducing any negative impact on requirements for statistical analysis. In reviewing item non-response, it is also important to check that errors in coding and entering data have not occurred, through rigorous, independent checking.

Unit and item non-response – interviews

Whether using telephone or face-to-face approaches, interviewers require a high level of interpersonal and technical skills to ensure that they access the population of interest effectively, achieve recruitment and conduct an interview which yields quality data in terms of the survey purpose. Factors which can impact positively on interview unit non-response apart from interviewer interpersonal skills include cash incentives, letters sent in advance of the study, interview guidelines and protocols and effective interviewer training related to telephone and face-to-face situations. High levels of contacts are usually necessary to recruit to telephone interviews. As described earlier in this chapter, computerized systems are now commonly used to record structured telephone (CATI) and personal interviews (CAPI); errors in data entry can lead to item non-response, hence the needs for training and institution of quality procedures to monitor response rates and check the reliability of data entry. In-depth information on effective interviewer selection, training and monitoring is provided in Fowler (2009) and Czaja and Blair (2005).

Differences in response styles

In the responses to questionnaires utilizing Likert scales, it should not be assumed that all respondents base their answers solely on the question content: in fact, responses can also be affected by participants' response styles. 'Response style' has been defined as 'the systematic inclination of responders to answer questions based on some unknown effect other than the content of the question (Paulhus 1991: 19). Common examples of response styles include acquiescence and disaquiescence – that is, a tendency to agree or disagree with an item irrespective of the content. In contrast, extreme and middle response styles are the respective tendencies to use extreme end points of scales or only the middle rating points. An unwanted consequence of response styles is that they can confound interpretations of scores and introduce bias. Differences in response style have been attributed to age, gender, personality, scale format and item ambiguity (Baumgartner and Steenkamp 2001).

The influence of personality traits on response styles has been investigated in a number of studies, and models have been developed to explain relationships between response styles and psychological traits: Bolt and Johnson (2009), for example, have proposed a multidimensional model which permits the investigation and control of response styles in ordered rating data to control bias. However, the potential for cultural characteristics also to influence response styles has been examined in a 26-country study by Harzing (2006); findings confirmed patterns of response styles noted in earlier studies, demonstrating that major differences existed between countries. Notably, country-level characteristics of power – distance, collectivism, uncertainty avoidance, and extraversion – all exerted a significant difference on acquiescence and extreme response styles. The language in which questionnaires were presented was also shown to influence response styles: more extreme responses were associated with a participant's native language while those presented in the English language elicited greater middle response styles. Harzing (2006) has drawn attention to the challenges these findings pose for researchers conducting cross-cultural surveys using questionnaires.

Approaches to remove or reduce the effects of response styles have included standardization methods used to remove bias associated with scale response: 'standardization is a process of data transformation which involves correction of scores of estimated attributes or cases using either means, or standard deviations or both' Pagolu and Chakraborty (2011: 2). Fischer (2004) has appraised different standardization methods and drawn attention to the challenges inherent in using them. Other approaches have included attention to questionnaire design, for example: to consider using ranking statements instead of Likert scales where ordering is appropriate; using a mix of positive and negative statements which requires participants to think more carefully about the question to reduce acquiescence/disaquiescence; and attenuating the effect of extreme response styles by extending the number of categories in Likert scales. Translation issues are also important: Harzing (2006) has drawn attention to the point that scale anchor terms can be difficult to translate and that translations may not result in metric equivalence – careful investigation of this is vital for researchers using questionnaire translations in different cultural settings.

Conclusion

This chapter has reviewed a range of issues relevant to the planning, design and conduct of a survey, with a focus on the use of quantitative methods. Contemporary survey approaches encompass cross-sectional and longitudinal studies which can utilize a diverse range of quantitative methods, including questionnaires and structured interviews. Modes of delivery can now include email and website, in addition to postal, telephone and face-to-face approaches. Whatever the methods and delivery modes chosen, conducting a survey can be challenging: error, and more specifically bias, can arise in relation to sampling and recruitment, attrition, response rates, respondents' characteristics and behaviours. Many of these challenges can be minimized at the outset through rigorous planning which addresses quality, legal and ethical issues, selection of appropriate data-collection methods and mode, together with the development of strategies to maximize access to the study population and minimize bias.

Key concepts

- **Survey approaches:** cross-sectional and longitudinal approaches can be either retrospective or prospective; cross-sectional design precludes the attribution of causality, whereas sample attrition, ageing, increased funding costs and the Hawthorne effect can pose challenges for longitudinal design.
- **Validity and reliability:** in relation to method, establishing internal validity (content, criterion-related, construct), external validity (generalizability of findings based on sampling framework, approach and size) and reliability (consistency, stability, dependability) are intrinsic to achieving a high-quality, rigorous design.
- **Error and bias:** these can arise, for example, where a sample obtained is not representative of the population of interest, or through unit and item non-response, response styles and interviewer skills. Effective planning, conduct of pilot studies, construction of a rigorous sampling framework, probability sampling, implementing measures to reduce statistical error, use of cognitive interviewing, attention to methodological design and creation of incentives are vital.
- **Response styles:** differences in response styles can confound interpretation of survey data; standardization, attention to elements of questionnaire design and translation (where appropriate) can reduce the impact of response styles.

Key readings on survey research

- R. Czaja and J. Blair, *Designing Surveys: A Guide to Decisions and Procedures*, 2nd edn (London: Pine Forge Press, 2005)
  Good resource on survey design and decision making through all stages of design implementation.
- F.J. Fowler, *Survey Research Methods* (London: Sage, 2009)
  Good overview on survey design, mainly quantitative methods.
- E. Saris and I.N. Gallhofer, *Design, Evaluation and Analysis of Questionnaires* (Chichester: Wiley, 2007)
  Invaluable resource on questionnaire design.
- N. Watson and M. Wooden, *Methodology of Longitudinal Surveys* (Chichester: John Wiley, 2009)
  An excellent guide to developing and completing different types of longitudinal surveys.

Examples of studies utilizing cross-sectional or longitudinal survey designs

- L.H. Aiken, W. Sermeus, K. Van den Heede, D.M. Sloane, R. Busse, M. McKee, L. Bruyneel, A.M. Rafferty, P. Griffiths, M.T. Moreno-Casbas, C. Tishelman, A. Scott, T. Brzostek, J. Kinnunen, R. Schwendimann, M. Heinen, D. Zikos, I. Strømseng Sjetne, H.L. Smith and A. Kutney-Lee, Patient safety, satisfaction and quality of hospital care: Cross sectional surveys of nurses and patients in 12 countries in Europe and the United States, *British Medical Journal*, 344 (2012), e1717
- M. Ashworth, J. Medina and M. Morgan, Effect of social deprivation on blood pressure monitoring and control in England: A survey of data from the Quality and Outcomes Framework, *British Medical Journal*, 337 (2008), a2030
- C.S. Brewer, C.T. Kovner, W. Greene, M. Tukor-Shuser and M. Djukic, Predictors of actual turnover in a national sample of newly licensed registered nurses employed in hospitals, *Journal of Advanced Nursing*, 68(3) (2012), 521–38
- E. McCaughan, O. McSorley, G. Prue, G. Parahoo, B. Bunting, J.O. Sullivan and H. McKenna, Quality of life in men receiving radiotherapy and neoadjuvant androgen deprivation for prostate cancer: Results from a prospective longitudinal study, *Journal of Advanced Nursing* online (2012), doi:10.1111/j. 1365-2648.2012.05987x
- G.J. Rubin, R. Amlot, L. Page and S. Wessely, Public perceptions, anxiety and behaviour change in relation to swine flu outbreak: Cross sectional telephone survey, *British Medical Journal*, 339 (2009), b2651
- N. Steel, M. Bachmann, S. Maisey, P. Shekelle, E. Breeze, M. Marmot and D. Melzer, Self reported receipt of care consistent with 32 quality indicators: National population survey of adults aged 50 or more in England, *British Medical Journal*, 337 (2008), a957

Useful websites

- http://www.nationalarchives.gov.uk
- http://www.nationalarchives.ie
- http://www.domesdaybook.co.uk
- http://www.manstatsoc.org
- **http://booth.lse.ac.uk/static/a/2.html**
- http://unstats.un.org/unsd/demographic/sources/surveys/Handbook23June05.pdf
- **http://the-sra.org.uk.resources/research-ethics/ethics-guidelines**
- **http://the-sra.org.uk/wp-content/uploads/safety_code_of_practice.pdf**
- http://www.bps.org.uk/publications/policy-guidelines/research-guidelines

References

Baird, C. (2000) Taking the mystery out of research: The pilot study, *Orthopaedic Nursing*, 19(2): 42–3.

Barnett, V. (1974) *Elements of Sampling Theory*. London: English University Press.

Balter, K.A., Balter, O., Fondell, E. and Lagerros, Y.T. (2005) Web-based and mailed question-naires: A comparison of response rates and compliance, *Epidemiology*, 16(4): 577–9.

Bartlett, J.E., Kotrlik, J.W. and Higgins, C.C. (2001) Organisational research: Determination of sample size in survey research, *Information Technology and Performance Journal*, 19(1): 43–53.

Baumgartner, J.E.M. and Steenkamp, H. (2001) Response style in marketing research: A cross national investigation, *Journal of Marketing Research*, 38(2): 143–56.

Bergman, M. (2008) *Advances in Mixed Methods Research: Theories and Applications.* London: Sage.

Bohannon, R.W., Maljanian, R. and Landes, M. (2004) Test–retest reliability of short form SF-12 component scores of patients with stroke, *International Journal of Rehabilitation Research*, 27(2): 149–50.

Bolt, D.M. and Johnson, T.R. (2009) Addressing score bias and differential item functioning due to individual differences in response style, *Applied Psychological Measurement*, 33(5): 335–52.

Borkan, B. (2010) The mode effect in mixed mode surveys, *Social Science Computer Review*, 28(3): 371–80.

Brannen, J. (2008) The practice of a mixed methods research strategy: Personal, professional and project considerations, in M. Bergman (ed.) *Advances in Mixed Methods Research: Theories and Applications.* London: Sage, pp. 53–65.

British Household Panel Survey (2011) http://www.iser.essex.ac.uk/bhps [Accessed November 2011].

British Psychological Association (2007) *Conducting Research on the Internet: Guidelines for Ethical Practice in Psychological Research.* Leicester: The British Psychological Society. Available at http://www.bps.org.uk/publications/policy-guidelines/research-guidelines [Accessed February 2012].

Brown, T.A. (2006) *Confirmatory Factor Analysis for Applied Research.* New York: The Guilford Press.

Cohen, J. (1988) *Statistical Power Analysis for Behavioural Sciences*, 2nd edn. New York: Academic Press.

Cooper, C., Blanchard, M., Walker, Z., Blizzard, R. and Livingston, G. (2009) Abuse of people with dementia by family carers: A representative cross sectional survey, *British Medical Journal*, 338, bmj.b155.

Cresswell, J.W. and Plano Clark, V.L. (2007) *Designing and Conducting Mixed Methods Research.* Thousand Oaks, CA: Sage.

Cronbach, L.J. (1951) Coefficient alpha and the internal structure of tests, *Psychometrica*, 16(3): 297–334.

Curtis, E. and Redmond, R. (2009) Survey postal questionnaire: Optimizing response and dealing with non-response, *Nurse Researcher*, 16(2): 76–88.

Czaja, R. and Blair, J. (2005) *Designing Surveys: A Guide to Decisions and Procedures*, 2nd edn. London: Pine Forge Press.

Department of Health (2011) *National Diet and Nutrition Survey.* London: Department of Health. Available at http://www.dh.gov.uk/en/Publicationsandstatistics/Publications/Publications Statistics/DH_128166 [Accessed November 2011].

De Vellis, R.F. (2003) *Scale Development: Theory and Applications.* Thousand Oaks, CA: Sage.

Dillman, D.A. (2007) *Mail and Internet Surveys: The Tailored Design Method*, 2nd edn. New York: John Wiley.

Drennan, J. (2002) Cognitive Interviewing: Verbal Data in the Design and Pretesting of Questionnaires, *Journal of Advanced Nursing*, 42(1): 57–63.

Edwards, P.J., Roberts, I., Clarke, M.J., DiGuiseppi, C., Wentz, R., Kwan, I., Cooper, R., Felix, L.M. and Pratap, S. (2008) Methods to increase response to postal and electronic questionnaires, *Cochrane Database of Systematic Reviews*, 3 MR000008, doi: 1002/1465858.pub4.

Fischer, R. (2004) Standardisation to account for cross cultural response bias: A classification of score adjustment procedures, *Journal of Cross Cultural Psychology*, 35(3): 263–82.

Fowler, F. J. (2009) *Survey Research Methods*. London: Sage.

Guise, V., Chambers, M., Valimaki, M. and Makkonen, P. (2010) A mixed mode approach to data collection: Combining web and paper questionnaires to examine nurses' attitudes to mental illness, *Journal of Advanced Nursing*, 66(7): 1623–32.

Haw, S.J. and Gruer, L. (2007) Changes in adult non–smokers' exposure to secondhand smoke in public and private places, *British Medical Journal*, 335: 549.

Harpham, T., Huttly, S., Wilson, I. and De Wet, T. (2003) Linking public issues with private troubles: Panel studies in developing countries, *Journal of International Development*, 15(3): 253–363.

Harzing, A. (2006) Response styles in cross national survey research, *International Journal of Cross Cultural Management*, 6(2): 243–66.

Hill, Z. (2004) Reducing attrition in panel studies in developing countries, *International Journal of Epidemiology*, 33(3): 493–8.

Huntington, A., Gilmour, J., Schluter, P., Tuckett, A., Bogossian, F. and Turner, C. (2009) The internet as a research site: Establishment of a web-based longitudinal study of the nursing and midwifery workforce in three countries, *Journal of Advanced Nursing*, 65(6): 1309–17.

Kelley, K., Clark, B., Brown, V. and Sitzia, J. (2003) Good practice in the conduct and reporting of survey research, *International Journal for Quality in Health Care*, 15(3): 261–6.

Lyratzopoulos, G., Barbiere, J.M., Greenberg, D.C., Wright, K.A. and Neal, D.E. (2010) Population-based time trends and socioeconomic variation in use of radiotherapy and radical surgery for prostate cancer in a UK region: A continuous survey, *British Medical Journal*, 340, bmj.c1928.

Medical Research Council National Survey of Health and Development (2009) http://www.nshd.mrc.ac.uk/nshd.aspx [Accessed November 2011].

Morgan, D.L. (2007) Paradigms lost and pragmatism regained: Methodological implications of combining qualitative and quantitative methods, *Journal of Mixed Methods Research*, 1(1): 48–76.

Musselwhite, K., Cuff, L., McGregor, L. and King, K.M. (2007) The telephone interview is an effective method of data collection in clinical nursing research: A discussion paper, *International Journal of Nursing Studies*, 44(6): 1064–70.

Ostlund, U., Kidd, L., Wengstrom, Y. and Rowa-Dewar, N. (2011) Combining qualitative and quantitative research within mixed methods research designs: A methodological review, *International Journal of Nursing Studies*, 48(3): 369–83.

Pagolu, M.K. and Chakraborty, G. (2011) *Eliminating Response style Segments in Survey Data via Double Standardization Before Clustering*. Paper 165, SAS Global Forum on Data Mining and Text Analytics, USA. Available at http://support.sas.com/resources/papers/proceedings11/165-2011.pdf [Accessed February 2012].

Paulhus, D.C. (1991) Measuring and correcting respondent behaviour, in J.P. Robinson, P.R. Shower and L.S. Wrightman (eds) *Measures of Personality and Data Transformation Methods: Social and Psychological Attitudes*, vol 1. San Diego: Academic Press.

Polit, D.F. and Beck, C.T. (2006) *Research Manual for Nursing Research: Generating and Assessing Evidence for Nursing Practice*. Philadelphia: Lippincott Williams & Wilkins.

Price, J.H., Dake, J.A., Murran, J., Dimming, J. and Akpanudi, S. (2005) Power analysis in survey research: Importance and use for health educators, *American Journal of Health Education*, 36(4): 202–7.

Ritter, P., Lorig, K., Laurent, D. and Mathews, K. (2004) Internet versus mailed questionnaires: A randomized comparison, *Journal of Medical Internet Research*, 6(3): 29e.

Robinson, S. and Marsland, L. (1994) Approaches to the problem of respondent attrition in a longitudinal panel study of nurses' careers, *Journal of Advanced Nursing*, 20(4): 729–41.

Robinson, S.M., Mackenzie-Ross, S., Campbell-Hewson, G., Egleston, C.V. and Prevost, A.T. (1998) Psychological effect of witnessed resuscitation on bereaved relatives, *Lancet*, 352(9128): 614–17.

Rothberg, M., Arora, A., Visintainer, P., Herman, J., Kleppel, R. and St Marie, P. (2010) Phantom vibration syndrome in medical staff: A cross sectional survey, *British Medical Journal*, 341, bmj.c6914.

Salant, P. and Dillman, D. (1994) *How to Conduct Your Own Survey*. New York: John Wiley.

Sale, J.E.M., Lohfeld, L.H. and Brazil, K. (2002) Revisiting the quantitative–qualitative debate: Implications for mixed methods research, *Quality and Quantity*, 36(1): 43–53.

Sapsford, R. (2007) *Survey Research*. London: Sage.

Saris, E. and Gallhofer, I.N. (2007) *Design, Evaluation and Analysis of Questionnaires*. Chichester: Wiley.

Scheidel, N. (2009) *Rome and China: Comparative Perspectives on Ancient World Empires*. Oxford: Oxford University Press.

Schonlau, M., Fricker, R.D. and Elliot, M. (2002) *Conducting Research Surveys via E-mail and the Web*. Santa Monica: RAND.

Shih, T. and Fan, X. (2008) Comparing response rates from web and mail surveys: A meta-analysis, *Field Methods*, 20(3): 249–71.

Streiner, D.L. and Norman, G. R. (2008) *Health Measurement Scales: A Practical Guide to Development*, 4th edn. Oxford: Oxford University Press.

Smith, E.M. (2005) Telephone interviewing in healthcare research: Summary of the evidence, *Nurse Researcher*, 12(3): 32–41.

Social Research Association (2003) *Staying Safe: A Code of Practice for the Safety of Social Researchers*. Available at http://the-sra.org.uk.resources/research-ethics/ethics-guidelines [Accessed March 2013].

Stewart, S. (2003) Casting the net: Using the internet for research, *British Journal of Midwifery*, 11(9): 543–6.

Twitchett, D., Loewe, M. and Fairbank, J.K. (1986) *The Cambridge History of China: The Ch'in and Han Empires 221BC–AD220*. Cambridge: Cambridge University Press.

United Nations Statistics Division (2005) *Designing Household Survey Samples: Practical Guidelines*. Series F 98. Department of Social and Economic Affairs Statistics Division. Available at http://unstats.un.org/unsd/demographic/sources/surveys/Handbook23June05.pdf [Accessed February 2012].

van Teijlingen, E.R., Rennie, A.M., Hundley, V. and Graham, W. (2000) The importance of conducting and reporting pilot studies: The example of the Scottish births survey, *Journal of Advanced Nursing*, 34(3): 289–94.

Watson, N. and Wooden, M. (2009) *Methodology of Longitudinal Surveys*. Chichester: Wiley.

Watts, G. (2011) In for the long haul, *British Medical Journal*, 342, bmj.d942.

Weitzel, M.H. (1990) Cutting the costs of survey research: Third class bulk and business reply mail, *Applied Nursing Research*, 2(2): 80–3.

Westerlund, H., Vahtera, J., Ferrie, J.E., Singh Marona, A., Pentti, J., Meldicor, M., Johela, M., Leinweber, C., Siegrist, J., Goldberg, M., Zins, M. and Kirimaki, M. (2010) Effects of retirement on major chronic conditions and fatigue: The French GAZEL occupational cohort study, *British Medical Journal*, 341, bmj.c6149.

Whittaker, A. (2009) *Research Skills for Social Work*. Exeter: Learning Methods.

Willis, G.B. (2005) *Cognitive Interviewing*. California: Sage.

11 Quasi-experimental and retrospective pretest designs for health care research

Jonathan Drennan

Chapter topics

- Quasi-experimental designs
- Internal validity
- Quasi-experimental designs in health care research
- Patient-reported outcomes
- Self-reports of change
- Pretest–posttest designs
- Response shift in health care research
- Controlling response shift
- Retrospective pretest designs

Introduction

Increasingly, health care interventions and treatments are becoming more complex and researchers need to have access to designs that will allow them to effectively measure and evaluate these innovations. This chapter discusses two designs that researchers can use when it is not feasible or ethical to use a randomized controlled trial (RCT). These designs are quasi-experimental designs and the retrospective pretest design. Both designs are approaches that can be used in the field and are increasingly being used in health care research.

The first section discusses quasi-experimental designs. This design is similar in many respects to randomized controlled trials, the fundamental difference being that subjects are not randomly allocated to the intervention or control group. This section of the chapter provides an overview of the design as well as outlining the various types of quasi-experimental designs that are available to health care researchers. In understanding the advantages and disadvantages of quasi-experimental designs it is important to have an understanding of the concept of internal validity and how threats to the internal validity of a study can impact on claims made about the outcomes of an intervention. Therefore, the threats to internal validity are also discussed. Examples of quasi-experimental designs used in health care research are provided throughout the chapter.

The second section reports on an approach that is increasingly being used in health care research to measure the extent to which patients change over the course of a treatment. This approach is known as the retrospective pretest design and is sometimes used in conjunction with a quasi-experimental design. This section also outlines the concept of response shift as it pertains to patient change. An understanding of response shift is important in understanding the rationale for using retrospective pretests. This section also provides an overview of the growing recognition of taking response shift into account when measuring patient change, and provides examples of response shift identified in health care research. Examples of how retrospective pretests, also known as thentests, are used in health care research are also outlined.

Quasi-experimental designs

This section outlines a design that can be used when it is not feasible or ethical to use a randomized control design (see Chapter 8). This design is known as a quasi-experimental design and, although similar in many respects to a true experimental approach, has a number of limitations, especially in relation to threats to the internal validity of a study (see Box 11.1 below). However, a well-constructed quasi-experimental study can provide evidence of the effect of an independent variable on an outcome. At a fundamental level, a quasi-experimental design differs from a true experimental design or randomized controlled trial in that there is no random assignment of subjects to a treatment or control group. As in randomized controlled trials, the independent variable is manipulated in quasi-experimental designs. The effect of this manipulation is then measured on the dependent or outcome variable (Shadish et al. 2002).

Shadish et al. (2002: 13–14) outline both the similarities and fundamental difference between quasi-experimental designs and true experiments:

> Quasi-experiments share with all other experiments a similar purpose – to test descriptive causal hypotheses about manipulative causes – as well as many structural details, such as the frequent presence of control groups and pretest measures, to support a counterfactual inference about what would have happened in the absence of treatment. But, by definition, quasi-experiments lack random assignment.

The fact that subjects are not randomly assigned to an intervention or control group could mean that groups differ on a number of factors (for example education level, social class or health status) and it is these factors rather than the intervention that explain the outcome.

Take, for example, two groups of surgical patients. One group, the intervention group, in Ward A, received an innovative pain control measure post-operatively. The second group, the control group, in Ward B, received the usual pain control care post-operatively. Patients were **not** randomly assigned to Ward A or B. If the intervention group at the end of the study report lower pain scores than the control group, can we say this occurred as a consequence of the intervention, or did other factors intervene? What other factors might have impacted on the observed outcome? Take a few minutes to write down these factors and then compare them to those in Box 11.1. Would these issues have occurred if we had randomly allocated patients to either the control or intervention groups? Probably not, as randomization would have ensured, to a greater or lesser extent, that both groups were equal.

Shadish et al. (2002: 105) highlight that causal relationships, including those measured through quasi-experimental designs, must meet three criteria: 'that cause precede effect, that cause covary with effect, and that alternative explanations for causal relationships are implausible'. This last aspect can be difficult to discern in quasi-experimental designs due to the fact that subjects are not randomly allocated to an intervention or control group; as Pedhazur and Schmelkin (1991: 277) state, 'the researcher is faced with the task of identifying and separating the effects of the treatment from the effects of all other factors affecting the dependent variable'. The main issue with quasi-experimental designs are the threats that can occur to the internal validity of a study through the use of this approach. This is an important aspect of quasi-experimental design and it is therefore important before we discuss these designs in detail to have an understanding of the concept of internal validity.

Internal validity

Internal validity 'refers to the validity of assertions regarding the effects of the independent variable(s) on the dependent variable(s)' (Pedhazur and Schmelkin 1991: 224). In effect the internal validity of a study answers the following question: was it the manipulated intervention or treatment (independent variable) that resulted in the observed outcome (dependent variable) or was the outcome caused by variables other than those manipulated?

As would be expected, due to the fact that in experimental and quasi-experimental research variables are manipulated, these types of studies have greater internal validity than non-experimental designs (Pedhazur and Schmelkin 1991). The principal reason that quasi-experimental designs have greater threats to internal validity than RCTs is, among other things, the lack of random allocation of subjects to either the intervention or control group. When randomized controlled trials are compared to quasi-experimental designs, by their very nature RCTs make a stronger case that the independent variable resulted in the observed change in the dependent variable than do quasi-experimental studies (Gliner et al. 2009). There are a number of threats to internal validity, and these are outlined in Box 11.1. An understanding of these will help in understanding the strengths and weaknesses of various quasi-experimental designs available to researchers.

Box 11.1 Threats to the internal validity of a study (Pedhazur and Schmelkin 1991; Shadish et al. 2002)

History 'refers to all events that occur between the beginning of the treatment and the posttest that could have produced the observed outcome in the absence of that treatment' (Shadish et al. 2002: 56). Take an example of an educational programme to encourage appropriate attendance at emergency departments among the general public. At the same time as the programme is launched, but not part of the intervention, a monetary charge is introduced for patients who attend an emergency department with a minor injury or illness. At the end of the study we find, when pretest and posttest scores have been compared, that there has been a drop in inappropriate attendances. However, to what extent was the change in attendance a result of the intervention or the introduction of the charge? The introduction of the monetary charge was a threat to the internal validity of this study. In effect, events external to a study can affect observed outcomes.

Maturation: participants in a research study naturally change and mature over time. Examples of changes include growing older, becoming more experienced or changes in a person's living situation. These changes could, rather than the treatment or intervention, affect the observed outcome. Take, for example, a health programme to facilitate the development of coping skills for adolescents with type 1 diabetes. Teenagers, as they mature, may develop skills to cope with their diabetes even without an intervention.

Testing: exposure to a test during the pretest phase of a study may impact on responses collected at the posttest phase. Take, for example, an intervention to reduce incidences of elder abuse in care settings. Exposure to questions during the pretest phase may change respondents' perceptions of what constitutes elder abuse at the posttest phase. It was exposure to the pretest questionnaire that led to attitude change and not the intervention. To counter this, Shadish et al. (2002) suggest using the Solomon Four Group Design where some participants receive a pretest and others do not. In this way it can be assessed whether the pretest impacted on the results of the posttest.

Instrumentation: the method or way an instrument is administered during a study may change over time. In addition, the instrument itself may change between the pretest and posttest. For example an instrument used to collect physiological data, such as heart rate, may be recalibrated between the pretest and posttest, leading to non-comparable measures. Data collectors may become more efficient in using an instrument over time and their ratings of behaviour become more proficient.

Regression towards the mean 'is a statistical phenomenon that occurs between any two imperfectly correlated variables' (Sweeney 2004: 945). Basically, observations that are high (or low) on one variable are also likely to be high (or low) on the second variable, but less so. We often select subjects for an intervention because they perform well or, as is most often the case, lowly on a measure (for example a group of patients who have very poor compliance with long-term medication). If patients who were measured as being poorly compliant at time 1 are then measured again at a later point in time, it is likely that their compliance scores will not be as poor as those measured at time 1 – even without an intervention. It is important to note that regression to the mean tends to occur when we choose subjects with extreme scores on the variable of interest. For example, if we choose patients with severe psychological distress to be part of our study, their distress may lessen over time even without an intervention.

Selection: this refers to how participants are selected for both the treatment and control groups. If the characteristics of participants in one group are different from those in the other, the differences observed at the end of an intervention may be due to these group differences rather than the treatment. Take again, for example, an educational programme to facilitate glycaemic control in adolescents with type 1 diabetes. Participants in the intervention group (that is, those who receive the educational programme) are chosen from clinic A and those in the control group (those who receive standard care) are from clinic B; participants are not randomly assigned to either group. The characteristics of participants in clinic A could be different from those in clinic B in that they have a higher education level, better social support, diet and higher family income. Due to this selection bias, participants in clinic A may achieve better glycaemic control than those in clinic B, even without the intervention. This form of selection bias can be

controlled for through random assignment to either treatment or control groups. However, as we shall see, random assignment does not occur in quasi-experimental designs
and selection is a threat to the internal validity of quasi-experimental studies.

   Attrition: refers to participants who drop out of a study; this is more likely to be seen
in longitudinal studies. For example, a study to facilitate glycaemic control in patients
with type 2 diabetes may find that subjects with poor control are more likely to drop
out of the study; therefore only those patients who are motivated remain. The results
identified in the posttest could be due to the attritional rates and the profile of those who
remain in the study and not the intervention.

Types of quasi-experimental designs

There are several types of quasi-experimental designs; these include:

- one-group pretest–posttest design[1]
- non-equivalent control group designs[1]
- interrupted time series design[1]
- regression discontinuity design – the researcher uses 'a cut-off score on a
  measured variable to determine eligibility for treatment, and an effect is
  observed if the regression line of the assignment variable on outcome for the
  treatment group is discontinuous from that of the comparison group' (Shadish and Clark 2004: 899)
- case-control design – 'one participant is observed repeatedly over time while
  the scheduling and dose treatment are manipulated to demonstrate that
  treatment controls outcome' (Shadish and Clark 2004: 899)

One-group pretest–posttest design

This is probably the most straightforward of all quasi-experimental designs. The format for this type of design is outlined in Figure 11.1.

$$O_1 \qquad X \qquad O_2$$

Figure 11.1   One-group pretest–posttest design (Shadish et al. 2002).

   The notation in Figure 11.1 is as follows: O_1 is the observation of the outcome of
interest prior to the intervention (pretest); X is the intervention or treatment; and O_2

---

[1]The discussion of all types of quasi-experimental designs is beyond the scope of this book;
therefore only the three most common designs – one-group pretest–posttest design, the non-
equivalent control group design and the interrupted time series design – will be discussed.
Interested readers are referred to Shadish et al.'s (2002) excellent book that covers in detail the
various types of quasi-experimental designs used in research.

is the measurement of the dependent variable (outcome) after the intervention (post-test). In theory, if there is a statistical difference between O_1 and O_2, the intervention had an effect; however, as we will see later, there are a number of problems with this conclusion. The subjects at time 1 (O_1) can be the same subjects as those at time 2 (O_2) (this is known as a 'within-participants' design), or they can be different (known as a 'between-participants' design) (Shadish et al. 2002).

As can be seen in the notation in Figure 11.1, this quasi-experimental design lacks a control group and the only comparison on the effectiveness or otherwise of the intervention is between pretest (O_1) and posttest (O_2). Therefore, it may not be the intervention that had an effect on the outcome of interest but a multitude of other factors, or confounding variables could have intervened (Shadish et al. 2002; Gliner et al. 2009). The main threats to the internal validity of this type of design are history, regression to the mean, instrumentation and maturation (Shadish et al. 2002; Kirk 2009; Reichardt 2009); that is, the outcome observed at O_2 may not have occurred as a result of the treatment but due to some other factor or confounding variable.

In spite of the limitations of this design, it is in many cases the only approach available to researchers; however it is recommended that results from these studies be treated with caution (Eccles et al. 2003). Shadish et al. (2002) recommend that the one-group pretest–posttest design can be improved by adding an extra pretest; therefore the design would look like that outlined in the notation in Figure 11.2.

$$O_1 \qquad O_2 \qquad X \qquad O_3$$

Figure 11.2 One-group pretest–posttest design with an added pretest (Shadish et al. 2002: 110).

There are a number of examples of one-group pretest–posttest designs used to evaluate health outcomes in the literature. For example, Vrijhoef et al. (2002) used this type of quasi-experimental design to evaluate the effect of a diabetes nurse specialist on a number of patient outcomes, including glycaemic control, patient satisfaction and quality of life for patients with type 2 diabetes in a primary care setting (see Box 11.2). A similar design was used by Waters and Raisler (2003) to measure the effectiveness of ice massage to reduce labour pain. Calabro et al. (2002) also used a one-group pretest–posttest design to evaluate the effectiveness of a training programme for mental health care workers in managing and preventing patient violence. In this study staff completed a pretest followed by the training (the intervention), following which they undertook a posttest. The authors defended their approach, highlighting that the nature of the training did not allow for the availability of a comparison or control group. The main question to ask with the above studies is: was it the intervention that led to the change or was it some other factor? For example, were patients already improving their glycaemic control before the intervention, or did some other factor improve staff management of violence in mental health settings other than the educational intervention? These questions can be answered by improving the type of quasi-experimental design, such as using a non-equivalent control group or interrupted time series designs.

Box 11.2 Evaluation of nurse specialist as main care provider for patients with type 2 diabetes – an example of a one-group pretest–posttest design

---

Vrijhoef et al. (2002) evaluated the effect a diabetes nurse specialist, as the main care provider in a shared care model for people with type 2 diabetes, had on a number of patient outcomes. Prior to the treatment (care provided by a nurse specialist), patients received routine care for their diabetes from their GP and, in some cases, an endocrinologist. The treatment was then introduced, which consisted of the diabetes nurse specialist becoming the main provider of care for people with diabetes as opposed to the GP. The authors outlined that it was not feasible to undertake this study with a control group and therefore used a one-group pretest–posttest design. Acknowledging the limitations of this design, the researchers in the study also compared the treatment group with other groups of patients with diabetes. A number of outcomes were measured including glycaemic control, patient satisfaction, quality of life and illness-related knowledge and behaviour. Data were collected over three time periods: baseline, six months and twelve months. During the course of the study, attrition of patients was a problem; there were 155 patients at baseline, 122 at six months and 103 at twelve months. Patients who were lost from the study had worse glycaemic control and a longer history of diabetes than those who completed the study. The study found that patients who received care from a diabetes nurse specialist improved over time in relation to glycaemic control and other physiological indicators such as diastolic blood pressure and cholesterol levels; no change was identified in the outcome variables that measured quality of life and satisfaction.

There are a number of threats to internal validity highlighted in this study, including maturation and history. Maturation may have affected the outcome in that, regardless of the intervention, over time patients may have improved their glycaemic control as they learned to live with their diabetes. History is a threat as health professionals other than the diabetes nurse specialist may have affected the extent to which patients cared for their diabetes. It is acknowledged in the study that, as well as contact with the diabetes nurse specialist, patients came in contact with their GP and, at times, endocrinologist. Attrition was also another threat to internal validity; patients who had better glycaemic control were more likely to complete the study. Those who were poorly engaged with their diabetes care may have dropped out of the study. Vrijhoef et al. (2002) were aware of the threats to the internal validity of their study and highlighted these in the limitations section. The authors also outlined the steps they took to control for these limitations, such as collecting data on several occasions and using a comparative group where feasible.

Non-equivalent control group designs

This type of quasi-experimental design is more robust than the one-group pretest–posttest design, mainly for the reason that it also contains a control or comparison group. However, in keeping with quasi-experimental designs, participants are not randomly assigned to either the intervention or control group. It is the most frequently used quasi-experimental design (Shadish et al. 2002). Figure 11.3 diagrammatically outlines this design.

NR	O_1	X	O_2
NR	O_1		O_2

Figure 11.3 Non-equivalent control group design (Shadish et al. 2002).

In the notation in Figure 11.3 'NR' means that participants are not randomly assigned to either the intervention or control group. Data are collected from both groups on the outcome of interest at pretest (O_1), followed by which only one group receives the intervention (X). Following the intervention, both the treatment group and the control/comparison group are measured again at posttest (O_2) on the same dependent variable measured during the pretest phase. If there is a statistically significant difference between the comparative and treatment groups this is assumed to have occurred as a result of the treatment or intervention (Eccles et al. 2003).

The pretest phase in this design is important for a number of reasons, including:

1 It allows us to form a baseline to compare both the intervention and control groups.
2 Due to the fact that participants are not randomly assigned to groups, it identifies differences that may impact on the outcome measured in the post-test phase. That is, it allows the researcher to identify the extent to which selection bias is present.
3 It facilitates statistical analysis in identifying the impact of the treatment on outcomes.

(Pedhazur and Schmelkin 1991; Shadish et al. 2002).

Shadish et al. (2002: 136) highlight that the use of 'carefully selected comparison groups facilitates causal inference from quasi-experiments'; however, they point out that 'such control groups are of minimal advantage unless they are also accompanied by pretest measures taken on the same outcome variable as the posttest'. One of the main problems with this type of design is the difficulty in identifying a control group that is comparable to the intervention group (Eccles et al. 2003).

Take, for example, a new education programme for young people with type 1 diabetes. The programme is introduced in clinic A (treatment group) but not in clinic B. Patients who attend clinic B will be used as the comparison group (remember, patients have not been randomly allocated to the intervention or control groups – this is what makes the design quasi-experimental). Prior to the intervention (education programme), both groups of patients are measured on the primary outcome or dependent variable – in this case, knowledge of glycaemic control. If we find that the intervention group have a higher prior knowledge score than the control group at the pretest phase, that is before the intervention, we may have encountered a selection bias. It is important to note that the participants have not been randomly allocated to the two groups and are therefore identified as being non-equivalent (Gliner et al. 2009). An example of a non-equivalent control group design is outlined in Box 11.3.

Box 11.3   Hospital-based palliative care teams improve the symptoms of cancer patients – an example of a non-equivalent control group design

Jack et al. (2003) used a non-equivalent control group design to identify the effect of a specialist palliative care team on symptom control of patients diagnosed with cancer. Patients who were referred to the specialist care team received the intervention (advice, support, symptom control); patients who were not referred to the team received standard care and acted as the control or comparison group. It can be seen that this is a quasi-experimental design due to the non-random allocation of research subjects to the intervention and comparison group. The authors point out that the reason for using a non-equivalent control group design was that it would not have been ethical to randomly allocate patients to either the palliative care intervention or standard care. This is an issue when undertaking research with vulnerable patients. Patients were assessed on their symptoms over three time points. The authors pointed out that 24 patients (12 each from the treatment and comparison groups) were lost to the study for various reasons. The authors provided baseline data for both patient groups – this highlights the extent to which the threats to the internal validity of the study are present. There were a number of differences at baseline: the treatment group (those patients that received care from the palliative team) had higher levels of nausea and insomnia and lower constipation scores than the comparison group; the authors acknowledged this as a weakness in the study. The study found that, although both the treatment group and the comparison group's symptoms improved over the course of the study, patients allocated to the palliative care team demonstrated a statistically significant greater level of improvement on a number of outcomes.

There are a number of threats to the internal validity (see Box 11.1 above) of this study, including: selection bias – there were a number of differences between the treatment and intervention group at baseline; attrition – a number of patients withdrew from the study prior to completion of data collection; maturation – participants may have developed coping skills without the intervention; and history – participants in both groups may have had input from other health care professionals outside the study that could have affected the outcomes.

Interrupted time-series design

In an interrupted time series design, data are 'collected at multiple time points before and after the intervention' (Grimshaw et al. 2000: S12). This approach allows a trend over time to be discerned. The pattern observed in the pretest is then compared to the pattern following the intervention (posttest). It is recommended that there are a number of measures before the intervention, with Gliner et al. (2009) recommending at least three pre-intervention measures to allow a baseline to be established. Interrupted time series designs have been identified as being useful for evaluating the introduction of national health care guidelines (see Box 11.4 below for an example) and the effectiveness of health-related media campaigns (Eccles et al. 2003). Eccles et al. (2003: 52) outline the advantage of using an interrupted time series design to evaluating the effectiveness of an intervention:

> The multiple time points before the intervention allow the underlying trend and any cyclical (seasonal) effects to be estimated, and the multiple time points after the intervention allow the intervention effect to be estimated while taking account of the underlying secular trends [secular trends are trends that occur over time separate to the intervention and may affect an outcome].

Figure 11.4 diagrammatically outlines an interrupted time series design in which there are five observations (O_1 to O_5) prior to, and five observations (O_6 to O_{10}) following, an intervention (X).

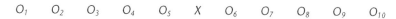

$$O_1 \quad O_2 \quad O_3 \quad O_4 \quad O_5 \quad X \quad O_6 \quad O_7 \quad O_8 \quad O_9 \quad O_{10}$$

Figure 11.4 Interrupted time series design (Shadish et al. 2002).

The interrupted time series design is identified as being more robust than the one-group pretest–posttest design, especially in relation to the internal validity threats of maturation, regression to the mean and testing; however, it is still susceptible to the threats of history, instrumentation and attrition (Reichardt 2009). Shadish et al. (2002) identify that history is the greatest threat to the internal validity of interrupted time series designs. As highlighted in Box 11.1, history is a threat to the internal validity of a study when factors other than the intervention or treatment influenced the outcome. Remember the example of the intervention to educate the public on the appropriate use of emergency departments when at the same time, separate to the study, the health service introduces new monetary charges for patients using an emergency department. If you discovered over time a drop in the number of attendances to emergency departments, to what extent can we say it was the educational intervention or other factors that led to the reduction? Researchers need to be aware that when using interrupted time series designs, factors other than the intervention can impact on the outcome. Gliner et al. (2009) outline a number of advantages of the time series design, including its use in studies where it is not possible to identify a control group; for example, when a new model of nursing care is being introduced to a hospital, measures of patient satisfaction can be taken for a time prior to the intervention as well as following the intervention.

There is evidence that interrupted time series designs are increasingly being used in health care research and that they are an effective design for measuring the effectiveness of health-related interventions. A specific example of an interrupted time series design in the evaluation of a health care intervention is outlined in Box 11.4.

> **Box 11.4** Evaluation of the national *cleanyourhands* campaign to reduce *staphylococcus aureus* bacteraemia and *Clostridium difficile* infection in hospitals – an example of an interrupted time series design

Due to concern within the National Health Service in the UK on the rates of methicillin-resistant *staphylococcus aureus* (MRSA) and *Clostridium difficile* infections in hospitals, a campaign was initiated to encourage staff to use best practice in hand hygiene to prevent the spread of hospital-acquired infections. This was named the *cleanyourhands* campaign. The campaign consisted of a number of interventions, including alcohol hand rubs at the patient's bedside, staff reminders and audits of compliance. Stone et al. (2012) used an interrupted time series design to evaluate the impact of the *cleanyourhands* campaign on the hospital purchase of alcohol hand rub and soap (used as an indicator of usage and hand cleaning compliance), trends in hospital-acquired infection rates and the association between infection rates and procurement of the hand rub and soap. The study took place over a four-year period. The authors pointed out that, due to the widespread and quick introduction of the initiative, it was not possible to undertake a randomized controlled trial. In addition, the researchers had to contend with a threat to the internal validity of the study through history (other infection-reducing initiatives were introduced at the same time as the *cleanyourhands* programme). Therefore, to control for these factors the research team chose an interrupted time series design to evaluate the initiative. Data were collected over three time periods: six months prior to the commencement of the campaign, during the roll-out of the initiative and 36 months following the campaign. The study found that rates of MRSA and *Clostridium difficile* infections fell over the course of the study and were associated with the increased procurement of soap and alcohol rub. The researchers were very aware of the threats to the internal validity of the study as there were other initiatives in place to reduce hospital-acquired infections; these threats or confounding variables were statistically controlled for by the research team in their analysis of the data. This is a very good example of an interrupted time series design and demonstrates how the authors identified and controlled threats to internal validity of the study results.

Summary of quasi-experimental designs

When answering research questions, it may not be feasible or ethical to randomly assign subjects to an intervention or control group; however the researcher still wishes to measure the effect or otherwise of an intervention. This is especially the case when working with complex interventions in health care settings. Quasi-experimental designs have developed to allow researchers do this. As pointed out, all quasi-experimental designs have strengths and weaknesses, some more than others. The main disadvantage of using a quasi-experimental design is the threat to internal validity of the study. Due to the fact that subjects are not randomly assigned to groups prior to the intervention, confounding variables that would normally be controlled for through randomization can affect the claims we make about the outcome. When using quasi-experimental designs in health care research, it is important that we design the study to reduce the threats to internal validity and, as much as possible, rule out alternative explanations for the outcomes identified.

Retrospective pretest designs

When we undertake research with patients, we often use respondents' self-reported measures of change to evaluate the progress of an illness or the impact of a therapeutic intervention on a number of patient-reported outcomes. Patients may self-report the extent to which they change over time on a number of outcomes associated with their illness, such as quality of life, pain or fatigue. Traditionally, the design used to measure impact of an intervention or change over time is to compare the study participant's pretest scores with their posttest scores (Shadish et al. 2002). The pretest–posttest design takes the difference between the patient's pretest score and their posttest score to provide a change score. In theory, if the posttest score is significantly different from the pretest score, it should indicate that change occurred on the variable of interest (for example: fatigue, pain, functional ability, quality of life). Traditional pretest–posttest measures work on the assumption that the respondent's conceptualization of the construct being measured will not change from the pretest to the posttest. However, the respondent's perception of a construct or internal frame of reference may change over time, leading to an under-reporting or over-reporting by the patient of any real change occurring between pretest and posttest. This change in perception is known as response shift (Howard et al. 1979; Howard 1980; Goedhart and Hoogstraten 1992).

A second problem with the standard pretest–posttest design is that it may also lead to the problem of a pretest sensitization effect, whereby taking a pretest affects the results on a posttest (Shadish et al. 2002). Pretest sensitization can influence the internal validity of an outcome (see Box 11.1) due to the respondent recalling their responses at the pretest stage; that is, the pretest can confound the treatment or intervention effect (Lam and Bengo 2002). Although a pretest–posttest design is seen as the best approach to measuring change, perversely the pretest itself may confound the treatment effect. Hoogstraten highlighted the fact that the 'biasing effect of pretesting cannot be neglected' (1980: 39). In addition to response shift and the pretest sensitization effect, another problem with using the pretest–posttest design is the inability of the researcher to collect pretest data due to the nature of the problem being investigated, time constraints and cost. To deal with the problems of response shift, pretest sensitization and the logistical problems of pretesting patients, the retrospective pretest design is a method that can be considered when measuring change.

Understanding response shift

Sprangers and Schwartz (1999: 1508) conceptualize response shift as 'a change in the meaning of one's self-evaluation of a target construct'. This change may occur due to a number of reasons, including: 1) recalibration: a change in 'the respondent's internal standards of measurement' and 2) reprioritization: a change in values or a reconceptualization of their illness and the construct of importance (for example, quality of life). Basically, a patient's concept of their illness, and factors associated with their illness such as pain or fatigue, changes over time. The metric or internal frame of reference that a patient used to assess an aspect of their illness (for example their level of fatigue) at the beginning of an illness may be very different from the one they use to assess this aspect of their illness following a series of treatments or a change in their illness. In addition, there may also be a difference between a patient's health status as measured through biomedical markers and a patient's own perception of their health and well-being (Sprangers and Schwartz 1999).

This reconceptualization of a construct may lead the patient to re-evaluate the outcome under investigation, for example fatigue, from a different perspective at the posttest stage from the one they held at the pretest stage. This change in perspective or internal frame of reference is as a result of the participant being exposed to the intervention, treatment or disease between the pretest and the posttest, leading to a shift in their response. This may result in the patient using a different metric to rate themselves at time 2 (posttest) than the one they used at time 1 (pretest), even though measurements at time 1 and time 2 are being taken using the same instrument. Patients may overevaluate or underevaluate their ability or knowledge in the early stages of their illness; however, as their illness progresses or they are exposed to treatments and therapeutic interventions they may realize that their perception of the construct at the beginning of their illness was very different than they estimated. This may be due to the fact that the value or meaning of a construct for the patient changes over time.

Although response shift can be identified in a number of health-related outcomes, the majority of work in this area relates to patients' perceptions of their quality of life. Sprangers and Schwartz (1999) have developed a theoretical model of how response shift affects health-related quality of life. There are five elements to the model: 1) a catalyst, 2) antecedents, 3) mechanisms, 4) response shift, and 5) perceived quality of life (QOL). Sprangers and Schwartz (1999: 1509) describe the catalyst as 'a change in a respondent's health status, that may or may not result from treatment'. The next element in the model, antecedents, refers to the demographic and psychosocial profile of the individual. Examples of antecedents include gender, level of education and self-esteem. The third element of the model, mechanisms, refers to approaches the individual uses to deal with the catalyst or the change in health status; in general, what coping styles and supports they use. The fourth element, response shift, is referred to by Sprangers and Schwartz (1999: 1059) as 'a change in the meaning of one's self-evaluation of QOL as a result of changes in internal standards, values and the conceptualization of QOL'. The final element, perceived quality of life, is viewed as incorporating a biopsychosocial perspective. Taken in totality, the model describes how perceived quality of life is impacted on by the person's illness, their sociodemographic factors, their mechanisms of support and coping and how, during the process of the illness, the patient recalibrates their understanding and meaning of quality of life – the response shift. Readers are referred to Sprangers and Schwartz (1999) for further details of the model; in particular the authors provide excellent examples of how the model can explain the process of response shift and how this impacts on quality of life. The value of the model is that it specifically incorporates response shift when measuring quality of life. This has merit in that it may provide an accurate identification of change occurring that may not have been identified when using measures where response shift has not been incorporated. Let us look at an example of response shift from the clinical literature (see Box 11.5).

Box 11.5   Magnitude and correlates of response shift in fatigue ratings in women undergoing adjuvant therapy for breast cancer – an example of response shift

---

Andrykowski et al. (2009), writing in the *Journal of Pain and Symptom Management*, provide a good example of response shift in a study measuring fatigue among women undergoing adjuvant chemotherapy and/or radiotherapy for breast cancer. Starting with the premise that the subjective nature of fatigue can lead to the meaning attributed to it by patients changing over time, the authors hypothesized that the meaning attributed to 'severe' fatigue can change according to the stage of illness or treatment the patient is experiencing. For example, Andrykowski et al. (2009) highlight that a rating of 5 on a 10-point scale measuring fatigue prior to treatment may not have the same meaning as 5 measured on the same scale following treatment, due to response shift. Women who had completed adjuvant therapy were asked to think back and rate their level of fatigue prior to commencing either radiotherapy or chemotherapy. Women tended to retrospectively lower their pre-treatment fatigue scores in comparison to their pretest scores taken prior to the treatments. In effect, when assessing their level of fatigue pre-treatment from the perspective of having completed either radiotherapy or chemotherapy (post-treatment), women concluded that their levels of fatigue were not as high as they had concluded at that time. Andrykowski et al. (2009: 348) concluded that the levels of response shift identified in the study were both 'statistically *and* clinically significant'. These results demonstrated that respondents reconceptualized or used a different internal frame of reference to conceptualize the meaning of fatigue following their treatment from the one they used just before their treatment commenced. Following the experience of fatigue after adjuvant therapy for breast cancer, women used that assessment to recalibrate their self-reports of fatigue prior to receiving their treatment. The respondents were, as would be expected, considerably more fatigued following their treatment than they were before their therapy; however, this led them to reconceptualize how they perceived their level of fatigue prior to the treatment. Therefore, patients' self-reported ratings of aspects of their quality of life, such as fatigue in the example above, at the beginning of an illness may be imprecise. What has occurred is that patients are rating their capability on a different dimension or metric at time 2 (posttest) than they did at time 1 (pretest) (Sprangers 1988).

Response shift is increasingly being acknowledged as an issue that needs to be taken into account when measuring change in patients, especially when undertaking research with people with long-term, life-limiting or chronic illnesses. Not taking response shift into account has been cited as a reason for underestimating or over-estimating change in patients' quality of life scores over time (Westerman et al. 2007; Barclay-Goddard et al. 2009). In a meta-analysis of research into response shift bias, Schwartz et al. (2006: 1540) concluded that 'response shifts are a common and significant phenomenon in QOL measurement, implying that people adapt their internal standards of QOL in response to a changing health state'. In effect, an individual's perception of what quality of life means to them changes throughout the course of their illness. This change may invalidate measures used to measure change as the patient is using a different frame of reference to rate their outcome at the posttest from the one they used at the pretest. It has been suggested that response shift theory can help to explain 'paradoxical and counter-intuitive findings' that may occur when researching the extent to which patients change over time (Sprangers and Schwartz 1999: 1058).

How do I know if a research participant has experienced response shift when measuring patient-reported outcomes? Response shift is detected by comparing the pretest and thentest ratings, using the retrospective pretest approach. To adjust for response shift, comparisons are made between respondents' posttest and thentest scores (Schwartz and Sprangers 2010). The next section describes this method, the retrospective pretest, which is both used to identify and control for response shift bias.

Controlling for response shift – use the retrospective pretest

The retrospective pretest, also known as the thentest, is increasingly being used in health care research to measure the extent to which patients change in relation to outcomes (for example pain, quality of life, functional status).[2] The retrospective pretest method differs from the traditional pretest–posttest design in that both post-test and retrospective pretest (thentest) measures of respondents are collected at the same time. Prior to the intervention or treatment, study participants complete, as normal, a pretest. Respondents then, following the intervention or treatment or after a period of time living with an illness or disease, are asked first to report on the outcome of interest now (posttest) and then asked at the same time to think back and rate themselves on the outcome before their illness or treatment for their illness commenced (thentest). Basically, the retrospective pretest design asks the respond-ent to recall a point in the past and compare it to where they are now. The collection of thentest and posttest ratings at the same time controls for the confounding effect of response shift bias due to the fact that the respondent is making the ratings regarding time 1 (thentest) and time 2 (posttest) from the same perspective (Howard 1980; Sprangers 1989). It is argued that a comparison of posttest and thentest scores provides a better indicator of patient change than comparing posttest and pretest scores (Schwartz and Sprangers 2010). Figure 11.5 provides a diagrammatic

---

[2]Readers are referred to Barclay-Goodard et al. (2009) for an overview of other research designs that can be used to address the issue of response shift when measuring self-reports of change.

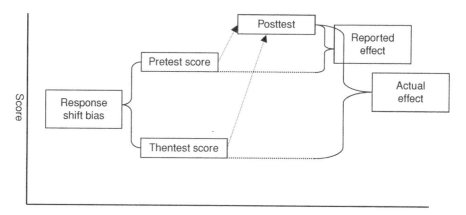

Figure 11.5   Diagrammatic representation of response shift bias (adapted from Sprangers et al. 1999).

representation of response shift and how the traditional pretest–posttest and retrospective pretest compare.

The theoretical assumption underlying the retrospective pretest method is that by asking the patient at the same time to rate where they are now in relation to the outcome under investigation *and* where they were prior to the intervention or treatment, they will be using the same internal frame of reference to rate the outcome. Furthermore, it is claimed that scores obtained from posttest minus thentest are more likely to show a valid effect than scores obtained from the traditional pretest–posttest method (Howard 1980; Sprangers 1988; Goedhart and Hoogstraten 1992; Drennan and Hyde 2008).

The thentest design can also be used to collect ratings retrospectively when pretest data are not available (Kreulen et al. 2002; Drennan 2012). For example, you may wish to ask a patient to retrospectively report on their functional or pain status prior to them experiencing their current disease or illness. Due to the fact that the illness has already occurred and it was not possible to collect pretest data, you can ask the patient to retrospectively assess their health prior to the illness occurring. Examples from the literature using this approach include Kreulen et al. (2002) who retrospectively measured patient satisfaction with their health status as a proxy for pretest satisfaction scores. Drennan (2012) also used a retrospective pretest in asking respondents who had completed a master's in nursing programme to retrospectively rate their leadership ability following completion of the programme.

A hypothetical example of what a retrospective pretest instrument may look like is provided in Table 11.1. The example is one that may be used to ascertain a patient's functional status following a treatment or intervention. The respondent is asked to report on each measure twice, allowing a comparison of their post-treatment scores with their pre-treatment scores. Because posttest scores and thentest scores are taken at the same time, they are being made from the same perspective or internal frame of reference.

Table 11.1 Hypothetical example of a self-report retrospective pretest instrument measuring functional ability (only three items are displayed)

	ABILITY													
	Circle the appropriate number where you see yourself _now_ following your treatment and where you saw yourself _prior_ to commencing your treatment. 1 = low ability through to 7 = high ability.													
	After the treatment ➡							**Before the treatment**						
Ability:	Low 1	2	3	4	5	6	High 7	Low 1	2	3	4	5	6	High 7
Ability to exercise	1	2	3	4	5	6	7	1	2	3	4	5	6	7
Ability to work	1	2	3	4	5	6	7	1	2	3	4	5	6	7
Ability to shop for groceries	1	2	3	4	5	6	7	1	2	3	4	5	6	7

Studies using retrospective pretests

Retrospective pretest designs were originally used to evaluate educational and training outcomes; these included leadership skills development courses (Rohs 1999), public health education programmes (Umble et al. 2000; Farel et al. 2001), courses in statistics and research methods (Drennan and Hyde 2008), and a healthy start programme designed to prevent child abuse (Pratt et al. 2000). The approach is increasingly being used in health care research, especially in the area of quality of life research. Some examples of the use of the retrospective pretest design include parent-reported quality of life in children with otitis media (Timmerman et al. 2003), quality of life in people with cancer (Sprangers et al. 1999; Oort 2005; Westerman et al. 2006) and satisfaction with health status of women with breast cancer (Kreulen et al. 2002). Box 11.6 provides another example of the use of the method in health care research which compared traditional pretest–posttest measures with the retrospective pretest method with patients diagnosed with advanced prostate cancer.

How do I analyse the results from retrospective pretest ratings? Due to the repeated measures aspect of the data and the fact that measures are dependent, depending on the number of time points, you can use paired t-tests or repeated-measures ANOVA for parametric data or Wilcoxon signed rank tests or Friedman's ANOVA for non-parametric data. It is important that when displaying your data, as well as comparison of outcome scores and effect sizes, the extent to which response shift is present should also be displayed. Bonferroni adjustment should also be applied to control for type 1 errors when multiple comparisons are involved (Drennan and Hyde 2008).

Box 11.6   Prospective vs retrospective assessment of lower urinary tract symptoms in patients with advanced prostate cancer – an example of response shift and retrospective pretests

---

Rees et al. (2003) undertook a study with patients diagnosed with advanced prostate cancer. Patients completed two instruments to assess their symptoms, the International Prostrate Symptom Score (IPSS) and the Symptom Problem Index (SPI), before treatment and three and six months after treatment. At three and six months, patients also completed a retrospective pretest. The retrospective pretest asked respondents to think back and 're-evaluate' their symptoms at the previous assessment from their current perspective. Findings indicated that the retrospective pretest scores identified a greater magnitude of improvement in patients' symptoms than those reported using traditional pretest–posttest ratings. Patients using the retrospective pretest method rated their symptoms as worse on both the IPSS and SPI than they had at pretest (time 1), indicating that response shift bias had occurred in patients' self-reports of symptoms. Rees et al. (2003) concluded that the retrospective pretest method could be used in conjunction with traditional pretests to give an accurate assessment of patient outcomes following treatment.

Criticism of retrospective pretests

Although identified as a method to control for response shift bias and provide an accurate identification of change that occurs over time, a number of criticisms have been levelled at retrospective pretesting as a method. Problems identified include social desirability and impression management, response bias, poor memory (Howard 1980; Lam and Bengo 2002), lack of a traditional pretest prior to the intervention (Shadish et al. 2002), regression to the mean (Pratt et al. 2000; Shadish et al. 2002), maturational effects (Pratt et al. 2000), and change in the context of actual stability (Conway and Ross 1984).

Social desirable responding in retrospective pretests occurs when respondents rate themselves after an intervention in terms of how much change should have occurred rather than what actually occurred. However, in a comparison of three retrospective methods of measuring change, post-then-only method, the post + perceived change method and the retrospective pretest method, Lam and Bengo (2002) identified that social desirable responding was less likely when the retrospective pretest method was used. One of the reasons postulated for this finding was the cognitive demands placed on respondents when using other retrospective methods to assess change.

Another criticism of retrospective pretests is that participants to an intervention may judge the intervention as beneficial, whereas the evidence may be to the contrary (Conway and Ross 1984). Psychological processes may be in play in convincing participants that an intervention was beneficial even if in actuality this was not the case. This may in itself lead respondents to overestimate their gains or outcomes as a consequence of intervention. This is especially so if participants have invested time, energy and money into an intervention (Conway and Ross 1984).

It is also argued that 'retrospective pretests should be a supplement to other design improvements, not used by themselves, and should be a method of last resort interpreted with great caution' (Shadish et al. 2002: 115). Howard et al. (1979), who provide the seminal writings in the area of retrospective pretests, recommend that the retrospective pretest should not be a replacement for the conventional pretest–posttest design but should be considered as an adjunct to other methods when response shift may be an issue in self-reported measures. It is also important to note that a number of threats to internal validity may influence the outcomes reported by participants on the retrospective pretest. For example, social desirability, 'thinking that change should have occurred' rather than it actually occurring, and memory biases; getting the respondent to think back to the beginning of the programme may, in some cases, lead to recall bias (Pratt et al. 2000). However, Howard reported higher correlations between social desirability responses for pretest scores than those associated with retrospective pretest scores: 'social desirability responding was actually diminished in utilizing the retrospective methodology' (1980: 102).

Howard (1980) recognizes that retrospective pretests are an important tool in the armoury of the researcher; however, the method is further strengthened when integrated with other objective and behavioural measures (Pratt et al. 2000). In the evaluation of a programme to help in the prevention of child abuse Pratt et al. (2000) used a variety of outcome measures as well as retrospective pretests. These measures included development assessment of infants, reports of child maltreatment and observations.

Conclusion

In health care research it is recognized that the gold standard for measuring the effectiveness of interventions is the randomized controlled trial. However, for a number of reasons, not least feasibility and ethical issues, it may not be possible to use this approach to measure the outcome of a treatment. In addition, health care interventions are increasingly complex and are being used with a variety of patient cohorts; therefore it is necessary that health care researchers have access to designs that can validly measure the complexity of interventions in the field. Both quasi-experimental and retrospective pretest designs provide viable and robust alternatives to the randomized controlled trial when researchers wish to measure outcomes from an intervention.

Quasi-experimental designs allow the researcher to measure the outcome of an intervention when it is not practicable to randomly assign subjects to treatment or control groups. This design has great utility in clinical practice where an intervention may have already commenced or patients are exposed to the intervention in one setting but not another. It is also argued that quasi-experimental designs are more 'natural' as they take place in the clinical setting as opposed to a laboratory setting. It is important to note, however, that quasi-experimental designs have weaknesses; even within the designs themselves there are strong and weak quasi-experimental designs, and some designs have fewer threats to internal validity than others.

The aim of using the retrospective pretest method is to reduce the problem of response shift bias, therefore allowing for the identification of actual change that may not be identified using traditional pretest–posttest designs. It has also been claimed that when using self-reported measurements of change the retrospective pretest method is superior to traditional pretest–posttest self-report measurement. Retrospective pretest scores may be a more accurate indicator of actual outcome when assessed against behavioural measures than when compared to the self-reported outcomes identified in traditional pretest–posttest designs. One of the main reasons postulated for the mismatch between traditional pretest–posttest scores and retrospective pretest scores is that participants change their frame of reference as a result of the effects of their illness. It is increasingly being suggested that researchers should, when measures of patient-reported outcomes are used, collect retrospective perceptions from respondents. Overall, retrospective pretesting can provide a more accurate indicator of the extent to which patients self-report change than that ascertained through using the traditional pretest–posttest design.

Both designs discussed in this chapter offer health care researchers methodological options when measuring health-related outcomes that may not be feasible with other designs. These designs, when carefully constructed, can provide evidence on the effect of an intervention or treatment on health-related outcomes and patients' self-reports of change.

Key concepts: Quasi-experimental designs

- Quasi-experimental designs can be used when it is not feasible or ethical to use a randomized control design.
- Quasi-experimental designs differ from randomized controlled trials in that they lack random assignment.
- Threats to internal validity are greater in quasi-experimental designs than randomized controlled trials; however, a well-constructed quasi-experimental study can provide evidence of the effect of an independent variable on an outcome.
- Quasi-experimental designs are increasingly being used in health care research to evaluate complex interventions.
- When using quasi-experimental designs in health care research, it is important to design the study so that threats to internal validity are reduced.

Key readings on quasi-experimental designs

- W. Shadish, T. Cook and D. Campbell, *Experimental and Quasi-experimental Designs for Generalised Causal Inference* (Boston, MA: Houghton Mifflin, 2002)
  If you read one book on quasi-experimental designs, it has to be this one. Building on the seminal work of Cook and Campbell in the 1960s and 1970s, this book comprehensively discusses research designs to identify causal inferences and relationships. It is essential reading for any student who wishes to use a quasi-experimental design in their research.

Examples of papers on quasi-experimental designs

The following papers provide an excellent example of the use of quasi-experimental designs in health care research.

- S. Stone, C. Fuller, J. Savage, B. Cookson, A. Hayward, B. Cooper, G. Duckworth, S. Michie, M. Murray, A. Jeanes, J. Roberts, L. Teare and A. Charlett, Evaluation of the national Cleanyourhands campaign to reduce *Staphylococcus aureus* bacteraemia and *Clostridium difficile* infection in hospitals in England and Wales by improved hand hygiene: Four year, prospective, ecological, interrupted time series study, *British Medical Journal*, 344 (2012), 1–11
- C. Smith, D. Nutbeam, L. Moore and J. Catford, Effects of the Heartbeat Wales programme over five years on behavioural risks for cardiovascular disease: Quasi-experimental comparison of results from Wales and a matched reference area, *British Medical Journal*, 16 (1998), 818–22

Key concepts: Retrospective pretest designs

- Traditionally, the design used to measure impact of an intervention or change over time is to compare the study participant's pretest scores with their posttest scores.
- Traditional pretest–posttest measures work on the assumption that the respondent's conceptualization of the construct being measured will not change from the pretest to the posttest.
- It has been found, however, that respondents' perception of a construct or internal frame of reference may change over time, leading to an under-reporting or over-reporting by the patient of any real change occurring between pretest and posttest. This change in perception is known as response shift.
- Response shift may lead a patient to re-evaluate an outcome being researched from a different perspective at the posttest stage from the one they held at the pretest stage.
- Response shift has been identified in health care research, especially in studies examining health-related quality of life.
- Response shift is increasingly being acknowledged as an issue that needs to be taken into account when measuring change in patients.
- Response shift can be identified by comparing pretest and thentest ratings using the retrospective pretest design.
- The retrospective pretest method differs from the traditional pretest–posttest design in that both posttest and retrospective pretest (thentest) measures of respondents are collected at the same time.
- The thentest works by asking respondents to think back to the time of the posttest and rate themselves on the outcome before their illness or treatment for their illness commenced.
- The theoretical assumption underlying the retrospective pretest method is that by asking the patient at the same time to rate where they are now in relation to the outcome under investigation *and* where they were prior to the intervention or treatment, they will be using the same internal frame of reference to rate the outcome.

Key readings in response shift and retrospective pretests

- C. Schwartz and M. Sprangers, Guidelines for improving the stringency of response shift research using the thentest, *Quality of Life Research*, 19(4) (2010), 455–64
  Sprangers and Schwartz have produced an admirable body of work on response shift and the retrospective pretest design and their papers are well worth reading for an in-depth discussion of work in the field. This paper provides guidelines on using the thentest in health care research when investigating the phenomenon of response shift. The authors provide a checklist for all the elements required when using the thentest, including the design of the study, identifying change and analysing the data.

- M. Sprangers and C. Schwartz, Integrating response shift into health-related quality of life research: A theoretical model, *Social Science and Medicine*, 48(11) (1999), 1507–15
  Another excellent paper by Schwartz and Sprangers. This paper provides a good overview of the theory that underpins response shift and how the concept is related to patient-reported outcomes. It outlines in detail a theoretical model that can be used to underpin research into response shift and how patients' perceptions change as a result of their illness.

Examples of papers on response shift and retrospective pretests in health care research

The following papers provide an excellent example of response shift and the retrospective pretest design in health care research.

- M. Andrykowski, K. Donovan and P. Jacobsen, Magnitude and correlates of response shift in fatigue ratings in women undergoing adjuvant therapy for breast cancer, *Journal of Pain and Symptom Management*, 37(3) (2009), 341–51

- M. Sprangers, F. Van Dam, J. Broersen, L. Lodder, L. Wever, M. Visser, P. Oosterveld and E. Smets, Revealing response shift in longitudinal research on fatigue: The use of the thentest approach, *Acta Oncologica*, 38(6) (1999), 709–18

- G. Kreulen, M. Stommel, B. Gutek, L. Burns and C. Braden, Utility of retrospective pretest ratings of patient satisfaction with health status, *Research in Nursing and Health*, 25(3) (2002), 233–41

Useful websites, conferences, resources

- Dr Lisa M. Lix, Associate Professor at the School of Public Health, has brought together resources from a workshop on analysing response shift in research. Many of the techniques described will be applicable to advanced researchers; however, there is a good link to a presentation on response shift – http://homepage.usask.ca/~lml321/Work shop%20Resources.html

- A presentation on response shift by Professor Lena Ring, Associate Professor of Pharmaceutical Outcomes Research at Uppsala University in Sweden – http://www.youtube.com/watch?v=jmrKBB2sRpQ

References

Andrykowski, M., Donovan, K. and Jacobsen, P. (2009) Magnitude and correlates of response shift in fatigue ratings in women undergoing adjuvant therapy for breast cancer, *Journal of Pain and Symptom Management*, 37(3): 341–51.

Barclay-Goddard, R., Epstein, J.D. and Mayo, N.E. (2009) Response shift: A brief overview and proposed research priorities, *Quality of Life Research*, 18(3): 335–46.

Calabro, K., Mackey, T. and Williams, S. (2002) Evaluation of training designed to prevent and manage patient violence, *Issues in Mental Health Nursing*, 23(1): 3–15.

Conway, M. and Ross, M. (1984) Getting what you want by revising what you had, *Journal of Personality and Social Psychology*, 47(4): 738–48.

Drennan, J. (2012) Masters in nursing degrees: An evaluation of management and leadership outcomes using a retrospective pre-test design, *Journal of Nursing Management*, 20(1): 102–12.

Drennan, J. and Hyde, A. (2008) Controlling response shift bias: The use of the retrospective pre-test design in the evaluation of a master's programme, *Assessment and Evaluation in Higher Education*, 33(6): 699–709.

Eccles, M., Grimshaw, J., Campbell, M. and Ramsay, C. (2003) Research designs for studies evaluating the effectiveness of change and improvement strategies, *Quality and Safety in Health Care*, 12(1): 47–52.

Farel, A., Umble, K. and Polhamus. B. (2001) Impact of an online analytic skills course, *Evaluation and the Health Professions*, 24: 446–59.

Gliner, J., Morgan, G. and Leech, N. (2009) *Research Methods in Applied Settings: An integrated Approach to Design and Analysis*. New York: Routledge.

Goedhart, H. and Hoogstraten, J. (1992) The retrospective pretest and the role of pretest information in evaluative studies, *Psychological Reports*, 70(3): 699–704.

Grimshaw, J., Campbell, M., Eccles, M. and Steen, N. (2000) Experimental and quasi-experimental designs for evaluating guideline implementation strategies, *Family Practice*, 17(Supp 1): S11–16.

Hoogstraten, J. (1980) The reactive effect of pretesting in attitude change research: General or specific, *Applied Psychological Measurement*, 4(1): 39–42.

Howard, G. (1980) Response shift bias: A problem in evaluating interventions with pre/post self-reports, *Evaluation Review*, 4(1): 93–106.

Howard, G., Schmeck, R. and Bray, J. (1979) Internal invalidity in studies employing self-report instruments: A suggested remedy, *Journal of Educational Measurement*, 16(2): 129–35.

Jack, B., Hillier, V., Williams, A. and Oldham, J. (2003) Hospital based palliative care teams improve the symptoms of cancer patients, *Palliative Medicine*, 17(6): 498–502.

Kirk, R. (2009) Experimental design, in R. Millsap and A. Maydeu-Olivares (eds) *The Sage Handbook of Quantitative Methods in Psychology*. Thousand Oaks, CA: Sage, pp. 23–45.

Kreulen, G., Stommel, M., Gutek, B., Burns, L. and Braden, C. (2002) Utility of retrospective pretest ratings of patient satisfaction with health status, *Research in Nursing and Health*, 25(3): 233–41.

Lam, T. and Bengo, P. (2002) A comparison of three retrospective self-reporting methods of measuring change in instructional practice, *American Journal of Evaluation*, 24(1): 65–80.

Oort, F. J. (2005) Using structural equation modeling to detect response shifts and true change, *Quality of Life Research*, 14, 587–98.

Pedhazur, E. and Schmelkin, L. (1991) *Measurement, Design and Analysis: An Integrated Approach*. New Jersey: Lawrence Erlbaum Associates.

Pratt, C., McGuigan, W. and Katzev, A. (2000) Measuring program outcomes: Using retrospective pre-test methodology, *American Journal of Evaluation*, 21(3): 341–9.

Rees, J., Waldron, D., O'Boyle, C., Ewings, P. and MacDonagh, R. (2003) Prospective vs retrospective assessment of lower urinary tract symptoms in patients with advanced prostate cancer: The effect of 'response shift', *BJU International*, 92(7): 703–6.

Reichardt, C. (2009) Quasi-experimental design, in R. Millsap and A. Maydeu-Olivares (eds) *The Sage Handbook of Quantitative Methods in Psychology*. Thousand Oaks, CA: Sage, Pp. 46–71.

Rohs, F. (1999) Response shift bias: A problem in evaluating leadership development with self-report pretest–posttest measures, *Journal of Agricultural Education*, 40(4): 28–37.

Schwartz, C. and Sprangers, M. (2010) Guidelines for improving the stringency of response shift research using the thentest, *Quality of Life Research*, 19(4): 455–64.

Schwartz, C., Bode, R., Repucci, N., Becker, J., Sprangers, M. and Fayers, A. (2006) The clinical significance of adaptation to changing health: A meta-analysis of response shift, *Quality of Life Research*, 15(9): 1533–50.

Shadish, W. and Clark, M. (2004) Quasi-experiment, in M. Lewis-Beck, A. Bryman and T. Liao (eds) *The Sage Encyclopedia of Social Science Research Methods*. Thousand Oaks, CA: Sage, pp. 898–902.

Shadish, W., Cook, T. and Campbell, D. (2002) *Experimental and Quasi-experimental Designs for Generalized Causal Inference*. Boston. MA: Houghton Mifflin.

Sprangers, M. (1988) *Response Shift and the Retrospective Pretest: On the Usefulness of Retrospective Pretest–Posttest Designs in Detecting Training Related Response Shifts*. Rotterdam: Het Instituut voor Onderzoek van het Onderwijs.

Sprangers, M. (1989) Response shift bias in program evaluation, *Impact Assessment Bulletin*, 7: 153–66.

Sprangers, M. and Schwartz, C. (1999) Integrating response shift into health-related quality of life research: A theoretical model, *Social Science and Medicine*, 48(11): 1507–15.

Sprangers, M.A., Van Dam, F.S., Broersen, J., Lodder, L., Wever, L. and Visser, M. R., Oosterveld, P. and Smets, E. (1999) Revealing response shift in longitudinal research on fatigue: The use of the thentest approach, *Acta Oncologica*, 38(6): 709–18.

Stone, S., Fuller, C., Savage, J., Cookson, B., Hayward, A., Cooper, B., Duckworth, G., Michie, S., Murray, M., Jeanes, A., Roberts, J., Teare, L. and Charlett, A. (2012) Evaluation of the national Cleanyourhands campaign to reduce *Staphylococcus aureus* bacteraemia and *Clostridium difficile* infection in hospitals in England and Wales by improved hand hygiene: Four year, prospective, ecological, interrupted time series study, *British Medical Journal*, 344: 1–11.

Sweeney, K. (2004) Regression toward the mean, in M. Lewis-Beck, A. Bryman and T. Liao (eds) *The Sage Encyclopedia of Social Science Research Methods*. Thousand Oaks, CA: Sage, pp. 945–6.

Timmerman, A.A., Anteunis, L.J. and Meesters, C.M. (2003) Response-shift bias and parent-reported quality of life in children with otitis media, *Archives of Otolaryngology – Head & Neck Surgery*, 129(9): 987–91.

Umble, K., Upshaw, V., Orton, S. and Kelly, M. (2000) Using the post-then method to assess learner change. Paper presented at the American Association of Higher Education Assessment Conference, North Carolina, June 2000.

Vrijhoef, H., Diederiks, J., Spreeuwenberg, C., Wolffenbuttel, B. and van Wilderen, L. (2002) The nurse specialist as main care-provider for patients with type 2 diabetes in a primary care setting: Effects on patient outcomes, *International Journal of Nursing Studies*, 39(4): 441–51.

Waters, B. and Raisler, J. (2003) Ice massage for the reduction of labor pain, *Journal of Midwifery and Women's Health*, 48(5): 317–21.

Westerman, M.J., The, A.-M., Sprangers, M.A.G., Groen, H.J.M., van der Wal, G. and Hak, T. (2007) Small-cell lung cancer patients are just 'a little bit' tired: Response shift and self presentation in the measurement of fatigue, *Quality of Life Research*, 16(5): 853–61.

12   Audit in health care

Corina Naughton

Introduction

Audit has become a feature of public and private sector organizations that are characterized by an ethos that emphasizes improvement, ongoing development and high standards in efficiency and performance. It is synonymous with transparency, for example the audit of public accounts, and the demonstration of quality and adherence to recommended standards and codes of practice, be they financial, legal, manufacturing or in health care. Audit in health care is perhaps one of the fastest growing areas of audit activity in any sector, and is viewed as an essential link in the quality improvement, change management and, more recently, the efficiency drive in health care (Burgess 2011).

This chapter aims to:

- define audit within a modern health care system
- examine the role of health care practitioners in relation to audit
- describe the audit process, including planning and audit design, and implementing and sustaining change.

Defining audit in health care

Clinical audit is the term traditionally used to describe audit activity in health care. Following its introduction in the early 1950s it had a specific focus on clinical practice, and was undertaken mainly by medical practitioners examining their own practice in the acute hospital setting. Audit in the medical profession was promoted as a means of improving and standardizing medical practice to ensure that patients received treatments based on the best evidence available (Baker et al. 1999). In recent years, audit has become established in nursing, pharmacy, physiotherapy and other health professions (Hammond et al. 2005; Dulko 2007; Montesi and Lechi 2009).

An early definition of audit stated that it is 'the process of critically and systematically assessing our own professional activities with a commitment to improve performance and ultimately the quality and/or cost effectiveness of patient care'

(Fraser 1982). This definition identifies the commitment to improved practice, but emphasizes the ownership of this process by the practitioners involved.

Audit in modern health care has extended beyond immediate clinical practice and increasingly involves aspects of the broader health care system such as administration, environment, resources and service utilization. There is confusion, however, as to what activity constitutes audit, and the term can be used to refer to any data collection on activity or performance rather than an explicit attempt to measure performance against pre-specified standards as part of an action plan to improve the quality of care or of a service (Loughlan 2011).

Another feature of audit in health care today is that practitioners are often external to the audit process and may no longer have ownership of it, especially in the case of multisite or national audits (Johnston et al. 2000). National or large-scale regional audits have increased in number and scope in recent years. In this type of audit, individuals or teams external to the care environment carry out the evaluation, or alternatively practitioners submit information to a central office and the results are reported directly to health service management rather than to the practitioners or units who were the subject of the audit.

A more recent definition of clinical audit reflects that of the National Institute for Health and Clinical Excellence (NICE) (NICE 2002), refines the concept of audit as a measure against criteria but reflects the broader application of audit in health care systems:

> Clinical audit is a quality improvement process that seeks to improve patient care and outcomes through systematic review of care against explicit criteria and the implementation of change. . . clinical audit is about measuring the quality of care and services against agreed standards and making improvements where necessary. (Burgess 2011: 6)

In essence, from the practitioners' view point, there are two tiers of audit in health care. The first level is clinical audit, carried out by health care practitioners within their immediate health care setting to inform their own practice or local unit activity. See Box 12.1 for an example of a practitioner-led audit and clinical practice change initiative.

Box 12.1   Practitioner-led audit and clinical practice change initiative (Shinners et al. 2012)

A nurse-led project involved the implementation of four care bundles (collections of evidence-based practice criteria) for urinary catheters, venous catheters, central venous catheters and enteral feeding across three departments. Once the evidence-based practice guidelines were agreed and circulated, ward champions in each department undertook monthly point-prevalence audits (all patients audited on a particular day) and reported the results back to the participating ward. Over a 12-month period, average compliance levels in the four care bundles' criteria improved from 58 per cent to 98 per cent.

The second level is audit carried out on behalf of management teams, regulators, or government bodies such as the Health and Information Quality Authority in Ireland (HIQA) or the Health Quality and Improvement Partnership (HQIP) in England and Wales. The focus is on monitoring performance in relation to contracts, comparing performance with other areas, benchmarking and ranking units or institutions (see Box 12.2).

Box 12.2 Report on Hand Hygiene Compliance in HSE Acute Hospitals (HSE 2011)

The Health Service Executive in Ireland undertook a national hand hygiene compliance audit in 36 acute hospitals in 2011. In each hospital, seven randomly selected wards were identified and 30 opportunities for hand hygiene per ward were observed, involving all health care personnel. A national target of 75 per cent compliance was set. An average compliance rate of 74 per cent hand hygiene compliance was reported, with tables identifying individual hospitals' performance. This audit is set to run on a biannual basis.

Both types of audit have as their goal improved quality and/or efficiency in health care; however, ownership of the data and control over implementing the audit recommendations rest at different levels in the organization.

Audit and professional practice

Clinical audit in professional practice is one of the primary methods of demonstrating adherence to evidence-based practice and achieving quality improvement. Clinical audit in medical practice is well established and is embedded into medical education, training and standards for professional competency (GMC 2009; Medical Council (Irish) 2011). In other health care professions it is at an earlier stage of development and it is not as explicit or visible in either education or practice (Cheater and Keane 1998; Turner et al. 1999; Dulko 2007). However, this is changing, especially with the expansion of the scope of practice of a number of health professions and the need to demonstrate evidence-based practice.

The current emphasis in health care on evidence-based practice carries with it an expectation that individual practitioners or professional groups engage in audit. However, there are challenges and variable views among practitioners towards audit (Johnston et al. 2000; Nettleton and Ireland 2000). Nonetheless, in line with the trend towards multidisciplinary or interprofessional management of complex medical and surgical conditions, the recommendation is that a multidisciplinary approach to audit is put in place (NICE 2002). It is increasingly recognized that multidisciplinary audit is more effective in introducing and sustaining change, as well as contributing to improved interdisciplinary communication and functioning (NICE 2002; Cheater et al. 2005; Waldron et al. 2011). An example of multidisciplinary audit impacting on practice is the UK National Sentinel Stroke Audit 2010 (http://www.rcplondon.ac.uk/resources/national-sentinel-stroke-audit). The audit measures adherence to national guidelines for stroke, standards and quality of stroke services, and tracks individual health care trusts' performance over time. This audit process has demonstrated improvements in many areas of practice in stroke care and continues to make recommendations to drive improvements in organizational structures and clinical practice (Intercollegiate Stroke Working Party 2010). A similar comprehensive audit of stroke services was also carried out in Ireland (Horgan et al. 2011).

Audit versus research

A long-standing debate concerns what is research and what is audit? The distinction is more conceptual than actual, as they share similar design principles, methodologies and data-analysis strategies, and both have the shared aim of generating reproducible, reliable and valid data. Research is concerned with producing new knowledge or confirming the generalizability of existing knowledge or evidence, whereas audit measures current practice against the best available research evidence (Baker et al. 1999). Benjamin (2008: 1241) sums up the difference as: 'research asks the question, what is the right thing to do? Whereas clinical audit asks, "are we doing the right thing in the right way?"'

In its purest sense, audit has two characteristics that distinguish it from research: 1) explicit criteria, based on current evidence are identified from the outset and data are collected to gauge performance against these criteria; and 2) implementation of change in response to the assessed performance is an integral part of the audit process. However, there is overlap between research and audit – for example, in areas where there are no agreed criteria or standards against which to measure practice, there may be an initial evaluation of practice from which recommendations or standards are developed, and this is seen as part of the audit process.

It is a misconception among practitioners and managers that audit is an easier or less rigorous process than research, and it is perhaps this misconception that has resulted in audits of variable quality, that have produced poor to moderate improvements in health care (Grimshaw et al. 2001; Jamtvedt et al. 2006; Bowie et al. 2007). Clinical audit, rather than being the poor relative of research, requires the same rigorous approach to design, methodology, analysis and dissemination as any survey or randomized controlled trial (RCT) and, in addition, requires that equal attention is given to change management.

Audit process

The audit process is traditionally represented as a cycle with a number of stages or phases. The most recent publication from HQIP in collaboration with NICE describes four stages (Burgess 2011):

1   Preparation and planning
2   Measuring performance
3   Implementing change
4   Sustaining improvement including re-audit

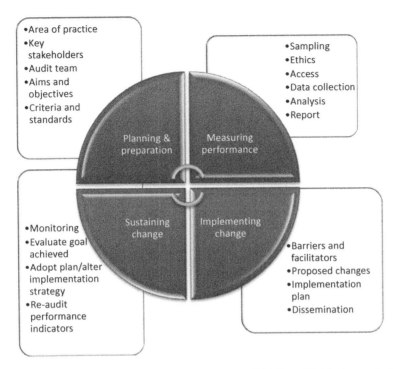

Figure 12.1 The audit cycle, adapted from Burgess (2011), with kind permission from Healthcare Quality Improvement Partnership (HQIP) and Radcliffe Publishing.

This overarching description of the stages underlines the complexity and challenge of collecting clinically credible and valid data on which to base practice changes followed by change management strategies that will result in a sustained change in human behaviour. Within each stage of the audit cycle, there are a number of steps that require careful consideration, decision making and action (Figure 12.1).

Stage I: Planning and preparation

The first stage of the audit process has the greatest potential to impact on the success or failure of the audit project. There can be a tendency to rush this stage and start data collection as soon as possible. This is nearly always a mistake, and can result in a poorly defined problem, aims and objectives that are too ambitious, results that lack validity or reliability – and that can lead to an unworkable solution. On the other hand, if this process is too slow and there is a lack of effective decision making, staff may lose enthusiasm and the project may eventually run out of momentum.

Identify the topic

The starting point for any research or audit project is to identify a topic. In some situations it is immediately clear what area of practice to concentrate on, especially if it is in response to a critical incident. This, however, should be the exception rather than the rule; in any organization a strategic planned audit activity rather than a reactionary approach to quality improvement is required. Increasingly, the selection of an audit topic is driven by national priorities but it is also important that practitioners, in collaboration with senior management, set priorities within their own organization. This does not preclude local unit, individual or uniprofessional audit activity, but there must be cognizance of the time, resources and cost involved that include implementing and embedding the recommendations into practice and the need to re-audit. A more efficient and effective approach is to identify a small number of carefully selected priorities and to complete the audit cycle, rather than selecting a larger number of topics that may be partially completed, resulting in marginal impact on practice and adding to the workload of already busy staff. Ashmore et al. (2011: 26) focuses on the feasibility of undertaking an audit and outlines a number of questions that should be asked before commencing the process:

1   Does the topic lend itself to the audit process or are different approaches more appropriate or efficient e.g. case series review, root cause analysis, activity or workload analysis?
2   Is the problem concerned amenable to change?
3   How much scope is there for improvement?
4   What are the potential benefits of undertaking this audit?

Identify the audit team

Identifying the project team is driven by the complexity and the scope of the audit topic. In some cases the audit is undertaken by a team external to the organization; in other cases it is the role of a defined unit within the health care setting. In the case of local or unit audits, the team is likely to be formed by staff working directly in that area. To be effective, members of the team need to share a commitment to resolving the problem that is the focus of the audit.

The complex nature of many health care problems means the team should normally be drawn from the relevant professional and support staff that have direct involvement in the problem area. Take as an example delays to theatre schedules, which are an ongoing issue in many hospitals. Unidisciplinary professions have undertaken audits to identify the causes of theatre delays (Haiart et al. 1990; Iver et al. 2004; Saha et al. 2009); however, despite this, delays remain a significant problem in health care (Marjamaa et al. 2008). Many such audits have lacked the involvement of key stakeholder groups in the audit team during the planning phase. Such a project, therefore, should consider representation from surgical teams, anaesthetic teams, surgical wards, theatre and recovery room teams, as well as service and administrative staff and hospital management; in a number of cases audit may also extend to patient groups.

Managing a collaborative project of this nature increases the complexity of the project management in terms of scheduling meetings, disseminating information and establishing effective team working patterns. However, this additional effort and time commitment should be viewed in the context of the overall change management process, not just the audit data collection.

Involving stakeholders

Once the audit topic is identified, it is important to consider who is affected by the problem. In essence, all parties that directly or indirectly experience the problem will be affected or involved in the initiative to improve the situation. Consideration needs to be given to involving patients or service users, clinical staff, support staff, managers and relevant external groups such as other departments or services external to the organization, including patient advocacy groups (Ashmore et al. 2011). Many of the problems in health care are broad and multifaceted; obtaining the views of the various stakeholders can help frame the problem, break it down into its component parts and facilitate the development of clear goals and objectives.

In the past, audit projects have lacked this wider consultation. In particular, patients or service users and their families were not involved in the planning stage and were simply viewed as a source of information (Kelson 1998; Oliver et al. 2004). In addition, with the increased focus on national audit, there is a risk that front-line health staff can experience audit as an external process that they have little influence over. The full consequence of this may not be realized until the change management phases of the audit process are initiated, with staff sceptical about the audit results and, due to their lack of involvement, even more so about the proposed changes. An approach that builds collaboration at the early planning stage is more likely to succeed and lead to better working and communication arrangements between health care professional and non-professional groups and health care administrators.

There is a growing body of research into meaningful methods of involving stakeholders in research that is also applicable to audit (Minogue and Girdlestone 2010; Franx et al. 2011; Pickard et al. 2011). Methods of involving stakeholders can include one-to-one conversations, small group meetings, workshops, focus groups and the potential of Web2 technology such as discussion boards, online surveys or forums (Légaré et al. 2011).

Project aims and objectives

Defining the aims of the project is the next significant step for the audit team; this involves defining the scope, breadth and depth of the subsequent data collection and determines the extent of the change. This step should not be rushed; careful consideration can avoid the collection of unnecessary information or information that lacks sufficient detail to design a feasible solution to the problem.

If the problem is complex and multifaceted it may be useful to use approaches from project management to gain a clearer picture of the different elements that contribute to the problem. The fishbone diagram or cause and effect charts are perhaps some of the best known tools from project management that can be used to graphically illustrate the problem (Baker et al. 1999; Grol et al. 2005). As well as identifying the individual factors, these factors can be categorized into core factors such as systems, people and environment, and material factors. Figure 12.2 illustrates the use of a fishbone diagram to identify possible factors that may impact on emergency

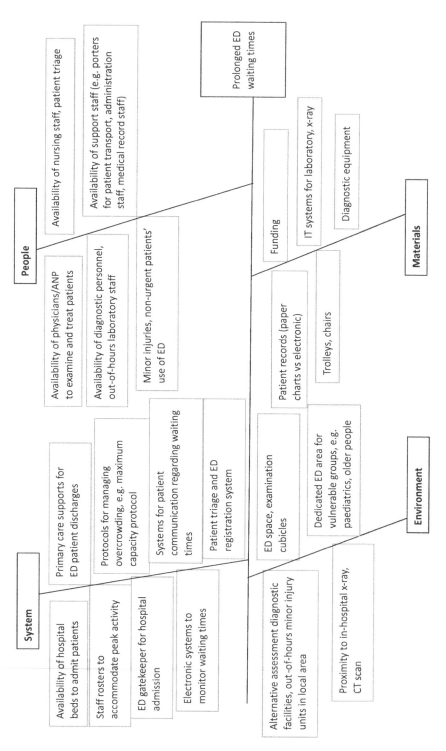

Figure 12.2 Fishbone diagram of factors that may impact on emergency department waiting times (Note: this is not intended to be an exhaustive list of factors).

department (ED) waiting times. These factors can be identified from a combination of the literature on this topic and local expertise (Rowe et al. 2006).

In terms of clarifying the project aims and objectives, such a diagram illustrates how each of the factors in their own right, for example availability of hospital beds, availability of physicians to review patients, speed of obtaining x-ray or laboratory results, may require a number of sub-audits within a larger audit. The scope of such a project is determined by the level of urgency and priority an organization places on this topic. If it is a high-level organizational priority with dedicated staff and resources available for audit, including change management, then several factors that are amenable to change may be selected for investigation. However, if the support is primarily confined to the ED staff then a single factor that is suitable for audit and amenable to change (such as delays in obtaining x-rays or increasing non-urgent patients' knowledge of alternative resources before attending ED) is all that may be feasible.

Clarifying the project title and aims

Once the scope of the project is agreed, it is useful to give the project a working title that clearly identifies the subject of the audit (who) and the object (what) that is to be audited. For example: 'an audit of non-urgent emergency department attendees' is broad and open to individual interpretation; in contrast: 'an audit to improve non-urgent emergency departments attendees' knowledge, and increase use of alternative health care facilities' provides a clearer focus for the project team and stakeholders.

The above title also articulates the overall aim of the study. In writing the aims of an audit project the emphasis is on the change to be achieved, unlike research where the aim reflects the exploration of a particular phenomenon. In audit, change-related verbs are often used, such as 'to increase', 'to decrease', 'to enhance'; while in research, aims are more often written using exploratory verbs. Table 12.1 contains examples of the difference in how aims are constructed for audit compared to research.

Table 12.1 Example of project aims for audit compared to research

Audit aims	Research aims
To improve communication with patients regarding ED waiting times	To identify patient information needs during ED visits
To increase efficiency in obtaining x-ray results	To assess the appropriateness of x-ray requests
To increase the proportion of patients in ED seen within four hours	To identify the predictors of prolonged (> six hours) ED visits
To enhance patient privacy during ED consultations	To gain a deeper understanding of people's experience of privacy during ED consultations
To decrease non-urgent ED attendances during peak ED activity	To test the hypothesis that an increase in availability of alternative out-of-hours health care facilities will reduce non-urgent ED attendances

As in research, the overall audit aim needs to be stated clearly. This usually involves identifying the target of the audit and the change to be achieved. The clarity of the audit aim is increased by developing a small number, usually between two and four, of more specific audit objectives (Box 12.3). These objectives operationalize how the aim will be achieved and specify indicators to enable assessment of how well the change was implemented: in other words, did the audit process succeed in addressing the original problem?

Box 12.3 Example of an audit aim and objectives

Overall aim: To improve communication with patients regarding ED waiting times.
   Specific objectives:

* To implement a system/protocol to provide information on waiting times for patients.
* To reduce by 50 per cent the incidence of patients waiting more than two hours without receiving updates on potential waiting times.
* To record patient feedback regarding the communication system.
* To reduce complaints from patients by 15 per cent regarding lack of information on waiting times.

Standards and criteria

Criteria and standards are key distinguishing features of an audit. A primary function of audit is to compare current practice to best practice as indicated in guidelines, international norms of practice or performance targets. Such guidelines, norms or targets are the basis for developing the audit criteria and standards. The audit team need to apply systematic methods to select the appropriate review criteria, which should be explicitly reported in the audit protocol (Hearnshaw et al. 2003). However, there is confusion surrounding the meaning of the terms 'standard' and 'criteria' and, at times, these terms may be used interchangeably. Ashmore et al. (2011: 33) suggest that criteria are 'measurable statements of what should be happening', while standards are 'explicit and quantifiable performance levels expressed as percentages'. These two elements can be stated separately or they can be combined into a single statement; an essential point is that the audit team are clear about what they are measuring and what level of performance is desirable. This is illustrated with an example of how clinical practice guidelines for cardiovascular disease prevention can be written as both criteria and standards for audit (see Box 12.4).

Based on the guidelines outlined in Box 12.4, practitioners in primary or secondary care can develop a set of criteria that describe what actions should be carried out at the individual patient level. They can also specify a standard that indicates what level of performance they hope to achieve at the patient population level.

Box 12.4   Example of international clinical practice guidelines

---

The European guidelines on cardiovascular disease (CVD) prevention in clinical practice (European Society of Cardiology 2007) indicate best practice in relation to cardiovascular risk reduction in people with both diagnosed and undiagnosed cardiovascular disease. The following is an example of specified physiological targets for management of established CVD:

European Society of Cardiology Guidelines on CVD Prevention (2007)
To achieve more rigorous risk factor reduction in high-risk subjects, especially those with established CVD or diabetes:

- blood pressure under 130/80 mmHg if feasible
- total cholesterol <4.5 mmol/L (−175 mg/dl) with an option of <4 mmol/L (−155 mg/dl) if feasible
- LDL cholesterol <2.5 mmol/L (−100 mg/dl) with an option of 2mmol/L (−80mg/dl) if feasible
- fasting blood glucose <6mmol/L (−110 mg/dl) and HbA1c <6.5% if feasible
- to consider cardioprotective drug therapy in these high-risk subjects, especially those with established atherosclerotic CVD

(Please see the complete guideline for a more comprehensive overview on this topic: http://www.escardio.org/guidelines-surveys/esc-guidelines/GuidelinesDocuments/ guidelines-CVD-prevention.pdf).

Criterion 1: Patients with a high-risk or established CVD will have a blood pressure check every six months.
  Standard: 80 per cent of patients.
Criterion 2: If a patient's B/P is >130/80 mmHg on more than three occasions or after 24-hour monitoring, then in consultation with the patient, anti-hypertensive medication will be started or existing anti-hypertensive therapy will be reviewed.
  Standard: 95 per cent of high-risk patients with elevated B/P.

It often makes more sense to combine the criteria and the standard into a single statement.

Practice standard 1: 80 per cent of patients with high-risk or established CVD will have a blood pressure check every six months.
Practice standard 2: 95 per cent of high-risk patients with persistently elevated B/P >130/80 mmHg (on more than three occasions or after 24-hour B/P monitoring) will be prescribed anti-hypertensive medication or have existing anti-hypertensive therapy reviewed.

Similar criteria and standards can be developed for the remaining guidelines on cholesterol, blood glucose, and lifestyle management.

Types of criteria

Criteria can be categorized as structural, process or outcome criteria; this approach aligns the audit process with Donabedian's view of quality in health care (Donabedian 1966).

Structural criteria are those that relate to environmental or resource factors. For example, using the CVD scenario, a structural criterion may be the establishment of a nurse-led CVD clinic for monitoring high-risk patients within six months, investment in new IT software to increase efficiency in patient data recording and retrieval, or training for staff on a new IT system.

Process criteria relates to specific actions and determines how a broad guideline is operationalized within individual health care settings. The two criteria mentioned above, measuring blood pressure and prescribing medication in CVD, are examples of process outcomes.

Outcome criteria have a narrow focus on patient outcomes and concentrate on the achievement of therapeutic goals, modification of behaviour or impact on mortality, morbidity or quality of life. For example, an outcome criterion related to CVD would be that 40 per cent of high-risk CVD patients have a blood pressure <130/80 mmHg at three consecutive readings, or that 30 per cent of high-risk CVD patients reported that they were not smoking at six months following a quit smoking intervention. Patient outcome criteria can be more difficult to measure, but should be built into re-audits. This level of information is the only real way to gauge the success or otherwise of an intervention to change practice and justify sustaining the change. Audit has being criticized for treating structure criteria (such as purchasing IT systems) and process criteria (increasing adherence to guidelines) as endpoints in themselves and ignoring the impact on patient outcome criteria (Hearnshaw et al. 2003; Dassow 2007).

What standard to specify?

Practitioners often wonder what standard (level of performance or target) to specify. There is no single answer. Sometimes the performance target may be set by an external body – for example, in the UK the Department of Health specified a target stating that 95 per cent of patients should wait no longer than four hours in ED (Woodcock et al. 2012), or in primary care performance targets for GP practices are outlined in the national Quality and Outcomes Framework (QOF) (NHS 2012).

Higher performance standards, up to 80 per cent or 90 per cent, may be set for structural or process criteria. These are criteria that practitioners have more control over compared to patient outcome criteria, which may be affected by socio-economic, environmental, educational, psychological or physiological factors. The performance levels in patient outcome criteria may be small or modest, such as a 5–10 per cent change in behaviour, compliance or physiological markers.

In the case of clinical guidelines, such as the CVD guidelines, the performance target may be based on previously published studies, national or regional averages or the current level of performance in the clinic or practice. The target may be set to achieve a specific benchmark such as 80 per cent or a percentage change, for instance

10–20 per cent increase in performance. For example, at baseline 50 per cent of high-risk patients had six-monthly blood pressure checks; a GP practice may set a performance target of 60 per cent of high-risk patients having a six-monthly blood pressure check within 12 months based on resources and feasibility of obtaining these targets. It is rarely advisable, or in some cases feasible, to specify a target of 100 per cent as patients have the right to self-determination and can choose to attend appointments, commence or adhere to medication or adopt changes in lifestyle.

Sources of guidelines and audit criteria

Increasingly patient care guidelines, criteria and professional standards of practice are developed by national and international organizations rather than by local practitioners; however, the criteria, and especially the performance targets, may be modified for local application. Examples of guidelines and audit criteria include professional standards and patient care guidelines, such as those produced by professional regulatory bodies and governmental organizations.

Professional standards

Professional standards, codes or scopes of practice are mandated by professional regulatory bodies such as medical councils, nursing boards and, in the case of allied health professions, the Health Professions Council. These bodies specify standards in relation to professional behaviour and competency, including areas such as patient confidentiality, record keeping, documentation, and prescribing and medication management.

Patient care guidelines and criteria

Developing original evidence-based guidelines requires considerable skill, training and time to source and synthesize the information and achieve expert consensus (Hearnshaw et al. 2003; Turner et al. 2008). In the last number of years, there has been a proliferation in the number of sources as well as the actual number of health care conditions for which guidelines have been developed. For busy front-line staff it is often more efficient and robust to use existing guidelines from established reputable sources to audit performance (Benjamin 2008). However, a growing difficulty is choosing between different conflicting guidelines for the same condition and assessing their quality (Chenot et al. 2008; Navarro Puerto et al. 2008). Below is a brief description of the most widely known and accessible sources.

Professional bodies and societies

One of the primary sources of information in relation to the management of specific patient conditions are guidelines produced by professional bodies that have a lead role in treating the condition. Increasingly, there is a move towards developing international standardized guidelines and audit criteria; an example is the European cardiovascular disease prevention guidelines, which are based on a consensus of professional opinions from different specialities across Europe (European Society of Cardiology 2007). Other examples include The National Clinical Audit of Falls and

Bone Health in Older people (http://www.rcplondon.ac.uk/resources/national-audit-falls-and-bone-health-older-people) and the National Sentinel Stroke Audit (http://www.rcplondon.ac.uk/resources/national-sentinel-stroke-audit), both coordinated by the Royal College of Physicians. In nursing, the Royal College of Nursing (RCN) have published guidelines in relation to pressure ulcer management, venous leg ulcer and other patient care issues (http://www.rcn.org.uk/development/practice/clinicalguide lines). Similarly, the Royal Society for Charted Physiotherapists and the Society and College of Radiographers also provide practice guidelines for their members.

Government health departments/health care providers

Government health departments and government-funded health care providers, such as the National Health Service (NHS) in the UK, or the Health Service Executive (HSE) in Ireland, are an important source of national guidelines for the management of common health care conditions. In England, the National Quality and Outcomes Framework in primary care utilizes criteria and performance standards based on clinical guidelines to promote adherence to evidence-based practice across a number of common clinical conditions (Gillman 2011; NHS 2012).

Quality health improvement agencies

There are a number of influential organizations, usually publicly funded, that synthesize existing research, professional consensus and economic evaluations to develop practice guidelines. These groups strongly influence the development of national guidelines and performance targets.

- *National Institute for Health and Clinical Excellence (NICE)*: In the UK and in Europe the National Institute for Health and Clinical Excellence (http://www.nice.org.uk) is one of the most widely known and influential organizations in health care. NICE has developed comprehensive sets of clinical guidelines related to specific patient groups, conditions or topic areas. For front-line practitioners it is perhaps one of the most valuable and accessible sources of synthesized health care information available. An equivalent organization in Scotland is the Scottish Intercollegiate Guidelines Network (SIGN).
- *Health and Information Quality Authority (HIQA):* In Ireland, the Health Information and Quality Authority (HIQA) has a primary role in establishing standards across primary, secondary and residential care settings. Recent standards include the National Standards for the Prevention and Control of Healthcare Associated Infections and National Quality Assurance Criteria for Clinical Guidelines (http://www.hiqa.ie/publications/).
- *National Guideline Clearing House (NQMC):* This is a public resource for evidence-based clinical practice guidelines and quality measures (http://guide-line.gov/). It is primarily a repository for practice guidelines from prominent professional bodies, societies and health care organizations, mainly from the United States and Canada but also Europe and Australia. Guidelines are submitted on a voluntary basis, and where there are comparable guidelines there is an attempt to compare and synthesize evidence and recommendations.

Time schedule and resources

Budget, time and the availability of resources are often the limiting factors that decide the scope of an audit. Clinical staff undertaking audit, especially if not supported by dedicated personnel, need to be realistic about what they can achieve, especially in relation to their own time. Bearing this in mind, audit is a highly recommended and often compulsory component of many clinical roles.

The audit team should draw up a realistic timeline for each stage of the audit process, identify potential sources of delay in advance and identify strategies to overcome these difficulties. Potential sources of delay may include: issues in gaining ethical approval, access to the target population, resistance to data collection, and low response rates.

Stage II: Measurement of performance

The second stage of the audit process is measuring performance. This phase is driven by the aims and objectives of the audit and the criteria and standards of performance specified. Clearly articulated aims and objectives will identify the target population and the type of data required to evaluate performance against the selected criteria.

Qualitative or quantitative methodology

The vast majority of audits involve a quantitative methodology. In the design the emphasis is on calculating a sample size, random sampling, and collecting quantifiable representative data that can be generalized to the wider patient population. However, with an increased awareness of involving service users and other stakeholders, qualitative approaches can be incorporated as an element of the evaluation process through the use of focus groups or semi-structured one-to-one interviews.

Ethical considerations

In the past ethics in relation to audit was a grey area. A commonly held belief was that audit did not require ethical approval (Dixon 2009). The changes to legislation on data protection in many countries mean this view is no longer valid and each project, whether described as research or audit, needs to be assessed from an ethical perspective. Today, the majority of institutions have guidelines on whether a project requires full ethical approval or exemption from ethical approval. Even if a project does not require ethical approval the protocol may have to be submitted for consideration to an ethics committee or institutional review board. At the very least, most institutions require that all audit projects are registered centrally for internal quality approval purposes (Dixon 2009).

It is the responsibility of the audit team to be aware of and implement local and national guidelines on consent, confidentiality and data protection (Dixon 2009). If in doubt whether or not an audit project requires ethical approval it is always best to seek the advice of the local audit office or ethics committee.

Do patients need to be informed? This is the subject of much debate within audit and there is no single answer. Patients or their guardians who are approached directly for interview or survey need to give consent (or assent) to participate, as would happen in a research study. It is less clear in relation to the review of clinical patient records; one of the key considerations is whether the information collected is identifiable (can be traced back to the patient or service user) or potentially identifiable. Many institutions alert patients through standard information leaflets or notices that their medical records may be the subject of routine clinical audit.

Sample selection and size

The target population should be clear from the audit aims. In the case of complex audits there may be more than one target population. For example, an audit to reduce ED waiting times may include patients as well as physicians, ED nurses, porters, x-ray or laboratory staff. The subject of the audit may be at a more micro level, for example ordering of a diagnostic test, prescription of medication or referral to a particular service.

The target population is defined through explicit inclusion and exclusion criteria, with a clear rationale for these criteria. The population in an audit study needs to reflect the normal variation found in the patient population; for example, exclusion criteria seen in research studies based on age, gender, or mental capacity may not be appropriate in an audit study.

As audit is being increasingly used as part of a strategy to drive more substantial and large-scale change in clinical practice, there is now greater attention given to calculating sample size and obtaining representative samples through use of random sampling methods (Benning, Dixon-Woods et al. 2011). In the past a sample size of 30–50 cases was regarded as adequate for audit purposes; for local units and small-scale changes to practice this may still be acceptable. However, audit that is designed to influence clinical practice and patient outcomes at an institutional, regional or national level requires the rigorous sampling methodologies of research projects.

The final step is to devise a random sampling strategy. In a single unit or institution the most frequently used method is either simple random sampling or systematic sampling.

In simple random sampling each patient in the sampling frame (list of patients) is assigned a number, e.g. 1–300, then using a random number table or random number-generation software (http://www.random.org/) a set of random numbers is generated and the corresponding patient record is selected.

Systematic sampling is also frequently used in audit; for example, every third or fifth patient in the sampling frame is selected until the required sample size is obtained. When using systematic sampling, it is important to avoid sampling bias; for example, a sampling frame based on the date the patient first registered with the practice rather than a sampling frame based on alphabetical order of names or date of birth may result in a more representative sample of the practice population.

Audit has been strongly criticized for inadequate sampling designs, relying mainly on small convenience samples. This often had the effect of producing results and subsequent recommendations that clinical practitioners did not trust and were easily discredited. If time, effort and resources are going to be invested in carrying out audit it is essential that every aspect, especially the sampling design, can stand up to close scrutiny (Bowie et al. 2007). If possible, expert advice should be sought in relation to calculating a sample size and selecting an appropriate random sampling strategy (see Chapter 9 for further detail on calculating sample size).

Data collection

Data collection in audit projects predominately uses the same approaches as that found in quantitative research. The focus in audit is on assessing and quantifying performance and/or quality of care or services, often against predefined criteria. The specific audit objectives dedicate the data-collection methodologies. The most frequently used approaches are surveys using questionnaires (see Chapter 15) or data extraction from existing databases, medical records or administration data such as waiting lists. The following are the steps and issues involved in data collection.

Define variable

At this stage a key step is to precisely define the variables that are required to meet the audit objectives. There is always the temptation to collect more data than required or to collect data that are readily accessible but do not meet the audit objectives.

A good exercise is to clearly identify under each objective the information required: what variables are to be measured and the possible sources of information. This exercise should help to keep the focus on the audit objectives and identify common sources of information on different variables. Box 12.5, again using the example of CVD, provides an example of how to define variables for measurement.

Box 12.5   Example of defining variables for measurement

Criterion 1: 80 per cent of patients with high risk or established CVD will have a blood pressure check every six months.

Variable to be collected	Variable1: Documented record of B/P measurement
	Answer format: Yes/No
	Variable 2: Recorded date within six months of current data
	Answer format: Yes/No or the actual date
Sources of information	Electronic patient record, patient charts

Criterion 2: 95 per cent of high risk patients with persistently elevated B/P >130/80 mmHg (on more than three occasions or after 24 hours of B/P monitoring) will be prescribed anti-hypertensive medication or have existing anti-hypertensive drug therapy reviewed.

Variable to be collected	Variable 3: B/P above or below criteria
	Answer format: Yes/No or actual B/P values
	Variable 4: Prescribed anti-hypertensive medication
	Answer format: Yes/No or name of drugs and dose
	Variable 5: Review date of antihypertensive medication
	Answer format: Yes/No or the actual date
Sources of information	Electronic or paper patient records, pharmacy database

---

The exercise outlined in Box 12.5 allows the audit team to clearly define the variables they need to collect and decide the level of detail they need to record, for example do they need to know the name of the anti-hypertensive medication or is it enough to indicate that anti-hypertensive medication was prescribed. Such decisions are influenced by the purpose, aims and objectives of the audit, the time available and the skill set of the team to be able to code and analyse the data.

Prospective versus retrospective data collection

The data collected can be retrospective (already recorded, requires data retrieval) or prospective (data are not yet recorded, require collection). In the case of retrospective data the audit team may have to design a data-extraction form to allow the systematic collection of data from existing records. Prospective data collection can involve the use of questionnaires to collect data directly from the sample population or it may involve the collection of data from existing records from some point in the future over a specific time period.

Sources of data

Audit projects should utilize existing sources of data where possible. Common sources of such data include:

- electronic or paper medical patient records
- GP practice records
- pharmacy and prescribing databases
- admission and discharge data
- emergency department records
- mortality records
- disease registries
- laboratory data
- theatre lists
- outpatient or day surgery records of attendance.

Designing data-collection instruments

The principles of designing data-collection instruments for audit are similar to those outlined in designing questionnaires for research purposes (see Chapter 15). Ashmore et al. (2011) outline a number of guidelines that should be considered when designing audit data-collection instruments:

- Only collect data on variables that are required.
- Patient demographic characteristics such as age and gender are often collected to allow for comparability between the audit sample and the target population, however this may not always be necessary.
- As already mentioned, patient identification information should not be recorded unless it is essential to the audit process.
- Layout should be clear and logical with sufficient space for data entry.
- If qualitative entries are required there should be sufficient space to allow the capture of verbatim quotes.

Researcher ID	Prescribing site study ID	Participant RNP study ID	Patient study ID

	Yes	No	Provide details
Patient age			Record age
Patient gender			Record gender
Evidence of PRN patient assessment			
Date of assessment (record)			
Time of assessment (record)			
Identifies primary complaint			
Record of presenting symptoms			
Record of duration of symptoms			
Record of past medical history			
Record of current medication prescribed			
Record of over-the-counter medication			
Record of known allergies (if yes), nature of allergy			
Explores family history			
Record of physical examination			
Record of final diagnosis			
Request diagnostic tests			
Interprets diagnostic tests			
Evidence of treatment/action plan			
Evidence of PRN patient review/ reassessment			

Figure 12.3 Registered nurse prescriber (RNP) audit data-extraction proforma. Adapted from the nurse prescribing observation schedule developed by Latter et al. (2007).

- The sequencing of the data-collection items on the data-extraction form should match the format of original data entry. For example, an audit to assess the appropriateness of drug prescribing involved extracting data on the clinical consultation from the patient's record (Naughton et al. 2012). The data-extraction form was designed to resemble the flow of a typical patient consultation found in the clinical notes (see Figure 12.3).
- If a number of criteria are to be assessed it may be beneficial, especially for data entry, to structure the form according to the different audit criteria.

- The date and time the data is collected should be recorded, along with the name of the person recording the information. This is particularly the case if multiple data collectors are involved.

Validated instruments

The audit data-collection form may be designed to collect data to facilitate the use of validated research instruments. For example, the audit of the appropriateness of prescribing involved the use of the Medication Appropriateness Index (MAI) tool (Drennan et al. 2009). The audit of bed utilization in Ireland involved the Appropriateness Evaluation Protocol (AEP) (HSE 2007). If such instruments are used, the audit team should conduct a literature search on the validity and reliability of the instruments prior to inclusion in the audit. Ideally, if there is sufficient statistical support available to the team, the validity and reliability of the instrument should be tested in relation to the current audit.

Training and piloting

As in research studies, piloting the data-collection instrument and the training of those involved in the data collection are essential to ensure the collection of reliable and accurate data. Sufficient time and resources should be allocated, especially if clinical staff are asked to collect the data. Inter-rater reliability should be tested if more than one person is involved in the data-collection process (see Chapter 16). During data collection it is essential to monitor the quality of the data collected in real time; data collectors should be supported and be able to clarify any issues with their supervisors or directly with the audit team to avoid inconsistencies in the data-collection procedure.

Data analysis and presentation

Once the data have been collected, the next step for the audit team is analysis of data. The depth and complexity of the analysis is determined by the purpose of the audit and the intended audience. National or regional audits, where there are comparisons made between institutions or practices, may require that in the analysis there is adjustment for case mix, hospital capacity, patient acuity and speciality.

At a local level, the primary statistic that should be reported is the percentage (proportion) of cases that meet the performance target; a 95 per cent confidence interval, to reflect the accuracy of this estimate, should also be calculated. Inferential statistics such as the chi-square tests, t-tests or Mann-Whitney U tests may be used to assess significant changes in performance from previous audits or against similar units (further details on data entry and analysis are outlined in Chapter 18).

As audit data are often intended for distribution to staff or service users who may not be familiar with statistics, visual presentation of the data is important. Such graphs may be produced in statistical software such as SPSS or using Microsoft Excel or equivalent packages (see Chapter 20 for further information on data presentation).

Qualitative data

The limited impact of audit on professional practice is largely not attributed to incorrect measurement of performance or lack of available evidence, but to a lack of understanding of the complexity of the organizational environment and the motivation of individuals in that environment (Grol et al. 2005; Charani et al. 2011). This realization has prompted the use of a mixed-methods approach to audit, whereby, in association with quantitative methodologies to measure performance, qualitative methodologies are used, such as focus groups or semi-structured interviews with practitioners and/or patient/client groups. The purpose of the qualitative data is to provide deeper insight into the needs, perspectives and constraints of the people targeted in any subsequent intervention or action plan to change behaviour (Polit and Beck 2012; Charani et al. 2011). This information is used in development and adapting change strategies to local circumstances. Such qualitative data may also be collected at subsequent re-audits to evaluate the impact of the intervention on practitioners or clients (Grol et al. 2005).

Sampling

The sampling in the qualitative element of an audit project is different from the quantitative. The qualitative element is interested in the person and contextualizing their practice or experience. The aim is to recruit practitioners or clients who are deeply embedded in the practice or experience and who can provide diverse perspectives (Polit and Beck 2010).

Two particular sampling strategies that may be used are:

1   **Snowball sampling**: the researcher starts with one participant and asks that participant to identify other potential participants. This method is especially useful in difficult-to-reach populations.
2   **Purposive sampling**: the researcher deliberately selects participants based on a particular characteristic or experience. In an audit context the researcher usually wishes to explore variation and diversity in practice; for example, in prescribing cholesterol-lowering medications in high-risk populations, the researcher may wish to interview practitioners who have high levels of compliance and practitioners who have lower levels of compliance based on the results from the quantitative audit data.

Data collection and analysis

To explore the contextual issues related to a particular practice, the two main qualitative data-collection approaches are one-to-one semi-structured interviews and focus group interviews. The focus group can be an efficient data-collection method and generates a discussion that can provide useful insight into different perspectives and motivations within an organization.

Analysis of the qualitative data for the purpose of informing the design of a change intervention often involves developing a descriptive category scheme or thematic analysis, whereby the data, following transcription, are organized into categories and allocated codes, and subsequently re-categorized into broader themes (Polit and Beck 2010). The categories or themes that emerge from this process in audit are often quite descriptive and concrete; however, more sophisticated analyses have been reported (Dixon-Woods et al. 2011). An example of a qualitative element in a larger evaluation project is that reported by Rapport et al. (2012), where multidisciplinary focus group interviews were conducted to explore professionals' views of changes to gastroenterology service organization and delivery, including participants' perspectives on barriers and facilitators to the change.

A qualitative data phase used in the audit process can be used to develop a deeper understanding of existing practice and help design change strategies.

Report writing

The final step of the performance measurement stage is to create a written record in the form of an audit report. The report can be constructed under the following headings:

- description of problem or area for review
- aims and objectives
- criteria and performance standards
- methodology, including target population, sample size, data-collection and analysis strategy
- results
- comparison with evidence base literature
- recommendations for practice

The final two steps in the report-writing process, comparison with current evidence base and recommendations for practice, provide the basis for implementing change in the organization based on the results of the audit.

Stage III: Implementing change

Implementing and sustaining change are the most complex stages in the audit cycle; a full discussion on implementing change in the audit cycle is outside the scope of this chapter, however this section will provide an overview of the primary literature that discusses this phase of the audit process.

Implementation model

Phases three (implementing change) and four (sustaining change) of the audit cycle are underpinned by theories related to change management and human and organizational behaviour; in turn, these theories are operationalized through implementation models (Grol et al. 2005). One such implementation model widely used in health care organizations is that proposed by Grol and Wensing (2005) (Figure 12.4).

The steps in the implementation of this change model overlap that of the audit cycle. The change management process starts with identifying and defining the research findings, guidelines or the area of practice under review, the formation of a team and the involvement of key stakeholders, followed by the clear articulation of the aims, objectives and measurement of performance.

Formation of an action plan for change

An action plan may be formulated by the audit team based on the data collected in the field; however, it is recognized that broader discussion with key stakeholders, especially

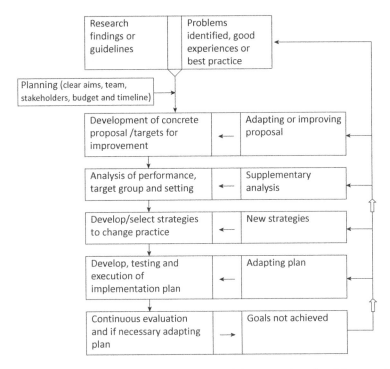

Figure 12.4 Implementation of change: a model (reproduced with permission of Richard Grol 2005).

groups directly affected by the proposed changes, is more likely to overcome resistance to the change process and result in greater levels of cooperation (Dixon-woods et al. 2011). If the action plan involves funding and resource issues, then people who are in a position to make such decisions should be consulted and involved. In formulating audit recommendations for changes in practice, it is vital these are actionable and realistic and that individuals assigned responsibility for implementing the changes have the position and authority to drive the change process (Hysong et al. 2006).

Barriers and facilitators to change

Data collection in the audit cycle concentrates on performance measurement against explicit criteria. In addition, Grol and Wensing (2004) recommend that the audit team simultaneously examine the organizational context and the characteristics, including attitude and motivation of the target group, to gain an understanding of the barriers and incentives for achieving change in practice. Grol and Wensing (2004) broadly categorized barriers or incentives to change, including: characteristics of the innovation, the professional group and the user group, and the social, organizational, economic and political context in which the change takes place (see Box 12.6).

Box 12.6   Perceived barriers to implementing guidelines (Grol and Wensing 2004; Charani et al. 2011; Franx et al. 2011; Hetrick et al. 2011)

Innovation

Awareness of the advantages in practice of the change
Feasibility, credibility, accessibility, attractiveness of the change
Poor applicability of guidelines to problems in everyday practice
Insufficient or unconvincing evidence base

Professional

Awareness among staff of the change (guidelines not read or accessible)
Lack of knowledge and skill to apply guidelines
Guidelines too rigid
Requires too much time
Motivation (implementing guidelines incurs costs)
Staff perception that change is imposed on them
Impact of change on patient–health care professional relationship
Lack of multidisciplinary approach to recommended change

Patient

Knowledge, skills, attitude, compliance
Lack of user involvement in developing guidelines
Lack of endorsement by patient advocacy groups

Social context

Opinions of colleagues (disagreement among physicians/experts)
Culture of the network, collaboration, leadership

Organizational context

Organization of care processes
No support from management
Heavy workloads
Lack of staff
Inadequate or lack of IT systems
Lack of support or specialist services
Inadequate integration of primary, secondary and tertiary care

Economic and political context

Financial arrangements (compensation, uncertain cost reimbursement) , regulations, policies

---

This information can be gathered through one-to-one and focus group interviews, observation, and a needs analysis in terms of resources and staff skills. The gathering and analysis of such information should be an explicit part of the project design and used to develop an action plan for change (Benning, Ghaleb et al. 2011).

Strategies for dissemination and implementing change

The aim of a change strategy is to enable the target group to modify work processes and overcome individual and organizational barriers to adopting the evidence-based guidelines or practices. In turn, the guidelines or new practices need to be sufficiently flexible to be adaptable to the local environment (Grol and Wensing 2005; Dixon-Woods et al. 2011). In designing the implementation strategy, it is important to select interventions to address the barriers in the local context. Additionally, due to the complexity of health care environments, it is suggested that multifaceted interventions, combining a number of the approaches outlined in Box 12.7, may be more successful than single interventions in changing practitioner behaviour.

Box 12.7   Implementation strategies highlighted as effective following systematic review

---

Printed protocols, guidelines and educational material

Dissemination of printed material is one of the most widely used and inexpensive interventions to change practice; it aims to raise awareness, increase knowledge and change attitudes of practitioners. A systematic review by Farmer et al. (2008) included 23 studies and concluded that this strategy can have a small positive impact on practitioner practice; however, there was no evidence of an effect on patient outcomes.

Audit and feedback

Audit and feedback continue to be the most frequently used interventions to modify practitioner behaviour across a broad range of clinical areas. The aim is to persuade practitioners to change behaviour through alerting them to aspects of their practice that may be at variance with peers or accepted guidelines. Jamtvedt et al. (2006) reviewed 118 studies and reported variable results including a decrease in compliance with recommended guidelines. When audit and feedback had a positive impact, the improvement in practitioner behaviour was small to moderate (ranging from 0.05 per cent to 16 per cent). Audit and feedback appeared to be most effective when baseline adherence was low and with higher intensity in delivering the intervention (Jamtvedt et al. 2006). A study by Hysong et al. (2006) sought to explain some of the variability in the effectiveness of audit and feedback as a strategy for changing behaviour. The authors suggested that timely, individualized and non-punitive feedback to practitioners about their adherence were characteristics of organizations with more successful adherence to guidelines.

Academic detailing or educational outreach visits (EOV)

One of the more recent innovations in this field is academic detailing or educational outreach visits. This involves a peer or another health care professional visiting a practitioner in their clinical environment and discussing aspects of their practice, including individualized audit and barriers to guideline adherence. O'Brien et al. (2007) evaluated 69 studies and concluded that EOV alone, but especially when combined with other interventions such as audit and feedback, had a small additional impact on practice compared to audit and feedback alone. Consistent but small changes in prescribing practices were identified, while small to moderate changes were identified in other areas of practice such as ordering screening tests.

Education meetings and workshops

Educational meetings, including conferences, workshops, symposiums, short courses, lectures and seminars, are widely used as forums for introducing and disseminating new knowledge, innovation and improved practice in the health care professions. Forsetlund et al. (2009) evaluated 81 trials and concluded that educational meetings, alone or when combined with other interventions, can result in a small to moderate (5–10 per cent) improvement in practitioner behaviour and a small (3 per cent) improvement in patient outcomes. Features of more successful interventions were combining didactic lecturers with interactive workshops, higher levels of attendance, and when outcomes were perceived as serious and involved changing less complex behaviours (Forsetlund et al. 2009).

Local opinion leaders

Use of influential local opinion leaders to change the behaviours of peers, although widely used on an informal basis, has only been formally evaluated in a small number of studies. Flodgren et al. (2011) identified 18 studies that used opinion leaders either in isolation or as part of a wider intervention. The median change in practitioner compliance, measured as the risk difference in compliance, was a 12 per cent increase across the 18 studies. However, study heterogeneity and limitation in design means there is ambiguity around the most effective approach to designing opinion leader interventions.

Computer reminders

Increasing computerization of health care settings has seen the introduction of on-screen computer reminders (pop-ups) to act as a prompt for recommended practices, especially in relation to prescribing, vaccinations or ordering tests. Shojania et al. (2009) reviewed 28 studies and concluded that computer reminders achieved a small to moderate improvement (on average a 4 per cent change) in practitioner behaviour and a small (3 per cent) positive impact on patient outcomes.

Multifaceted interventions

Multifaceted interventions are increasingly used to modify health practitioners' behaviour. This involves the combination of two or more interventions with the aim of increasing compliance above that which can be achieved by using a single-strand intervention. However, the evidence on the effectiveness of multifaceted interventions is variable (Grimshaw et al. 2004; Grindrod et al. 2006; Boaz et al. 2011) and unlike other interventions outlined here has not be subjected to an extensive systematic review. Nutley et al. (2007) suggested that the overall impact of multifaceted interventions can be unpredictable and may act in a non-linear fashion to modify practitioner behaviour; the author concluded that the combination of interventions used must be tailored to the specific circumstances. Boaz et al. (2011) undertook a review of systematic reviews on the effectiveness of interventions in implementing research into practice. The evidence suggests that single-strand interventions have some impact but it is likely that 'promoting the use of evidence-based practice requires complex multifaceted interventions' (Boaz et al. 2011: 6); the authors also caution that the recommended practice change should be explicitly based on the best available evidence.

Stage IV: Sustaining change

Sustaining change can be regarded as an ongoing rather than the final stage of the audit process, and may be more challenging than other stages in the process. At an individual level the change has to be assimilated into routines, and at an organizational level it needs to be embedded into the organization rather than just added on (Grol and Wensing 2004). Stage III may have involved a limited roll-out of the change among more progressive or willing units; however, in Stage IV, the change may have to be implemented across diverse clinical areas or patient groups. This stage is characterized by reminders, monitoring, feedback, revaluation and modifying the implementation strategy to achieve the standards of performance set at the audit planning phase (Ashmore et al. 2011).

Part of the strategy to sustain the change is re-audit. In the re-audit a smaller number of criteria or performance indicators may be measured, compared to previous data and reported back to clinical staff to evaluate progress. Monitoring of these key indicators often needs to become part of routine practice to ensure sustained improvement. As well as monitoring performance, there needs to be critical analysis of why targets are not being met, why there is variation in performance between similar units, and how interventions can be tailored to overcome specific barriers (Bosch et al. 2007). Sustaining the change and aiming for higher levels of performance requires the type of quantitative and qualitative data collection and reporting already described in this chapter. In addition, this process should reinforce commitment and build lateral networks among front-line staff to sustain the changes in practice and behaviour independent of the audit team.

Our understanding of how and why some implementation strategies to improve practice work in some settings and fail in others, and why there are regional and organizational variations in quality indicators such as infection rates, waiting times, patient morbidity and mortality that are not explained by patient factors (Wennberg 2011), is only starting to emerge through process evaluation of change implementation strategies. Dixon-Woods et al. (2011) used an ex-post theory approach to explain the initial and sustained success of a multifaceted programme to reduce sepsis associated with central venous catheters (CVC) in intensive care units. The authors describe complex social processes, that included: 1) isomorphic pressures for units to conform to agreed practices; 2) networked communities that exerted normative pressure; 3) reframing the problem of CVC sepsis as a social problem that could be tackled; 4) several interventions that functioned at different levels to shape a culture of 'doing better'; 5) harnessing data on infection rates as a disciplinary force; and 6) use of hard edges, such as perceived external scrutiny, or censure (Dixon-Woods et al. 2011). Mayer et al. (2011) has also reported a complex and sustained intervention to promote hand hygiene that combined behavioural modification theories and positive reinforcement with audit and feedback.

Theories that underpin implementation strategies in quality improvement in complex health care organizations and among professional groups are essential to develop effective and efficient strategies within limited resources. Front-line practitioners, as individuals and as part of multidisciplinary teams, are expected to have the knowledge and skills to evaluate practice in line with the best available evidence and where necessary to initiate and sustain changes that achieve the best outcomes for patients, service users and the wider community.

Clinical audit is situated within a broader framework of quality improvement, evidence-based practice and patient safety. The complexity of initiating and sustaining change at the individual and organizational level is becoming better understood and is regarded as an important new field of health service research (Grol et al. 2008). No single approach or intervention will be sufficient; it will require ongoing development of theoretical frameworks and adaptive models for quality improvement. However, it is likely that the principles of audit will continue to be useful to front-line practitioners within this quality improvement movement.

This raises a question regarding the place of audit and audit training in the undergraduate and postgraduate curriculum. Alternative assessments of students undertaking degrees, especially higher degrees, in the health sciences are being used (Smith et al. 2002). Knight (1997) has identified a number of alternatives to the dissertation. Taking the view that the thesis as a way of assessing an understanding of research in professional master's programmes is artificial, Knight argues that there is a need to devise other types of projects that are more appropriate to the student's area of professional practice. Suggestions made to replace the traditional thesis include action research projects, evaluation studies and audits, with the emphasis placed on applicability to professional practice.

Conclusion

Clinical audit skill is recognized as a core or highly recommended competency for health care professionals by their professional or regulatory bodies and health care funders. Clinical audit has emerged as one of the enduring strategies in the evidence-based practice and quality improvement movements in health care. The early failure of clinical guidelines and audit to make an impact on practice can be attributed to a naive understanding of the barriers and enablers of change at different levels in health care organizations and how professional groups adopt new practices. If viewed as a simple data-collection exercise, clinical audit is likely to be a waste of time and resources, but if audit becomes part of a well-planned change-implementation strategy in clinical practice, it is a valuable tool. Thus high-quality audit, undertaken to improve clinical practice and patient outcomes, requires the same rigour, organization and methodological approach as any research project.

Key concepts

- Clinical audit has evolved from an isolated activity undertaken by individuals to become part of multifaceted strategies employed in the quality improvement movement in health care systems.
- Knowledge of and ability to undertake clinical audit to evaluate practice is increasingly recognized as a desirable, and in some cases compulsory, skill for health care practitioners.

- Current day clinical audit has moved beyond the measurement of performance against agreed criteria; audit now also mandates introducing change to address the deficits in practice and sustaining improvements over time.
- Well-designed audit projects need to recognize and address the sociocultural, environmental and individual motivation factors in sustaining change initiatives through the collection of both quantitative and qualitative data.
- For front-line practitioners, clinical audit and feedback remains one of the key mechanisms within their control to identify areas of practice for improvement, introduce achievable change initiatives and sustain improvement over time through re-audit and feedback.

Key readings on audit in health care

- R. Burgess, *New Principles of Best Practice in Clinical Audit*, 2nd edn (Oxford: Healthcare Quality Improvement Partnership/Radcliffe Publishing, 2011)
- R. Grol, M. Wensing and M. Eccles, *Improving Patient Care: The Implementation of Change in Clinical Practice* (London: Elsevier, 2005)
- G. Jamtvedt, J.M. Young, D.T. Kristoffersen, M.A. O'Brien and A.D. Oxman, Audit and feedback: Effects on professional practice and healthcare outcomes, *Cochrane Database of Systematic Reviews*, 2:CD000259, 2006
- National Institute for Health and Clinical Excellence (NICE), *Principles for Best Practice in Clinical Audit* (Oxford: Radcliffe Medical Press, 2002)

References

Ashmore, S., Ruthven, T. and Hazelwood, L. (2011) Preparation, planning and organisation of clinical audit, in R. Burgess (ed.) *New Principles of Best Practice in Clinical Audit*, 2nd edn. Oxford: Radcliffe Publishing.

Baker, R., Hearnshaw, H. and Robertson, N. (1999) *Implementing Change with Clinical Audit*. Chichester: Wiley and Sons.

Benjamin, A. (2008) Audit: How to do it in practice (The competent novice), *British Medical Journal*, 336(7655): 1241–5.

Benning, A., Dixon-Woods, M., Nwulu, U., Ghaleb, M., Dawson, J., Barber, N., Franklin, B.D., Girling, A., Hemming, K., Carmalt, M., Rudge, G., Naicker, T., Kotecha, A., Derrington, M.C. and Lilford, R. (2011) Multiple component patient safety intervention in English hospitals: Controlled evaluation of second phase, *British Medical Journal Online*, 342:d199, doi: 10.1136/bmj.d199.

Benning, A., Ghaleb, M., Suokas, A., Dixon-Woods, M., Dawson, J., Barber, N., Franklin, B.D., Girling, A., Hemming, K., Carmalt, M., Rudge, G., Naicker, T., Nwulu, U., Choudhury, S. and Lilford, R. (2011) Large scale organisational intervention to improve patient safety in four UK hospitals: Mixed method evaluation, *British Medical Journal* Online, 342:d195, doi: 10.1136/bmj.d195.

Boaz, A., Baeza, J., Fraser, A. and European Implementation Score Collaborative Group (EIS) (2011) Effective implementation of research into practice: An overview of systematic reviews of the health literature, BMC Research Notes, 4:212. Available at http://www.biomedcentral.com/1756-0500/4/212 [Accessed 30/01/2012].

Bosch, M., van der Weijden, T., Wensing, M. and Grol, R. (2007) Tailoring quality improvement interventions to identified barriers: A multiple case analysis, *Journal of Evaluation in Clinical Practice*, 13(2): 161–8.

Bowie, P., Cooke, S., Lo, P., McKay, J. and Lough, M. (2007) The assessment of criterion audit cycles by external peer review – when is an audit not an audit?, *Journal of Evaluation in Clinical Practice*, 13(3): 352–7.

Burgess, R. (2011) *New Principles of Best Practice in Clinical Audit*, 2nd edn. Oxford: Radcliffe Publishing.

Charani, E., Edwards, R., Sevdalis, N., Alexandrou, B., Sibley, E., Mullett, D., Franklin, B. and Holmes, A. (2011) Behavior change strategies to influence antimicrobial prescribing in acute care: A systematic review, *Clinical Infectious Diseases*, 53(7): 651–62.

Cheater, K. and Keane, M. (1998) Nurses' participation in audit: A regional study, *Quality in Healthcare*, 7(1): 27–36.

Cheater, F., Hearnshaw, H., Baker, R. and Keane, M. (2005) Can a facilitated programme promote effective multidisciplinary audit in secondary care teams? An exploratory trial, *International Journal of Nursing Studies*, 42(7): 779–91.

Chenot, J.F., Scherer, M., Becker, A., Donner-Banzhoff, N., Baum, E., Leonhardt, C., Keller, S., Pfingsten, M., Hildebrandt, J., Basler, H. D. and Kochen, M. M. (2008) Acceptance and perceived barriers of implementing a guideline for managing low back in general practice, *Implementation Science*, 3(7): 1–6.

Dassow, P. (2007) Measuring performance in primary care: What patient outcome indicators do physicians value?, *Journal of the American Board of Family Medicine*, 20(1): 1–8.

Dixon, N. (2009) *Ethics and Clinical Audit and Quality Improvement (QI): A Guide for NHS Organisations*. London: Healthcare Quality Improvement Partnership. Available at http://www.hqip.org.uk/assets/Downloads/Ethics-and-Clinical-Audit-and-Quality-Improvement-Guide.pdf [Accessed 20 January 2012].

Dixon-Woods, M., Bosk, C., Aveling, E.L., Goeschel, C. and Pronovost, P. (2011) Explaining Michigan: Developing an ex post theory of a quality improvement program, *The Milbank Quarterly*, 89(2): 167–205.

Donabedian, A. (1966) Evaluating the quality of medical care. Reprinted 2005: *The Milbank Quarterly* 2005, 83(4): 691–729.

Drennan, J., Naughton, C., Allen, D., Hyde, A., Felle, P., O'Boyle, K., Treacy, M.P. and Butler, M. (2009) *National Independent Evaluation of the Nurse and Midwife Prescribing Initiative*. Dublin: University College Dublin.

Dulko, D. (2007) Audit and feedback as a clinical practice guideline implementation strategy: A model for acute care nurse practitioners, *Worldviews Evidence Based Nursing*, 4(4): 200–9.

European Society of Cardiology (2007) The European guidelines on cardiovascular disease prevention in clinical practice: Executive summary. Available at http://www.escardio.org/guidelines-surveys/esc-guidelines/Pages/cvd-prevention.aspx [Accessed 12 December 2011].

Farmer, A.P., Légaré, F., Turcot, L., Grimshaw, J., Harvey, E., McGowan, J.L. and Wolf, F. (2008) Printed educational materials: Effects on professional practice and healthcare outcomes, *Cochrane Database of Systematic Reviews*, 3:CD004398.

Flodgren, G., Parmelli, E., Doumit, G., Gattellari, M., O'Brien, M.A., Grimshaw, J., Eccles, M.P. (2011)Local opinion leaders: effects on professional practice and healthcare outcomes. *Cochrane Database of Systematic Reviews*, 8:CD000125.

Forsetlund, L., Bjørndal, A., Rashidian, A., Jamtvedt, G., O'Brien, M.A., Wolf, F., Davis, D., Odgaard-Jensen, J. and Oxman, A.D. (2009) Continuing education meetings and workshops: Effects on professional practice and healthcare outcomes, *Cochrane Database of Systematic Reviews*, 2:CD003030.

Franx, G., Niesink, P., Swinkels, J., Burgers, J., Wensing, M. and Grol, R. (2011) Ten years of multidisciplinary mental health guidelines in the Netherlands, *International Review of Psychiatry*, 23(4): 371–8.

Fraser, R. (1982) Medical audit in general practice, *Trainee*, 2: 113–15.

General Medical Council (2009) *Good Medical Practice: Guidelines for Doctors*. London: GMC.

Gillman, S. J. (2011) *Pay for Performance in UK General Practice – The Ambiguous Impact of the Quality and Outcomes Framework*. Rockville, MD: National Quality Measures Clearinghouse, US Department of Health and Human Services.

Grimshaw, J.M., Shirran, L., Thomas, R., Mowatt, G., Fraser, C., Bero, L., Grilli, R., Harvey, E., Oxman, A. and O'Brien, M.A. (2001) Changing provider behavior: An overview of systematic reviews of interventions, *Medical Care*, 39(8, Supp. 2): II2–45.

Grimshaw, J.M., Thomas, R., MacLennan, G., Fraser, C., Ramsay, C., Vale, L., Whitty, P., Eccles, M.P., Matowe, L., Shirran, L., Wensing, M., Dijkstra, R. and Donaldson, C. (2004) Effectiveness and efficiency of guideline dissemination and implementation strategies, *Health Technology Assessment*, 8(6): 1–84.

Grindrod, K., Patel, P. and Martin, J. (2006) What interventions should pharmacists employ to impact health practitioners' prescribing practices?, *Annals of Pharmacotherapy*, 40(9): 1546–57.

Grol, R. and Wensing, M. (2004) What drives change? Barriers to and incentives for achieving evidence-based practice, Medical Journal of Australia, 180(6, Supp.): S57–60.

Grol, R. and Wensing, M. (2005) Effective implementation: A model, in R. Grol, M. Wensing and M. Eccles (eds) Improving Patient Care: The implementation of Change in Clinical Practice. London: Elsevier, pp. 41–57.

Grol, R., Baker, R. and Moss, F. (2004) *Quality Improvement Research: Understanding the Science of Change in Healthcare*. London: BMJ Books.

Grol, R., Wensing, M. and Eccles, M. (2005) *Improving Patient Care: The Implementation of Change in Clinical Practice*. London: Elsevier.

Grol, R., Berwick, D.M. and Wensing, M. (2008) On the trail of quality and safety in healthcare, British Medical Journal, 336(7635): 74–6.

Hammond, R., Lennon, S., Walker, M.F., Hoffman, A., Irwin, P. and Lowe, D. (2005) Changing occupational therapy and physiotherapy practice through guidelines and audit in the United Kingdom, *Clinical Rehabilitation*, 19(4): 365–71.

Haiart, D.C., Paul, A.B. and Griffiths, J.M. (1990) An audit of the usage of operating theatre time in a peripheral teaching surgical unit, *Postgraduate Medical Journal*, 66(778): 612–15.

Hearnshaw, H.M., Harker, R.M., Cheater, F.M., Baker, R.H. and Grimshaw, G.M. (2003) Are audits wasting resources by measuring the wrong things? A survey of methods used to select audit review criteria, *Quality & Safety in Healthcare*, 12(1): 24–8.

Hetrick, S.E., Simmons, M., Thompson, A. and Parker, A.G. (2011) What are specialist mental health clinician attitudes to guideline recommendations for the treatment of depression in young people?, *Australian and New Zealand Journal of Psychiatry*, 45(11): 993–1001.

Horgan, F., McGee, H., Hickey, A., Whitford, D.L., Murphy, S., Royston, M., Cowman, S., Shelley, E., Conroy, R. M., Wiley, M. and O'Neill, D. (2011) From prevention to nursing home care: A comprehensive national audit of stroke care, *Cerebrovascular Disease*, 32(4): 385–92.

HSE (2007) *Acute Hospital Bed Review: A Review of Acute Hospital Bed Use in Hospitals in the Republic of Ireland with an Emergency Department*. Dublin: HSE.

HSE (2011) *Report on Hand Hygiene Compliance in HSE Acute Hospitals*. Dublin: HSE Health Protection Surveillance Centre (HPSC).

Hysong, S.J., Best, R. G. and Pugh, J.A. (2006) Audit and feedback and clinical practice guideline adherence: Making feedback actionable, *Implementation Science*, 28, doi:10.1186/1748-5908-1-9.

Intercollegiate Stroke Working Party (2010) *National Sentinel Stroke Clinical Audit (2010)*. London: Royal College of Physicians.

Iyer, R.V., Likhith, A.M., McLean, J.A., Perera, S. and Davis, C.H. (2004) Audit of operating theatre time utilization in neurosurgery, *British Journal of Neurosurgery*, 18(4): 333–7.

Jamtvedt, G., Young, J.M., Kristoffersen, D.T., O'Brien, M.A., Oxman, A.D. (2006) Audit and feedback: Effects on professional practice and healthcare outcomes, *Cochrane Database of Systematic Reviews*, 2:CD000259.

Johnston, G., Crombie, I.K., Davies, H., Alder, E. and Millard, A. (2000) Reviewing audit: Barriers and facilitators factors for effective clinical audit, *Quality in Healthcare*, 2(23): 23–36.

Kelson, M. (1998) *Promoting Patient Involvement in Clinical Audit: Practical Guidance on Achieving Effective Involvement*. London: College of Health and Clinical Outcomes Group.

Knight, P. (1997) Learning, teaching and curriculum in taught master's courses, in P. Knight (ed.) *Masterclass: Learning, Teaching and Curriculum in Taught Master's Degrees*. London: Cassell Education, pp. 1–15.

Latter, S., Maben, J., Myall, M. and Young, A. (2007) Evaluating the clinical appropriateness of nurses' prescribing practice: Method development and findings from an expert panel analysis, *Quality Safety Health Care*, 16(6): 415–21.

Légaré, F., Boivin, A., van der Weijden, T., Pakenham, C., Burgers, J., Légaré, J., St-Jacques, S. and Gagnon, S. (2011) Patient and public involvement in clinical practice guidelines: A knowledge synthesis of existing programs, *Medical Decision Making*, 31(6): E45–74.

Loughlan, C. (2011) Appendix 2: Clinical audit, impact and quality improvement: A discursive review, in R. Burgess (ed.) *New Principles on Best Practice in Clinical Audit*, 2nd edn. Oxford: Radcliffe Publishing, pp. 128–49.

Marjamaa, R., Vakkuri, A. and Kirvelä, O. (2008) Operating room management: Why, how and by whom?, *Acta Anaesthesiologica Scandinavica*, 52(5): 596–600.

Mayer, J., Mooney, B., Gundlapalli, A., Harbarth, S., Stoddard, G.J., Rubin, M.A., Eutropius, L., Brinton, B. and Samore, M.H. (2011) Dissemination and sustainability of a hospital-wide hand hygiene program emphasizing positive reinforcement, *Infection Control and Hospital Epidemiology*, 32(1): 59–66.

Medical Council (Irish) (2011) *Professional Competence: Guidelines for Doctors*. Dublin: Medical Council.

Minogue, V. and Girdlestone, J. (2010) Building capacity for service user and carer involvement in research: The implications and impact of best research for best health, *International Journal of Healthcare Quality Assurance*, 23(4): 422–35.

Montesi, G. and Lechi, A. (2009) Prevention of medication errors: Detection and audit, *British Journal of Clinical Pharmacology*, 67(6): 651–5.

National Health Service (NHS) (2012) *The Quality and Outcomes Framework 2010/11*. NHS Information Centre. Available at http://www.ic.nhs.uk/qof [Accessed 16 July 2012].

National Institute for Health and Clinical Excellence (NICE) (2002) *Principles for Best Practice in Clinical Audit*. Oxford: Radcliffe Medical Press.

Naughton, C., Drennan, J., Hyde, A., Allen, D., O'Boyle, K., Felle, P. and Butler, M. (2012) An evaluation of the appropriateness and safety of nurse and midwife prescribing in Ireland, *Journal of Advanced Nursing*, doi:10.1111/jan.12004.

Navarro Puerto, M.A., Ibarluzea, I.G., Ruiz, O.G., Alvarez, F.M., Herreros, R.G., Pintiado, R.E., Dominguez, A. R. and León, I. M. (2008) Analysis of the quality of clinical practice guidelines on established ischemic stroke, *International Journal of Technology Assessment in Healthcare*, 24(3): 333–41.

Nettleton, J. and Ireland, A. (2000) Junior doctors' views on clinical audit – has anything changed?, *International Journal of Healthcare Quality Assurance*, 13(6): 245–53.

Nutley, S., Walter, I. and Davis, H. (2007) *Using Evidence: How Research can Inform Public Service*. Bristol: The Policy Press.

O'Brien, M.A., Rogers, S., Jamtvedt, G., Oxman, A.D., Odgaard-Jensen, J., Kristoffersen, D.T., Forsetlund, L., Bainbridge, D., Freemantle, N., Davis, D.A., Haynes, R.B. and Harvey, E.L. (2007) Educational outreach visits: Effects on professional practice and health care outcomes, *Cochrane Database of Systematic Reviews*, 17(4): CD000409.

Oliver, S., Clarke-Jones, L., Rees, R., Milne, R., Buchanan, P., Gabbay, J., Gyte, G., Oakley, A. and Stein, K. (2004) Involving consumers in research and development agenda setting for the NHS: Developing an evidence-based approach, *Health Technology Assessment*, 8(15): 1–148, III–IV.

Pickard, A.S., Lee, T.A., Solem, C.T., Joo, M.J., Schumock, G.T. and Krishnan, J.A. (2011) Prioritizing comparative-effectiveness research topics via stakeholder involvement: An application in COPD, *Clinical Pharmacology & Therapeutics*, 90(6): 888–92.

Polit, D. and Beck, C. (2010) *Essentials of Nursing Research: Appraising Evidence for Nursing Practice*, 7th edn. Philadelphia: Lippincott Williams & Wilkins.

Polit , D. and Beck, C. (2012) *Nursing Research: Generating and Assessing Evidence for Nursing Practice*, 9th edn. London: Wolters Kluwer/Lippincott Williams & Wilkins.

Rapport, F., Seagrove, A., Hutchings, H., Russell, I., Cheung, I., Williams, J. and Cohen, D. (2012) Barriers and facilitators to change in the organisation and delivery of endoscopy services in England and Wales: A focus group study, *BMJ Open*, 2012;2:e001009, doi:10.1136/bmjopen-2012-001009

Rowe, B.H., Bond, K., Ospina, M.B., Blitz, S., Friesen, C., Schull, M., Innes, G., Afilalo, M., Bullard, M., Campbell, S.G., Curry, G., Holroyd, B., Yoon, P. and Sinclair, D. (2006) *Emergency Department Overcrowding in Canada: What are the Issues and What can be Done?* Technology overview no. 21. Ottawa: Canadian Agency for Drugs and Technologies in Health.

Saha, P., Pinjani, A., Al-Shabibi, N., Madari, S., Ruston, J., Magos, A. (2009) Why we are wasting time in the operating theatre?, *International Journal of Health Planning and Management*, 24(3): 225–32.

Shinners, E., Long, P., Tupas, A. and McGrane, L. (2012) Use of care bundles as a practice development initiative across three departments in a non-acute hospital setting, *Irish Journal of Medical Science*, 181(Supp. 7): S219.

Shojania, K.G., Jennings, A., Mayhew, A., Ramsay, C.R., Eccles, M.P. and Grimshaw, J. (2009) The effects of on-screen, point of care computer reminders on processes and outcomes of care, *Cochrane Database of Systematic Reviews*, 8(3): CD001096, doi: 10.1002/14651858. CD001096.pub2.

Smith, C., Erkel, E. and Stroud, S. (2002) Promoting scholarship in nurse practitioner programs, *Clinical Excellence for Nurse Practitioners*, 5(5): 25–30.

Turner, P., Harby-Owren, H., Shackleford, F., So, A., Fosse, T. and Whitfield, A. (1999) Audits of physiotherapy practice, *Physiotherapy Theory and Practice*, 15(4): 261–74.

Turner, T., Misso, M., Harris, C. and Green, S. (2008) Development of evidence-based clinical practice guidelines (CPGs): Comparing approaches, *Implementation Science*, 3: 45.

Waldron, N., Dey, I., Nagree, Y., Xiao, J. and Flicker, L. (2011) A multi-faceted intervention to implement guideline care and improve quality of care for older people who present to the emergency department with falls, *BMC Geriatrics*, 11: 6.

Wennberg, J.E. (2011) Time to tackle unwarranted variations in practice, *British Medical Journal*, 342:d1513.

Woodcock, T., Poots, A. and Bell, D. (2012) The impact of changing the 4 h emergency access standard on patient waiting times in emergency departments in England, *Emergency Medical Journal*, 13(3), doi:10.1136/emermed-2012-201175.

13 Evaluation research

Ruth Belling

Chapter topics

- Defining evaluation research
- Ethics and governance issues
- Purposes of evaluation
- Importance of evaluation in health care
- Importance of key stakeholders
- Types of evaluation

- Design principles
- Mixed methods
- Planning and conducting evaluation studies
- Report writing and feedback of evaluation findings

Introduction

Evaluation in its broadest sense seeks to identify and assess value, worth, merit, strengths and weaknesses, for a particular audience. Practically anything can be evaluated, from programmes to products, services to policies (World Health Organization 2007), people to organizations, providing sufficient motivation, skills and resources are invested (Stufflebeam 2001). Evaluation may be embarked on for a whole variety of reasons. In health care it is often driven by a need to improve outcomes and effectiveness (Clancy and Eisenberg 1998; Belling 2003). The evidence it provides can play a vital role in decision making, care provision and resource allocation (Smith et al. 2005; US Department of Health and Human Services 2005).

This chapter aims to introduce the concept and purposes of evaluation and its importance in health care research. It assumes no prior knowledge or experience of evaluation, but provides an overview of different types of evaluation, to inform and assist decision making about the appropriateness and feasibility of using these in health professionals' own individual and organizational contexts. The chapter will highlight and discuss the principles and choices underpinning evaluation study design as well as describe the practical stages of planning, implementation, report writing and feedback of evaluation findings. Since health professionals may reasonably contemplate evaluating any aspect of health care, this chapter raises issues and presents a generic set of steps and questions which can be applied at the outset of any evaluation, whether it concerns a treatment programme to reduce heart disease, a community clinic, implementation of a new care model, impact of a mental health policy or a mentoring programme for newly qualified nurses.

Defining evaluation research

There is no universally accepted definition of evaluation. Nor is there a single or right approach to designing and carrying out an evaluation study. However, the definitions of evaluation promoted by most national associations of evaluators have many similarities. (For links to the more established associations, see the list of useful websites at the end of this chapter.)

In essence, evaluation seeks to identify or ascertain the value, merit, worth, effectiveness or impact of something (products, programmes, services, policies, people or organizations), for a particular audience.

It follows, therefore, that any evaluation process must consider three areas:

- what is meant by value, merit, worth, effectiveness and impact, and how this will be determined
- defining what exactly is to be evaluated (and what is not)
- who the evaluation is for

The latter is, crucially, the most powerful but sometimes least considered influence.

What is 'value' and who decides?

It is always advisable to keep an open mind about terms such as 'value', which may mean different things to the various parties involved in shaping an evaluation study. What will it mean to the evaluation's primary audience? What does it mean to the evaluation's stakeholders and those of the programme, service or otherwise that will come under scrutiny? What does it mean to the evaluator or evaluation team responsible for carrying out the evaluation? Any good dictionary should highlight at least three meanings of 'value':

- merit, importance, significance, benefit, usefulness, desirability
- cost, monetary worth, price
- code of behaviour, ethics, moral standards, principles

Bear in mind that there are many evaluation approaches to choose from and some will only focus on one aspect of the above.

Evaluation, audit and research

Evaluation is sometimes confused with audit, monitoring and surveillance (National Patient Safety Agency 2010). In health care, audit seeks to systematically identify whether care meets a predetermined standard or set of criteria. Where audit tends to ask, 'Does this . . . ?' or 'Is this . . . ?', evaluation often addresses broader, more open questions not sufficiently answerable using audit techniques alone, such as 'How well . . . ?', 'How effective . . . ?', 'What outcomes . . . ?', or 'What impact . . . ?' Evaluations with multiple aims or methods may include audit to achieve a specific objective, but this is usually just one element within a broader, overall design. Surveillance is the continuous monitoring of or routine data collection on a number of factors over a regular interval of time. Data gathered as part of surveillance activities may be useful in an evaluation study, particularly where longer-term and population-based outcomes are of interest, but are unlikely to fully address evaluation questions which are tailored to a particular need or audience.

Is evaluation always considered to be research? Well, one of the main criteria for research is that it aims to produce new knowledge: that is, something not known before. Evaluation can result in new knowledge, much of which has practical relevance beyond the immediate context in which it was gained. Small-scale, localized studies, however, are sometimes criticized on the grounds that findings may lack generalizability to contexts outside the individual study's immediate setting. Like all forms of research, it has strengths and limitations depending on the purpose, approach and context in which it is applied (Bowling 2009). Perhaps a more helpful question is: when does it matter how evaluation is categorized? Arguably, it matters most when categorization influences whether or how a study can be carried out. Service evaluation as performed in the UK's National Health Service (NHS) may serve to illustrate this point. A study categorized as a service evaluation may allow evaluators to bypass what is often a lengthy and bureaucratic system for gaining ethical approval for research studies (National Patient Safety Agency 2010). Clearly, this may be of practical benefit to some, while others may find it means constraints elsewhere, for example in publishing results in some scholarly journals.

Ethics and governance issues

Perhaps in health research more than most fields where evaluation is applied, ethics and governance issues (how research is managed) play a significant role (Morris and Cohn 1993). Health care research in many countries is highly regulated, subject to legal requirements and/or policy restrictions, usually intended to protect patients and ensure that their participation in research is voluntary and based on informed consent. Anyone considering carrying out an evaluation study is strongly advised to make sure that they have the relevant permissions and ethical approval *before* they collect any data or try to recruit study participants.

Importance and purposes of evaluation in health care

Evaluation is vital in health care. Some of its many benefits include providing evidence and information to support decision making, service planning and resource allocation (Smith et al. 2005). Used effectively, it can improve the way health care is managed, organized and delivered, and improve outcomes for patients and service users. However, the (sometimes frustrating) reality is that evaluation is rarely considered seriously until an activity is under threat. By then it may be far too late to take appropriate action.

A common misconception about evaluation is that it occurs only *after* an activity has taken place, or once it is well established. The danger with this is that the vital thinking about and planning for evaluation is similarly delayed or avoided, resulting in weakened evaluation designs and missed opportunities to collect valuable data.

Of course, evaluation also has downsides. It can be costly, time-consuming, and may require specialist skills to achieve its aims. Before committing to such an investment, be sure it is feasible to achieve a study's aims and objectives within whatever resource constraints (timescale, funding, skills) apply.

So, where to begin? The first important step is to clarify the evaluation's purpose and what it intends to achieve. What are the evaluation's aims and objectives? Where there are several aims, which will take priority? This should be discussed, and the purpose, aims and objectives *agreed* with key stakeholders (individuals or groups with a vested interest in the evaluation and the activity or intervention being evaluated).

Importance of key stakeholders

Stakeholders can help (or obstruct) an evaluation at any point: before it goes ahead, while it is being carried out and after the findings have been produced and are ready for dissemination. Identifying which stakeholders are likely to influence the evaluation should be done at the outset and strategies for engaging their support incorporated into an evaluation plan (US Department of Health and Human Services 2005).

In identifying stakeholders, priority should be given to those who will:

- fund or authorize the evaluation
- provide or enable access to sources of required data
- be responsible for the activity to be evaluated
- be able to increase the credibility of the evaluation
- authorize or advocate the implementation of findings and recommendations
- be affected by the evaluation process and/or its findings, for example patients and service users, staff

Bear in mind, however, that each stakeholder group will have their own motivations and agendas, which are rarely made explicit. Although not written specifically for health researchers, Easterby-Smith (1994) has some useful material on the politics of carrying out evaluations.

One strategy, particularly useful if the evaluator or evaluation team are independent of the activity to be evaluated, is to consider setting up an advisory panel or steering group for the duration of the project. Provided such groups have clear terms of reference, they can have many advantages, for example in:

- focusing an evaluation's design
- gaining access to and information from data sources
- building consensus
- piloting data-collection tools and analysis strategies
- exploring strategies to disseminate findings or gain support for recommendations
- keeping stakeholders informed of progress

Types of evaluation

Many types of evaluation exist. These are sometimes categorized by purpose or by the research philosophies, methodologies or approaches which they employ. As with all forms of research, decisions as to the appropriateness of approach and choices of method should be driven by a study's aims, objectives and the needs of its primary audience/stakeholders.

Types of evaluation by purpose

There are two types: formative evaluation and summative evaluation.

Formative or process evaluation

Formative evaluation usually occurs during the formation of a programme, activity or service. It defines, explores and documents the processes and mechanisms that form or underpin a health care programme, activity or service (Saunders et al. 2005). Although the terms 'process' and 'qualitative' are sometimes used interchangeably, data can be both quantitative and qualitative. The aim is usually to *improve* processes, enabling changes to be made for the purpose of increasing effectiveness and/or efficiency. Process evaluation can be used to assess, for example, how a public health programme is currently operating or to document how a new service model has been or is being implemented (Tolma et al. 2009). In addition, researchers are recognizing the value of using process evaluations alongside randomized controlled trials (RCTs) and other large-scale or multisite studies (Oakley et al. 2006). Process evaluations have many benefits in this context. They may be used to explore how interventions are implemented and received, assist with the interpretation of findings on outcomes, investigate contextual factors which may influence an intervention, or help distinguish between interventions which are inherently faulty and those which are poorly delivered.

Summative evaluation

Summative evaluation approaches usually occur once a programme, activity or service has been implemented (Stufflebeam 2001). These determine an activity's merit or worth according to its end results. The aim is usually to assess effectiveness by evaluating whether goals and objectives have been achieved (Fain 2005). There are broadly two types: outcomes evaluations, which focus on immediate effects or shorter-term results, and impact evaluations, which focus on longer-term effects.

Types of evaluation by methodology

Disciplines such as education, accountancy, arts and social science have borrowed and adapted evaluation approaches, methods and processes to suit their particular contexts. These approaches may be categorized into three broad groups, differentiated by their overall stance on 'reality' and how to study it. Three groups of evaluation approaches are noted here: scientific, assisted sense-making and natural sense-making. In research terms these broadly equate to the philosophies of positivism, realism and constructivism respectively. To some extent these are artificial boundaries, and they are presented here to aid explanation rather than constrain choices. An evaluator may choose to work at any point on the underlying continuum. Indeed, on larger-scale projects involving mixed methods, it is not uncommon to simultaneously occupy different points along this spectrum. The reasons for categorizing evaluation approaches in this way, here and in the table below, are firstly to provide 'hooks' to research terminology with which readers may be more familiar, and secondly because of the variety of activities that may be evaluated in health care settings and the increasing participation of patients and service users in all aspects of evaluation in many westernized countries.

Table 13.1 summarizes and compares some of the key features and assumptions underpinning each of the three groups of evaluation approaches with regard to:

- their stance on 'reality' and how to study it
- their implications for the position of the evaluator
- some fundamental guidelines or principles appropriate to each set of approaches
- commonly used methods for gathering and analysing information

Economic evaluation

Economic evaluation involves comparative analysis of the costs and consequences of alternative treatments, programmes or interventions (Petrou and Gray 2011). They are typically concerned with additional costs and health benefits associated with new treatments compared to existing treatments, and are designed to address questions of whether particular interventions or treatments could lead to better outcomes and reduced costs (Knapp et al. 2006).

There are three main types of economic evaluation:

- cost–effectiveness analysis
- cost–utility analysis
- cost–benefit analysis

Which form of analysis is most suitable depends on the scope of the evaluation (whether it is intended for decision making at individual or case level, system level or across entire economies) and how outcomes will be measured. In cost–effectiveness analysis, for example, outcomes may be measured in units such as better functioning or fewer symptoms, whereas cost–utility analysis involves generic measurements combining quality and quantity of life, such as Quality Adjusted Life Years (QALYs).

Identifying treatment or service costs, however, can be difficult as these often go beyond direct costs of health care provision, and may include 'hidden' costs (Beecham et al. 2010) such as the support of unpaid carers or the impact of ill health on employment. Also, many interventions are designed to produce long-term benefits, hence long-term costs and outcomes must also be identified. Studies covering long time periods are notoriously problematic in terms of participant retention and continually changing contexts, so increasingly, economic evaluations make use of complex decision or simulation models to address knowledge gaps (Petrou and Gray 2011).

Table 13.1   Three groups of evaluation approaches: key features

Key features	'Scientific' approaches	'Assisted sense-making'	'Natural sense-making'
Nature of reality	External Objective	External Objective	Internal Subjective
Nature of 'social reality'	Examined in same ways as 'natural scientific' reality	'Social' reality constructed by participants	'Reality' is socially constructed
Relationship of evaluator to evaluation studies	Independent observer	Independent observer	Part of the phenomena
Purpose	Causation	Explanation	Negotiation
Design guidelines	Verifiable facts Search for fundamental laws	Meaning given to facts Search for underlying mechanisms generating patterns of meaning	Meaning Seeks to understand what is happening within its specific context
Testing and verification	Phenomena reduced to basic elements Hypothesis generation followed by testing and verification	Basic elements within context Propositions can be verified or falsified	Focus on whole situation/context Ideas and theory derived from data Focus on falsification
Methods	Specify concepts to enable measurement Empirical evidence Experiments/quasi-experiments Controlling variables	Identify and understand patterns of meaning Interviews Context specification	Multiple methods used to identify differing views of phenomena Fieldwork Specificity
Sampling	Large samples	Dependent on context Purposive sampling	Small, in-depth samples, over time
Generalization	To populations	To theory	To theory

Source: Ruth Belling (2000), unpublished

Programme theory/logic models

These approaches set out to describe or develop a logic model or theory about how a health care programme or service operates. Essentially, these approaches allow evaluators to map out what goes into a programme or service, what its processes are, its outcomes and effects. Once the underpinning logic or theory is outlined, the resulting flow chart can act as a guide for further evaluation and testing of the various connections and assumptions made. This approach has become popular in the USA, particularly in evaluating public health as well as social care programmes (Weiss 1998). The main purpose behind the use of such models is to determine whether a programme or activity is operating as intended and meeting the needs of those for whom it was introduced. Once the theory or logic is established, quantitative methods are most often used to test or refine it. A criticism of such approaches is their focus on intended or desired effects, to the exclusion of unintended outcomes or consequences. However, an evaluation study might, for example, use this focus constructively to create an alternative 'road map' of how a programme or service is operating in practice, which may then be compared against the intended vision.

Realist evaluation

Realist or realistic approaches to evaluation have philosophical roots in what may be termed 'assisted sense-making' (see Table 13.1). These share the same view of 'reality' as 'scientific' approaches (external and existing independently), but acknowledge the importance of human beings' attempts to make sense of the different contexts in which they live and work. There are many derivations of realist approaches, but two of the better known are those of Pawson and Tilley (1997), whose work traces its development from the natural science of Bhaskar (1979) and that of Mark et al. (2000), which draws on a 'common sense realism', which is highly pragmatic.

The main benefits of realist approaches are that they seek not only to identify patterns of meaning but to provide explanations. They are systematic and pragmatic approaches, which fit well with the practical orientation of evaluation in health care (Douglas et al. 2010). Both quantitative and qualitative methods of data collection and analysis can be used. Disadvantages, for some, are that the findings of individual evaluations can only be generalized to theory for verification in other contexts. Skills may be required in the use of both quantitative and qualitative methods.

Empowerment/user-led evaluation

In these approaches, the ultimate 'users', 'consumers' or 'stakeholders' of either the evaluation or the activity to be evaluated are intended to play a driving role in the evaluation at any or all stages (Fetterman et al. 1996). Such approaches go beyond stakeholder, patient or carer involvement in identifying the purpose and the questions an evaluation will address, or how the results will be used, to the more technical aspects of study design, data collection and analysis more traditionally carried out by trained and experienced evaluators and researchers.

Examples are often found in public health and social care settings, but these approaches are equally appropriate in other areas of health care. Indeed, in many countries, particularly Canada, the USA and UK, active participation in research by the ultimate users of health care products and services is encouraged at national governmental level – as evidenced by many national and private research funding bodies' requirements to demonstrate in funding applications how and to what extent users of health care (particularly patients and service users) will be involved in evaluation processes.

The benefits and drawbacks of empowerment/user-led approaches may depend on the extent to which health care users, consumers and stakeholders have control over and experience of an entire evaluation process. Some may, for example, have the desire, but not the expertise or the experience of designing and conducting evaluations, or some may only wish to be involved at certain stages. Issues to be addressed may include resources, training and development and potential bias, since these may influence success in achieving a study's goals.

At their best, empowerment approaches to evaluation are inclusive, equitable and driven by those who will benefit most from improvements to the activity to be evaluated. They prioritize and stress issues, concerns and needs of health care users, rather than those imposed by external individuals, organizations or policies. They focus on using the results and enabling participants to develop skills in evaluation for the future.

The main weaknesses are that processes can be lengthy and negatively political. Interpretation of differing views and values in a flexible, interactive way can be highly demanding and difficult. Inexperience or lack of skills may result in evaluations that are technically unsound, or too complex, broad and prone to continual change to be feasible for many health care organizations.

Design principles

Because evaluation study designs are tailored to specific evaluation questions and the nature of the activity or intervention to be evaluated, this may result in any number of individual designs. What follows, therefore, are some key design principles underpinning evaluation research.

As a guide, any evaluation design should address the following areas:

- Clarify the evaluation's purpose, aims and objectives.
- Develop relevant and specific evaluation questions.
- Select an appropriate evaluation approach or design for each evaluation question.
- Identify information/data sources needed to answer each question.
- Choose appropriate methods to collect this information.
- Plan how the information will be analysed to demonstrate that the evaluation questions have been answered.

Designing any evaluation study is an iterative process, where choices and decisions made in any one of the above areas influence what is appropriate or feasible in another. Evaluation questions should be specific and unambiguous. This makes it easier to identify the kinds of information necessary to answer them, and also helps determine how key stakeholders will know that the questions have been answered satisfactorily.

It may seem obvious to recommend that the evaluation questions should drive the choice of information sources and data-collection methods, rather than the other way around. But too often the design process starts with preconceived ideas about data-collection methods or the availability of certain kinds of information, rather than choices based on the most appropriate or effective way to answer a particular question. Instead, try to generate a number of options or alternative approaches. *Then* consider their feasibility given whatever resource constraints may apply, so alternative options are not dismissed too soon. Design choices may also involve the use of multiple and/or mixed methods – these will be addressed later in the chapter.

There are also important timing issues to consider. A problem for summative evaluations is in deciding when an activity is likely to produce effects. Measure outcomes too soon and there may be nothing to detect, thereby giving a potentially misleading impression. Pressures on evaluators and commissioners of evaluation studies to show results as soon as possible can create tensions which may be reflected in poor study designs. If it is uncertain when an intervention is likely to produce changes or effects, or how long these may last, then there is a strong case for measuring outcomes at multiple time points. Studies evaluating organizational changes in health care are particularly vulnerable to this, as stakeholders often underestimate how long it takes for changes to become embedded into practice.

Given that this particular book focuses on quantitative aspects of health research, some examples of overall study designs appropriate to 'scientific' evaluation approaches are provided in Table 13.2. For further information on realist study designs, see Pawson and Tilley (1997).

Multiple and mixed methods

Evaluators have access to a wide variety of research methods (Bowling 2009), both quantitative and qualitative, each with its strengths and limitations (other chapters in this book give more details on some of these). Complex evaluations may require multiple research methods to answer their questions, perhaps using one method to compensate for limitations in another (Greene et al. 1989). Mixed methods are those where both quantitative and qualitative methods are employed in a single study.

Other reasons for using mixed methods:

- To develop or inform the use of particular methods (Greene et al. 1989), such as carrying out individual or group interviews (e.g. focus groups) to inform development of constructs or items for quantitative surveys.
- To gain insight into different units or levels of analysis, by 'nesting' one method within another (Tashakkori and Teddlie 2003), for example by following closed response survey questions using a rating scale with an open question to obtain reasons for a particular response.

Table 13.2   Design examples for evaluating effectiveness of health care activities using 'scientific' approaches

Study design	Features	Appropriate for:
Process or implementation evaluation	Where set goals or performance criteria exist, consider using: • quality/performance indicators • legal requirements/policy guidelines • patient/service user needs/ expectations • productivity, efficiency or cost measures • national or regional bench-marks, including patient pathways Where no set goals, criteria or indicators exist, designs might map or establish current processes/ pathways, through: • document analysis, e.g. case notes, critical incidents, protocols • observation • mixed methods, e.g. interviews with key stakeholders	New, ongoing or mature health care programmes, services, delivery models Policy implementation monitoring and evaluation Evaluating adherence to treatment protocols/guidelines
Quasi-experiments	Measures outcomes before and after an intervention or activity: • may collect data at several time points • may include outcomes for intervention and comparison groups • comparison groups are matched on key characteristics, forming possible alternative explanations for outcome differences	Programme, service, policy and organizational/workforce development evaluations Where randomization is not ethical or feasible
Randomized experiments	Measures outcomes for randomly assigned intervention group and control groups Usually before and after intervention	Where randomization is both ethical and feasible

Source: Adapted from Bernholz et al. (2006)

Planning and carrying out evaluation research

Evaluations require careful planning. Planning is essential to highlight potential problems before they occur, identify possible solutions and keep studies on track to achieve goals within the desired timescale and budget.

Plans should include the following:

- resources – financial resources, people and skills required to carry out and oversee the evaluation study
- communication and feedback processes – how results and recommendations will be used and disseminated
- timescale – covering essential phases of the study, from set-up to completion
- contingency plans – assess critical aspects of the evaluation process, weigh up the risks and create alternative solutions, for instance how to overcome access issues to information sources, what to do if key members of the evaluation team are unable to continue work on the project

Resources

The time, money, skills and attitudes needed to conduct sound evaluation studies are frequently underestimated. Without adequate resources to see a study through to completion, any evaluation becomes infeasible and impractical. A key element of any evaluation plan will concern funding. How will the evaluation study be funded? From existing resources? Or will the evaluation plan need to include time and other resources dedicated to preparing funding or grant proposals? How much will the study cost, and over what period of time?

Who will conduct the evaluation? This may partly depend on whether the evaluation needs to be seen to be conducted independently, that is by evaluators who are neither responsible for any aspect of the activity being evaluated, nor employed by the activity's funders. Does the evaluator or evaluation team have the skills required? The Canadian Evaluation Society suggests six distinct areas where skills are required:

- ethics
- evaluation planning and design (including research design skills and contextual understanding)
- data collection
- data analysis and interpretation
- communication and interpersonal skills
- project management

In many organizational circumstances, one individual may not be able to supply the full range of skills and attributes required to conduct a particular evaluation. If it is a large or complex evaluation, it may be neither feasible nor desirable for one person to carry out the entire process.

Who will manage or oversee the evaluation? What arrangements will be in place to ensure accountability? If the evaluation team is to be independent of the evaluated activity, would the study benefit from having a steering or advisory group?

Communication and feedback processes

Communication and feedback processes are sometimes overlooked in conducting evaluation studies. They are especially important, however, when the evaluator(s) are independent and therefore physically or otherwise removed from key stakeholders and the activity being evaluated, and/or unable to directly access information sources or study participants without an intermediary. Again, a steering or advisory group can be helpful in managing communication, enabling evaluators to gain information from stakeholders, and in keeping stakeholders informed about progress.

The evaluation plan should also address how results will be communicated and used. For independent evaluators, influence on the use of results is often limited to suggestions or recommendations in presentations and written reports. Communication strategies should be appropriate to the interests of different stakeholder groups. The evaluation's funders, for example, may want a full written report, while health care providers and users of health care activities may require presentations, posters summarizing the evaluation, newsletter articles, talks or web-related material for a variety of audiences. These take time to prepare, so try to agree at the outset what should be included, to ensure sufficient resources are available when needed.

Timescales

What is the timescale for the evaluation – weeks, months, years? It is often helpful to create a timeline for the overall project, breaking it into discrete phases, and to mark on that timeline what needs to happen by when. Most evaluations have an end target or deadline. For example, a health service provider may want to make budget decisions before the end of their financial year. Let's assume their cut-off date is 31 December. The evaluation might therefore aim to present results a month before, to give stakeholders time to feed the information into budget discussions, giving the evaluation a targeted finishing date of 30 November. Work backwards from that date, allocating sufficient time to tasks to enable targets, deadlines and other key milestones to be met. This should enable the evaluator to spot potential problems before they occur, determine whether the study is actually feasible within the timescale given its available resources and, if necessary, to provide evidence on which to negotiate further resources.

There is a host of project-management tools and software which may be worth considering to provide an overview and help keep track of the whole evaluation process, particularly if the evaluation is complex, lengthy or has multiple collaborators or evaluators working on different aspects. Make sure at the outset that everyone involved is aware of key milestones and their impact on the overall evaluation process.

At their most basic level, evaluations have three distinct phases:

- preparatory phase – design and set-up (including gaining ethical approval and permissions)
- data collection and analysis phase (including drawing conclusions and making recommendations)
- feedback and dissemination phase

The amount of time needed for the preparatory phase (everything that needs to be in place before an evaluator can start collecting study data) will depend on the timescales of local governance systems and research ethics committees, which may only meet infrequently to process applications. Remember that most governance systems require sight of data-collection instruments and participant information sheets, so much of the practical detail of a study will need to have been worked out in advance. In addition, certain tasks may need to wait until permission to go ahead has been obtained, for example hiring skilled staff to work on the project or gaining access to study participants. The downside, of course, is that much effort and resources are required at the outset, with no guarantee that permission will actually be granted to carry out the study. Even for relatively straightforward evaluations it is not uncommon for this phase to take three to six months, longer if study funding also needs to be secured.

It may be possible during the data collection and analysis phase to carry out more than one task in parallel without compromising the design, particularly if it involves multiple data-collection methods. In one example involving document analysis of case notes and a staff survey, evaluation team members were able to carry out each of these simultaneously. Each method required three months of one person's time, so having two evaluators allowed the study to move into the dissemination phase within six months rather than the originally anticipated nine. Three months can make a big difference to stakeholders. In this case the time saving meant results were able to be presented at an important annual conference.

For the dissemination phase it is wise to gain some agreement from funders and other key stakeholders about what forms this will take, for which audiences, and over what period. The primary audience is those stakeholders for whom the evaluation was undertaken in the first place, so priority should be given to satisfying their information needs. In many cases this is likely to involve a written report (see following sections for more information) and/or a presentation summarizing the study and its key findings. There may also be papers for research and professional journals, newsletter articles, conference presentations, workshops or seminars, posters, web items and so on. Again, it is worth specifying and agreeing such commitments in advance, including roles, responsibilities, ownership of data/intellectual property and authorship.

Contingency plans

A key aspect of evaluation planning is to consider what risks or eventualities could jeopardize the success of the project and, where possible, to develop alternative solutions. Some funders may require applicants to carry out a formal risk assessment of the project before they will part with any money. After all, why spend valuable resources on a project that is unlikely to deliver to expectations? Even if no formal risk assessment is required by funders or governing bodies, evaluators should still give their study the best possible chance of achieving its objectives by asking themselves a few simple questions. What are the critical points in the evaluation process? Where is the evaluation most vulnerable? Access to study participants, for example, is often fraught with unexpected complications. If the design is survey-based, what impact will it have on the study's ability to answer the evaluation questions satisfactorily if insufficient numbers of respondents are recruited? How can the response rate be maximized? Would the design be stronger if multiple or mixed methods were used to supplement the survey? Perhaps most of the skills required to conduct the evaluation reside in one key person – how will those skills be replaced if that person, for whatever reason, is unable to work on the study?

Common problems encountered in evaluations often stem from not considering evaluation early enough, poorly specified or unachievable aims and objectives, stakeholder and accountability issues, insufficient resources, lack of planning and unrealistic timescales. Although no one can foresee every circumstance which may disrupt or set back an evaluation, time spent working through alternative strategies and weighing up their benefits and drawbacks *before* they may need to be implemented can mean the difference between success and failure.

Report writing and feedback of findings

Most commissioners of evaluation studies require some form of written report when the study is completed, and/or an oral presentation summarizing the key findings (see also Chapter 20). Some may stipulate a maximum word limit for reports, or request that material be formatted in a certain way, but often decisions about structure are left to the evaluator.

The most important thing is to write with the report's primary audience in mind. Make it as easy as possible for them to use the information without unintentionally altering the key messages. The evaluation set out to answer one or more questions, so the report should show how the study addressed those questions as well as answer them.

The report should be presented as clearly, legibly and professionally as possible. Reports littered with spelling mistakes are not only difficult to read, they send out unhelpful messages, casting doubt on a study's credibility and the professional standards of the evaluators. Spellcheckers might be frustrating, but they are also a report writer's friend. Don't be shy about using them. Alternatively, find a good proofreader.

Here are some of the elements that might be used to structure a report:

- Title page
- Acknowledgements
- Executive summary
- Table of contents
- Introduction/background to the study
- Purpose, aims and objectives of the evaluation
- Evaluation design and methodology
- Data collection
- Data analysis
- Results
- Discussion
- Limitations
- Conclusions and recommendations
- References
- Appendices

Funders and stakeholders of evaluation studies often need to be prepared by the evaluator for sensitive results and recommendations. This should be a major part of any evaluation's communication strategies, and therefore included in the evaluation plan. If the study has a steering group or advisory panel working closely with the project team, it is advisable to keep them informed of progress, and steering group meetings are a legitimate, useful and timely way of doing so. Not only are members thus forewarned about emerging findings, they also have the opportunity to comment on them and discuss appropriate ways forward. One strategy is to circulate a draft final report (minus the executive summary) to study funders, inviting feedback. Only then are final changes made and an executive summary added.

Everyone has their own writing style and level of personal organization. The report writing process can be creative and stimulating, but in more cases than not it may take longer than anticipated to achieve a full draft. Writing sections of a report as the research progresses is one way to overcome this.

Conclusion

Evaluation research seeks to identify value, merit, worth, effectiveness or impact for a particular audience. Done appropriately, it can provide robust evidence and information, making it a vital and powerful tool in effectively managing health care, allocating resources and supporting improvements in outcomes for patients and service users. There are many challenges in designing and conducting evaluation research studies. The very nature of evaluation, where goals are rarely pre-established and where there are often conflicting needs and priorities of different stakeholders, may make it difficult to balance pragmatism and methodological rigour. It is essential, therefore, to agree the evaluation's purpose, specific aims and constraints at the outset, allowing these to drive design choices and filter out inappropriate or infeasible alternatives. Incorporating these decisions into a plan should help highlight potential problems before they occur, enabling the researcher to identify possible solutions and keep studies on track to achieve goals within the desired timescale and budget. By doing so, many of the common pitfalls in evaluation research can be minimized or avoided and the benefits of engaging in evaluation strengthened. Good luck with your evaluation research study.

Key concepts

- Evaluation seeks to identify value, merit, worth, effectiveness or impact. What, how and why something is evaluated depends on the evaluation's context and stakeholders.
- Evaluation is vital in providing evidence and information to support health care management, decision making and resource allocation, and to improve delivery and outcomes for patients and service users.
- Many types of evaluation exist. These are sometimes categorized by purpose or by research methodologies and principles they employ.

- Complex evaluations may use multiple research methods and/or 'mixed' methods, collecting and analysing both quantitative and qualitative data to achieve their objectives.
- Planning is essential to highlight potential problems before they occur, identify possible solutions and keep studies on track to achieve goals within the desired timescale and budget.
- Common pitfalls are not considering evaluation early enough, poorly specified or unachievable aims and objectives, stakeholder and accountability issues, insufficient resources, lack of planning and unrealistic timescales.

Key readings in evaluation research

- R. Pawson and N. Tilley, *Realistic Evaluation* (New York: Sage, 1997)
  This is a seminal guide to evaluation design, data collection and analysis from a realist perspective. It also provides a brief and thought-provoking history of how evaluation has developed and some of the assumptions underpinning evaluation research.
- A. Bowling, *Research Methods in Health*, 3rd edn (Maidenhead: Open University Press, 2009)
  This book provides an excellent introduction to the range of research methods available to evaluators, with examples of application focused on health care.
- M. Easterby-Smith, *Evaluating Management Development, Training and Education*, 2nd rev. edn (Aldershot: Gower Press, 1994)
  This book has a good section on the influence of organizational politics on conducting evaluation studies.

Examples of evaluation studies in health care research

The following research papers and evaluation reports provide examples of evaluation studies carried out in health care practice and policy:

- World Health Organization, *Monitoring and Evaluation of Mental Health Policies and Plans* (Mental Health Policies and Service Guidance Package) (Geneva: World Health Organization, 2007)
- R. Belling, *User Views Evaluation of Reducing Teenage Pregnancy Project: Young Parents Project* (London: London South Bank University, 2003)
- M. Knapp, L. Thorgrimsen, A. Patel, A. Spector, A. Hallam, B. Woods and M. Orrell, Cognitive stimulation therapy (CST) for people with dementia, *British Journal of Psychiatry*, 188 (2006), 574–80
- J. Beecham, A. Ramsay, K. Gordon, S. Maltby, K. Walshe, I. Shaw, A. Worrall and S. King, *Realistic evaluation of mental health improvement partnerships in England* (UK: NIHR SDO, 2010)

Useful websites

Many countries worldwide have professional associations of evaluators. These country and regional websites contain much useful and freely available information, including checklists on how to conduct evaluations, ethical guidance and professional standards:

- American Evaluation Association (AEA) – http://www.eval.org
- Canadian Evaluation Society – http://www.evaluationcanada.ca
- European Evaluation Society – http://www.europeanevaluation.org
- UK Evaluation Society – http://www.evaluation.org.uk
- Author's own website – http://www.evaluationworks.co.uk

References

Beecham, J., Ramsay, A., Gordon, K., Maltby, S., Walshe, K., Shaw, I., Worrall, A. and King, S. (2010) Cost and impact of a quality improvement programme in mental health services, *Journal of Health Services Research and Policy*, 15(2): 69–75.

Belling, R. (2000) *Transferring managerial learning back to the workplace: The influence of personality and the workplace environment.* Unpublished PhD thesis, Cranfield University, UK.

Belling, R. (2003) *User Views Evaluation of Reducing Teenage Pregnancy Project: Young Parents Project.* London: London South Bank University.

Bernholz, E., Carra, J., Clark, P., Ginsburg, A., Habibion, M., Heffelfinger, J., Introcaso, D., Oros, C., Scheers, N.J., Shipman, S., Stinson, L. and Valdez, B. (2006) *Evaluation Dialogue Between OMB Staff and Federal Evaluators: Digging a Bit Deeper into Evaluation Science.* Washington, DC: US Government Accountability Office. http://www.fedeval.net/docs/omb2006briefing.pdf [Accessed 5 April 2013].

Bhaskar, R. (1979) *The Philosophy of Naturalism: A Philosophical Critique of the Contemporary Human Sciences.* Brighton: Harvester.

Bowling, A. (2009) *Research Methods in Health,* 3rd edn. London: Open University Press.

Clancy, C.M. and Eisenberg, J.M. (1998) Outcomes research: Measuring the end results of health care, *Science*, 282(5387): 245–6, doi:10.1126/science.282.5387.245.

Douglas, F.C., Gray, D.A. and van Teijlingen, E.R. (2010) Using a realist approach to evaluate smoking cessation interventions targeting pregnant women and young people, *BMC Health Services Research*, 10: 49–50.

Easterby-Smith, M. (1994) *Evaluating Management Development, Training and Education,* 2nd edn. Aldershot: Gower Press.

Fain, J.A. (2005) Is there a difference between evaluation and research? *The Diabetes Educator*, 31(2): 150–5.

Fetterman, D., Kaftarian, S.J. and Wandersman, A. (1996) *Empowerment Evaluation: Knowledge and Tools for Self-assessment and Accountability.* Aldershot: Gower Press.

Greene, J. C., Caracelli, V.J. and Graham, W.F. (1989) Toward a conceptual framework for mixed-method evaluation designs, *Educational Evaluation and Policy Analysis*, 11(3): 255–74.

Knapp, M., Thorgrimsen, L., Patel, A., Spector, A., Hallam, A., Woods, B. and Orrell, M. (2006) Cognitive stimulation therapy (CST) for people with dementia, *British Journal of Psychiatry*, 188: 574–80.

Mark, M.M., Henry, G.T. and Julnes, G. (2000) *Evaluation: An Integrated Framework for Understanding, Guiding and Improving Policies and Programs*, San Francisco: Jossey-Bass.

Morris, M. and Cohn, R. (1993) Program evaluators and ethical challenges: A national survey. *Evaluation Review*, 17(6): 621–42.

National Patient Safety Agency (2010) *Defining Research*. London: National Patient Safety Agency.

Oakley, A., Strange, V., Bonell, C., Allen, E. and Stephenson, J. (2006) Process evaluation in randomised controlled trials of complex interventions, *British Medical Journal*, 332(7538): 413–16.

Pawson, R. and Tilley, N. (1997) *Realistic Evaluation*. New York: Sage.

Petrou, S. and Gray, A. (2011) Economic evaluation alongside randomised controlled trials: Design, conduct, analysis and reporting, *British Medical Journal*, 342:d1548, doi: 10.1136/bmj.d1548.

Saunders, R. P., Evans, M.H. and Joshi, P. (2005) Developing a process evaluation plan for assessing health promotion program implementation: A how to guide, *Health Promotion Practice*, 6(2): 134–47.

Smith, S., Sinclair, D., Raines, R. and Reeves, B. (2005) *Health Care Evaluation (Understanding Public Health)*. London: Open University Press.

Stufflebeam, D.L. (2001) *Evaluation Models*, New Directions for Evaluation 89. San Francisco: Jossey-Bass.

Tashakkori, A. and Teddlie, C. (2003) *Handbook of Mixed Methods in the Social and Behavioural Science*. Thousand Oaks, CA: Sage.

Tolma, E.L., Cheney, M.K., Troup, P. and Hann, N. (2009) Designing the process evaluation for the collaborative planning of a local turning point partnership, *Health Promotion Practice*, 10(4): 537–48.

US Department of Health and Human Services (2005) *Introduction to Program Evaluation for Public Health Programs: A Self-study Guide*. Atlanta, GA: Centers for Disease Control and Prevention.

Weiss, C. (1998) *Evaluation*, 2nd edn. New Jersey: Prentice Hall.

World Health Organization (2007) *Monitoring and Evaluation of Mental Health Policies and Plans*, Mental Health Policies and Service Guidance Package. Geneva: World Health Organization.

PART 4

Measurement and data collection

14 Using cognitive interviewing in health care research

Jonathan Drennan

Chapter topics
- Problems with questionnaire design
- Cognitive psychology
- Survey methods
- Cognitive interviewing
- Think-aloud interviews
- Verbal probing
- Concurrent and retrospective interviews
- Process of cognitive interviewing
- Cognitive interviewing in health care research
- Critical evaluation of cognitive interviewing

Introduction

When we undertake quantitative research with patients we generally use questionnaires to measure an outcome. However, many of these instruments are designed from the perspective of the researcher rather than the patient. It is becoming increasingly recognized that patients may attribute different meanings to questions and questionnaires than those intended by a researcher. Therefore, prior to undertaking research with patients, especially patients or clients who may have difficulties understanding questions, it is recommended that individual questions and questionnaires are pretested. There is, however, generally a lack of advice on how to pretest a questionnaire prior to its use in the field (Presser et al. 2004). This chapter introduces a structured technique known as cognitive interviewing, a technique that is increasingly being used in health care research to pretest questionnaires. The chapter provides an overview of the theory underlying cognitive interviewing, the different formats of the technique that are used in the pretesting of survey questionnaires, and examples of how this approach has been used in health care research. The chapter concludes with a field guide on how to use cognitive interviewing to pretest a questionnaire.

Challenges for respondents in completing questionnaires

There are a number of cognitive steps a respondent must go through in attempting to answer a question on a survey (Tourangeau 1984; Willis 1999, 2005; Snijkers 2002). These include interpretation and comprehension – this relates to the extent to which a respondent understands a question or the words in a question. For example, in health care research terms on a questionnaire such as 'fasting', 'ligaments', 'incontinence', 'cancer', 'consultant' and 'abdomen' may have a different meaning to a patient than they do to a health care professional or researcher. Willis (2004) points out that it is this mismatch between the researcher's and patient's perceptions of the meaning of terms that lead to the majority of problems seen in survey questionnaires.

Another step in answering questionnaires is information retrieval – this relates to the respondent's ability to recall the information required to complete the question; can the patient recall dates, times, events and so on? Respondents also have to decide and judge questions; this relates to the extent to which the respondent engages with the items and provides valid responses to the questions.

As highlighted, questionnaires are generally developed from the perspective of the researcher rather than from the standpoint of the respondent; Willis (1999: 29) refers to this as 'the armchair crafting of survey questions'. Therefore, terms or concepts that are familiar to an academic researcher may have a different meaning or may be misunderstood by the subject. Adair et al. (2011) also report how assumptions made by researchers regarding the banality or usability of questions, especially when used with vulnerable populations, can be proven wrong when used in the field.

Willis (2004) provides an example of a commonly used question in health care research: '*In general, would you say your health is excellent, very good, good, fair or poor?*' This relatively simple question is widely used in research studies, especially those related to quality of life. Even though a researcher may perceive the question as relatively straightforward, Willis (2004) identifies issues that may arise with such a question; for example, does it refer to physical health, mental health, or a combination of both? If it refers to both, what weighting does the respondent give to each aspect of general health? Other terms that can cause issues for patients include terms such as 'regularly', 'difficulty', 'fasting' and 'income' (Drennan 2003).

To counter the problems associated with questions, cognitive interviewing is becoming increasingly recognized as a technique that can be used in conjunction with other approaches to pretest questionnaires prior to their use in the field.

Cognitive interviewing

Cognitive interviewing is an amalgamation of cognitive theory and survey methodology in the understanding of the processes respondents use in completing survey questionnaires (Drennan 2003). There has been an exponential growth in the use of the technique as a method of pretesting questionnaires, which is based on the think-aloud process described by Ericsson and Simon (1980). It is through the use of cognitive interviewing that the process a respondent uses to answer a question is understood.

Beatty (2004: 45) defines cognitive interviewing as:

> The practice of administering a survey questionnaire while collecting additional verbal information about the survey responses; this additional information is used to evaluate the quality of the response or to help determine whether the question is generating the sort of information that the author intends.

Basically, cognitive interviewing is used to measure a respondent's 'verbal reports about their thinking when answering questions' (Conrad and Blair 2004: 68). In effect, the method ascertains the thought processes respondents use to answer questions (Presser et al. 2004). This information is then used to construct questions that are understandable and valid for the population for which they were intended.

If questions are highlighted as problematic during the cognitive interviewing process they may be amended, or in some cases removed. However, sometimes removing a question or questions from a standardized instrument will affect its validity. In this case cognitive interviewing still has utility in that the preamble to the question may be altered to enable understanding or provide reassurance to the patient participating in the study. Adair et al. (2011) provide an example of this when pretesting questions on standardized instruments with homeless people with mental health problems. The authors decided, following cognitive interviewing and the feedback from respondents, to leave sensitive questions dealing with suicidal and homicidal ideation in the questionnaire but to add a preamble that would assure subjects of the confidentiality of responses and explain that there were a series of questions that dealt with subjects of a personal nature.

Cognitive interviewing in health care research

There are a number of reasons why cognitive interviewing is a useful methodological tool for health care researchers. These include making adjustments to or modifying particular questions that may be perceived as problematic to identify 'potential sources of response error' (Willis 2004), identifying questions that may be problematic for particular subgroups in a survey (Conrad and Blair 2004), testing the acceptability and usability of sensitive questions, pretesting respondents' understanding of medical terminology used in the survey, and identifying a respondent's ability to recall dates and times. For example, patients are often asked on surveys to provide specific answers: 'how many times in the last year have you visited your general practitioner?' or 'how many times have you experienced pain in the last three weeks?'

Pretesting the questionnaire with different subgroups before using it in the field is also useful. Miller et al. (2011) highlight that question wording can have different meanings not only in different cultural groups but also between urban and rural respondents. Cognitive interviewing is also useful for pretesting sensitive questions regarding lifestyle that are often used on patient surveys. These may include questions regarding drug or alcohol abuse and sexual practices. The method is also useful in identifying questions that at first hand may appear benign to researchers (such as descriptions of living arrangements or employment status), which, however, may be identified as sensitive or complex by respondents (Adair et al. 2011). This may lead the researcher to change the position of such items on the questionnaire, exchange a word on the questionnaire for a synonym or add a preamble to the question to aid clarification. For example, the term 'nausea' may be supplemented with 'feeling sick' (Murtagh et al. 2007: 89). Other issues that may be highlighted through cognitive interviews with patients include legibility and questionnaire layout, problems with skip patterns and time periods, question comprehension, word comprehension, response burden and social desirable responding (Drennan 2003; Murtagh et al. 2007).

Cognitive interviewing is particularly useful when developing or pretesting questionnaires for use with special populations such as children and adolescents, people with an intellectual disability, older people and people experiencing mental health problems. It is becoming increasingly evident that proxies for these groups, such as parents, relatives or health care staff, are no longer adequate to measure experiences and health-related outcomes (de Leeuw et al. 2004); therefore questions and questionnaires are being developed to directly measure the views, outcomes and attitudes of populations that may not have previously been researched.

Challenges in undertaking cognitive interviews with vulnerable groups in health care

There are challenges in undertaking cognitive interviews with special populations. For example, difficulties in using the cognitive interview technique when pretesting questionnaires with children and adolescents have been highlighted; however, there is support for the process. De Leeuw et al. (2004) outline that, in theory, children should be good candidates to partake in the cognitive interviewing process due to the way they verbalize their thoughts during play or in class. However, drawing on the literature, de Leeuw et al. (2004: 424) highlight that the cognitive interview process has not been successful with children or adolescents due to a lack of 'ability or the motivation to articulate their thought processes spontaneously'. A number of approaches have been recommended that should be used when using cognitive interview techniques with children and adolescents, including comprehensive verbal introductions provided to the child or adolescent about the process, using warm-up exercises, asking the child to read the question out loud, use of probes more frequently than those used in the process with adults, ensuring that a familiar or non-threatening environment is used, a parent or guardian being present at the interview, avoiding overuse of paraphrasing – keep the instructions concrete, use frequent reassurance, allow time for breaks during the process and observe non-verbal behaviours (de Leeuw et al. 2004). Examples of cognitive interviews reported in the literature with vulnerable populations are highlighted in Box 14.1.

Box 14.1 Examples of cognitive interviews with vulnerable groups

---

An example of cognitive interviewing used with children is provided by Irwin et al. (2009) who completed interviews with children and adolescents between the ages of 8 and 17 to ascertain their understanding of items measuring patient-related outcomes including: physical functioning, emotional health, social health, fatigue, pain and asthma – a disease that is prevalent in childhood. Irwin et al. (2009) reported that children as young as 8 years of age successfully participated in the cognitive interview process. The process also identified that children readily understand response options used in questionnaires but may have trouble with words that are familiar to adults such as 'difficulty' and 'irritability'.

Adair et al. (2011) also provide a good example of the use of cognitive interviewing with a special population. The aim of the study was to use cognitive interviewing to test the extent to which homeless individuals with mental health problems understood and responded to items on existing standardized instruments that measured physical and mental health, social contact, substance use and contact with services. The rationale for pretesting existing instruments was that they had not been previously used with this particular population or that the instruments were newly developed.

When to use cognitive interviewing in health care research

Cognitive interviewing can be used to pretest questions on newly developed instruments or as a means of ascertaining the utility and relevance of existing questionnaires when used in a new setting or with a different population. Adair et al. (2011), for example, used cognitive interviewing to pretest existing questionnaires such as the *Colorado Symptom Index* and the *Community Integration Scale* with a homeless population. The authors identified that the cognitive interview technique was most beneficial in highlighting the relevance of items and found through using the cognitive interview process that a number of items on the standardized instruments did not apply to the circumstances of the respondents.

Cognitive interviewing is increasingly being used in a number of health and social studies to ascertain the usability and relevance of questionnaire items developed for health surveys. For example, Brown et al. (2008: 942) undertook cognitive interviewing to test the construct validity of the *Anxiety Sensitivity Index*. In palliative care Ahmed et al. (2009: 667) used cognitive interviewing as part of a multidimensional approach to develop an instrument that is completed by patients to assist health care professionals 'to identify patients and families that would benefit from a referral to specialist supportive and palliative care'. Murtagh et al. (2007) used cognitive interviewing in the enhancement and further development of an instrument measuring symptoms in patients with end-stage renal disease. Cognitive interviewing has also been used to develop internationally comparable questions measuring disability (Miller et al. 2011). Other examples of the application of the technique that attest to its growing importance in health care research include: cancer care (Wu and McSweeney 2004), children's quality of life (Irwin et al. 2009), fatigue (Christodoulou et al. 2008), pain (Matter et al. 2009), mental health in homeless people (Adair et al. 2011), and elder abuse in the community (Naughton et al. 2012), to name but a few.

Process of cognitive interviewing

A cognitive interview, a form of semi-structured interview, is carried out between the researcher and a respondent who is representative of the sample to which the questionnaire being tested will eventually be administered. Throughout the process the interviewer elicits a verbal response from the participant; it is through these verbal responses that the investigator gains an insight into the thought processes that the respondent is using when responding to survey questions. Cognitive interviews are usually held face to face; however, cognitive interviews can also be undertaken over the telephone (Willis 1999). Although telephone-based cognitive interviews are useful, especially if it is intended that the final questionnaire is to be administered in this format, Willis (1999) recommends that face-to-face interviews are preferable as they allow the researcher to identify non-verbal cues that may arise during the interview process. There are a number of methods used in the interview process, but the two most commonly used are the think-aloud process and verbal probing (Beatty 2004; Willis 2004).

Think-aloud and verbal probing

When using cognitive interviewing, it is important to remember that not only are you testing a respondent's understanding of a research question, you are also ascertaining whether the answer is relevant to the question that has been asked (Willis 2004). In addition, the principal aim of cognitive interviewing is to test the questionnaire and identify problems and not to measure the respondent's answers to the question per se.

The think-aloud process used in cognitive interviewing allows us to develop an insight into the steps a respondent takes when answering a research question. When using the think-aloud process the respondent is asked to verbalize their thoughts as they respond to a question (Taylor 2000; Schuwirth et al. 2001; Willis 2004). The interviewer asks the respondent to tell them out loud what they are thinking as they read a particular item on a questionnaire. It is through this verbalization that an understanding of how the respondent comprehends a particular question is ascertained (Drennan 2003; Willis 2004).

Willis (1999) recommends that prior to the interview commencing the subject should be given a think-aloud exercise such as asking them to describe a room in their home. This will assist them in verbalizing their thoughts prior to the full interview commencing and helps them to be at ease.

The other approach commonly used in cognitive interviewing is verbal probing. During the cognitive interviewing process, the researcher asks the respondent a series of probing questions. Probing is used to further understand the cognitive processes the respondent is using when answering a particular item on a questionnaire. Probes could include statements such as: 'tell me what you were thinking while answering that question' or 'what does the term "health" mean to you?' Willis (1999) identifies different types of probes that can be used by the interviewer when testing the respondent's understanding of the questionnaire, including: comprehensive probes, recall probes, specific probes and general probes. Comprehensive probes are used to ascertain a respondent's understanding of terms used in a questionnaire, for example a respondent can be asked 'what does the word "diabetes" mean to you?' Willis (1999) also recommends that the respondent be asked to paraphrase the question: 'what does the question mean to you in your own words?' In addition, recall probes can be used: can the respondent recall dates or time periods? Specific probes ask the respondent why they chose a specific answer, whereas general probes relate to observing the behaviour of the respondent during the cognitive interview. An example of a general probe could be: 'I noticed you hesitated at that question – can you tell me why?' (Willis 1999: 6).

Prior to an interview a number of scripts should be developed (Willis 1999). These will help formulate questions that may be useful to explore during the interview process. Beatty (2004: 47), in testing a quality of life component of a questionnaire that required respondents to recall the number of days that someone was unwell, used pre-scripted probes such as: 'how did you decide on that number of days?', 'did you have difficulties in deciding whether days were good or not good?' It is recommended that the types of scripted probes used during the cognitive interview process be carefully considered beforehand as they can affect the process of the interview (Beatty 2004).

In addition, unscripted probes, which respond to the vagaries of the interview, can also be used. It is recommended that scripted probes be not rigidly adhered to but used as a guide to the interview process (Willis 1999; Beatty 2004). Beatty (2004) further advises that interviewers should be allowed to use their discretion during the cognitive interview in deciding which probes to use; following up on a respondent's answer is essential in exploring their thought processes when completing a questionnaire.

Probing may be also be concurrent (directly after each question or item) or retrospective (following completion of the questionnaire). Generally, concurrent probing is used as this allows the interviewer to ascertain what the respondent was thinking the moment they answered the question. Retrospective probing is recommended when pretesting self-administered questionnaires and when testing a questionnaire in the final phase of its development – just prior to it being used in the field (Willis 1999). Undertaking retrospective probing just prior to a questionnaire being used in the field is also beneficial as it approximates 'a more realistic type of presentation' (Willis 1999: 8). Willis (1999) further highlights that retrospective probing is useful when the researcher wants to see if the respondent can complete a self-administered questionnaire: for example, can they complete the response formats? Do they understand the skip instructions if questions do not apply? Do they skip sections of the questionnaire due to a poor design or layout?

Adair et al. (2011) found that probing was more beneficial and extracted more comprehensive data than the think-aloud process when testing questionnaire items with a vulnerable population. Probing is particularly beneficial in eliciting responses from respondents who may have a cognitive impairment and may find the think-aloud process difficult. What probes are trying to achieve is to encourage the respondent to verbalize their thought processes (Conrad and Blair 2004). For example, a respondent may be asked to report what they think the terms 'occupational therapist', 'physiotherapist' or 'nurse' mean to them. Drennan (2003) provides the example of how the term 'nurse' in a questionnaire can have multiple meanings to a respondent, including public health nurse, hospital nurse, midwife or a home help whom they view as providing 'nursing' care.

It is generally recommended that both think-aloud and verbal probing be used together in the cognitive interviewing process. In cognitive interview studies that have been undertaken with patients, generally both think-aloud techniques and probing are used simultaneously (Murtagh et al. 2007). In addition, the use of the think-aloud process and probing allows the researcher to view the questionnaire from the perspective of the intended recipient; this is especially useful if the questionnaire is being used to explore a health condition; the researcher may gain insight into the extent to which the questionnaire validly measures aspects of the condition from a person who is experiencing the illness (Willis 1999; Adair et al. 2011). For example, Adair et al. (2011) used a probe in a cognitive interview with people with mental health problems who were homeless to ask if there were any health problems that they or other people they knew had that were not included in the questionnaire.

Samples used in cognitive interviewing

The vast majority of studies that use the cognitive interview technique use purposive sampling (Ahmed et al. 2009; Irwin et al. 2009). The subjects recruited for the pretesting interview process should match as well as possible the characteristics of the intended sample that will be used in the field. Therefore, the instrument should be pretested on a cohort that is similar in age, gender and health status to the intended population. An example of this is from Adair et al. (2011), who undertook cognitive interviewing with people who were homeless and had mental health problems. Respondents were identified that matched the population; this included the use of purposive sampling in terms of gender and ethnic background. It is also important that participants in the cognitive interview process have experience of the construct being measured.

There is no set sample size for cognitive interviewing, with the number of respondents used varying according to the study. Willis (1999) recommends that a quota format be used, that is, ensuring the participants in the cognitive interview process are similar to the eventual sample that will complete the questionnaire in the field. As Willis (1999: 33) notes, 'one does not desire sample sizes large enough to supply precision in statistical estimates. Rather, we strive to interview a variety of individuals.' Willis (1999) suggests that between 12 and 15 cognitive interviews are adequate to identify problematic areas in the pretesting of a questionnaire. As the questionnaire is amended on the feedback obtained from this process, further interviews may be required to judge the effect of the changes. However, it may also be the case that difficulties are identified after only four or five interviews, and at this stage amendments should be made before continuing with the process. As in qualitative interviewing, data saturation may occur with the same problems arising again and again. At this stage amendments can be made to the questionnaire and further cognitive interviews completed.

Length of the cognitive interview

The length of time spent on the cognitive interview is determined by the length and complexity of the questionnaire being tested. However, it is important that the interviewer takes into account the burden on the respondent of the process, with the opportunity of breaks offered to the participant. Generally cognitive interviews last approximately one hour (Willis 1999), with similar time frames reported when the process is used with children (Irwin et al. 2009) and patients in palliative care (Murtagh et al. 2007).

Setting for cognitive interviews

Cognitive interviews can be carried out in a 'cognitive laboratory'; this is a special room or unit that contains recording and/or video equipment. However, the process can also be completed in other settings, including those that approximate the location in which the actual administration of the questionnaire will be undertaken. Examples of field settings where cognitive interviews have been completed include either the home or the clinic for patients with end-stage renal disease (Murtagh et al. 2007) and drop-in centres or night shelters when pretesting questionnaires with people with mental health problems that are homeless (Adair et al. 2011).

Data from cognitive interviews

The aim of analysis of the data that arise from cognitive interviews is to identify problems that the respondents encountered in the survey questionnaire and then to categorize those problems (Drennan 2003; Conrad and Blair 2004). The verbal reports from the respondents' think-aloud process are the data of the cognitive interview process, and data may be collected through video and/or audio recordings and/or written notes. It is also argued that the interviewer's comments during the process should also be considered data and there is a debate on the extent to which they should be used in the analysis (Conrad and Blair 2004). The physical demeanour of the respondent during the questioning process may also be considered as data. This may include, for example, actions such as frowning, hesitation, turning pages of the questionnaire back and forward, and these should also be included in the analysis. Generally, as the majority of data collected are narrative, qualitative analysis techniques such as content analysis are used in making sense of the data.

Due to the small sample sizes used in cognitive interviewing it is important to remember that the data collected may not be representative of the population who will eventually complete the questionnaire. Therefore, it is important that the interviewer uses their clinical judgement when deciding on the steps that need to be taken to amend the questionnaire following the cognitive interview process (Willis 1999). If there are a number of interviewers involved in the process, Willis (1999) recommends that interviewers' comments on each question tested are initially taken individually and then aggregated to provide an overview of the issues that arose during the process.

An excellent framework for analysing the data collected from a cognitive interview is provided by Conrad and Blair (2004); it is this framework that is used in the field guide to cognitive interviewing presented below.

Criticism of cognitive interviewing

Cognitive interviewing is not without criticism. One issue that has arisen is that, as the cognitive interview process is somewhat different from the reality of the administration of the questionnaire, problems may be identified that would not be encountered in the field (Beatty 2004). Beatty (2004) highlights that in a cognitive interview process each question or item may be preceded or succeeded by a discussion, which would not normally occur in the administration of the questionnaire in the field.

This, it is argued, can lead to problems being identified that would not normally occur. To prevent this issue occurring, Beatty (2004: 52) recommends that 'reorienting probes' (probes that encourage the respondent to give a specific answer) are used instead of 'elaborating probes' (probes that ask a respondent to provide information 'beyond the specific answers to the survey questions'). The rationale for this approach is that reorienting probes are more likely to be used in the field administration of a questionnaire. Beatty (2004) found that using only reorienting probes reduced the frequency of imprecise responses occurring. However, when respondents were asked to elaborate on their experience of completing the questionnaire they reported that they had provided responses, especially those requiring a precise numerical value, because interviewers expected them to do so. This led Beatty (2004: 56) to conclude that the interview process used in the field may '*actually* suppress the appearance of problems'.

The inconsistency with which the cognitive interviewing technique is applied has also been identified as problematic. There are differences in the experience level of interviewers, sample size, the extent to which probes are used either concurrently or retrospectively, and the techniques used to analyse the data (Presser et al. 2004).

Another issue is that the cognitive interview process is artificial and does not match the reality of the administration of the questionnaire in the field (Drennan 2003). In addition, the subjects who take part in the cognitive interview process may be substantially different from the respondents that will be surveyed in the field (Willis 1999). Analysis of the data collected through the cognitive interview process has also been criticized on grounds of its subjectivity (Drennan 2003). To overcome this subjectivity, a framework for analysing the data is recommended (Lessler and Forsythe 1996; Conrad and Blair 2004). The field guide outlined below shows how the data can be structured under various problem classifications that help the researcher add structure to the data collected from the cognitive interview. Although cognitive interviewing has been criticized as being artificial and subjective (Ericsson and Simon 1993; Conrad et al. 1999; Willis 1999), it can be an effective process when used to ensure the validity of survey instruments and questionnaires.

Example of a field guide for cognitive interviews in the pretesting of a survey questionnaire

The example provided here is hypothetical but is based on cognitive interviewing studies that the author has been involved in to pretest questionnaires prior to their use in the field. Remember, the overall aim of cognitive interviewing is to understand how respondents perceive and interpret questions on a survey and to identify potential problems that may arise when the questionnaire is used in the field. The process involves the analysis of respondents' verbal reports collected during the pretesting phase of instruments being distributed and used in the main data-collection stage of the study. Cognitive interviews used in this setting allowed the research team to gain insight into the cognitive processes that respondents used when completing a questionnaire through the respondents verbalizing their thoughts.

The field guide to cognitive interviewing includes the following resources:

- The process for completing a cognitive interview, including how to identify problematic questions.
- How to introduce the process to subjects involved in the cognitive interview process (see Box 14.2).
- Examples of probing questions to be used in the interview process (Box 14.3).
- Framework for classifying problematic questions identified through the cognitive interview process (Box 14.4).

Field guide for cognitive interviews

1. Retrospective semi-structured, tape-recorded interview. Usually one researcher and one respondent.
2. Interview should be undertaken in a room where disturbances will be kept to a minimum with subjects who match the characteristics of the proposed sample.
3. Interviewer administers the questionnaire and takes notes of any issues that occurred during its administration. Observations that would be of interest to researchers include:
   a. respondent skipping or not answering questions
   b. respondent hesitating or stating they do not understand a question (for example asking the interviewer to repeat the question)
   c. respondent providing the incorrect response to a question
   d. changes in respondent's appearance (for example frowning, hesitation, discomfort).
4. Use probing questions (see Box 14.3). Probes should be used to gain an understanding of the statements/questions from the respondent's perspective:
   a. Request respondents to paraphrase statements, especially those that seemed problematic: 'Can you repeat the statement in your own words?', 'How confident are you that you have understood the statement?'
   b. Ask them to define meanings of words used in questions.
   c. Ask the respondent about any statements they may have skipped: 'I'd like to ask you about this item [*point to it*] You didn't/refused to answer it. Was there a particular reason for that?'
   d. Ask respondents to explain their responses and identify areas of the questionnaire that posed difficulty in understanding, interpretation or completion of the questionnaire. For example, ask the respondent about the response options for 'importance' and 'frequency': 'Did you find it difficult to come up with an answer while keeping all of the response options in mind?'
   e. If the respondent frowned or hesitated at a question, ask them if there was a particular difficulty.
   f. Use a wrap up question: 'Do you have anything else you would like to tell us that you haven't had a chance to mention?'

5 Respondents are then interviewed retrospectively (after they have completed the questionnaire). Ask them what their overall perception was of the questionnaire, what did they think of the questionnaire? Could they follow the instructions? Was it easy to answer? What did they think of the length of time the questionnaire took to complete?

6 Make notes under each of the problem areas (Conrad et al. 1999):[1]

   a Identification of **lexical problems**:

      i Lexical problems are associated with respondents' comprehension and use of words and the context in which they are used on the questionnaire. Words that are familiar to one group of respondents (for example 'nausea', 'abdomen', 'fasting') may not be to another, or they may have a different meaning.

      ii After the respondent has completed the questionnaire ask them if there were any words they had particular problems with. For example: 'Did you understand the meaning of "therapeutic intervention"?' Write down the word that was problematic and the respondent's interpretation of it.

   b Identification of **inclusion/exclusion problems**:

      i Did the respondent answer all statements?

      ii What questions on the questionnaire did not particularly refer to them?

   c Identification of **temporal problems**:

      i Ask the respondent, following completion of the questionnaire, if they realized that the statements related to the last week/month/year etc.?

      ii Ask the respondent if they understood the response option categories: for example 'importance', 'frequency', 'agreement'?

      iii Did the respondent use a full range of scores on the response categories?

   d Identification of **logical problems**:

      i Did the respondent complete the entire questionnaire?

      ii Did the respondent become confused in answering what was expected of them?

      iii Did the respondent ask you to go back over a question to understand its meaning?

      iv How long did it take the respondent to complete the questionnaire?

      v How many questions were left unanswered?

   e Identification of **computational problems**:

      i Computational problems include those that do not fall into any other category. Examples of problems that may be included in computational categories include long-term memory recall, questions with complicated structure and those involving mental calculation.

---

[1]Adapted from Conrad et al. (1999).

Box 14.2   Process to be followed by each cognitive interviewer (adapted from Dillman (2000)

I am working on behalf of _____. We are carrying out a confidential survey to explore people's experience of their health. In a minute I'm going to ask you a number of questions. I'd like you to answer them in the same way you would if I asked them during your visit to the clinic. I will take you through the questionnaire step by step. When you have finished I would then like to ask you some questions about your thoughts and feelings about completing the questionnaire.

Now commence the questionnaire

Box 14.3   An example of probes that may included in the cognitive interview process (adapted from Conrad and Blair 2004; Christodoulou et al. 2008; Irwin et al. 2009; Ahmed et al. 2009)

- What was going through your mind as you tried to answer the question?
- You took a little while to answer that question. What were you thinking about?
- How would you make the instructions easier to understand?
- What does 'in the last week/month/year' mean to you?
- Do you think the time period is adequate to answer this question? Is it too long or too short?
- Tell me, in your own words, what do you think this question is asking?
- What does this question mean to you?
- What did you think of when answering this question?
- Were there any questions you did not want to answer?
- Were there any questions you found upsetting?
- Did you understand this question? If not, can you explain why?
- Are there any specific words that are difficult to understand?
- How would you change the words to make that question clearer?
- Was this item difficult to answer? If yes, why?
- How did you choose your answer?
- In your own words, what do you think this group of questions is asking about?
- How do you think these items are related?
- Are there any questions that don't belong in this group?
- What do you think about the response choices? Do you understand how to complete the responses? Why did you choose that response?
- In your experience, is this question relevant to you?
- Would this question/questionnaire be relevant to other patients?
- Would this question be relevant to other people with this condition?
- How would you make the response choices clearer or easier to understand?
- Are there things that we forgot to ask about that you think are important?
- What are your overall thoughts/opinions of the questionnaire?
- Was the questionnaire too long?

Box 14.4 Classification of problems identified in the cognitive interview (adapted from Conrad et al. 1999)

Problem	Problematic item	Respondent's perspective	Researcher's notes
Lexical problems (e.g. any words that the respondent had particular problems with)			
Inclusion/exclusion problems (what items were skipped/left unanswered?)			
Temporal problems (did the respondent understand the response options?)			
Logical problems (did the respondent complete the questionnaire in the order presented?)			
Computational problems (any other problems)			

Conclusion

When developing a new questionnaire for use with patients or using pre-existing questionnaires with new patient groups, especially those who are vulnerable, it is important that questionnaires are thoroughly pretested prior to their use in the field to ensure that they are valid, relevant and usable by the population for which they are intended. There is great variety in the operationalization of cognitive interviewing and readers are advised to read around the subject before deciding on an approach that best suits their research method. However, cognitive interviewing is increasingly recognized as an approach that can systematically identify potential problems with survey questionnaires. In addition, as it is becoming recognized that there is a need to include the voice of vulnerable groups in the research process, cognitive interviewing is a method that allows the questionnaire to be developed from their perspective rather than the perspective of the researcher.

Key concepts
- Non-response or non-completion of questionnaires is a major problem in survey research, leading to the collection of incomplete data.

- Problems with questionnaire response need to be identified prior to the distribution of questionnaires to the chosen sample.
- Cognitive interviewing, an amalgamation of cognitive psychology and survey research methodology, is a method that can be used to reduce non-completion and non-response of survey questions and questionnaires.
- Cognitive interviewing allows researchers to understand survey questionnaires from the respondent's rather than the researcher's perspective.
- Cognitive interviews are of most worth when used in association with other reliability and validity measures.
- Researchers should consider cognitive interviewing when developing survey questionnaires to investigate new or poorly described health concepts, researching and translating questionnaires for culturally diverse groups, and developing questionnaires for samples where questionnaire completion may pose particular problems.

Key readings in cognitive interviewing

- D. Dillman, *Internet, Mail and Mixed-Mode Surveys: The Tailored Design Method*, 3rd edn (New York: John Wiley and Sons, 2008)
  An invaluable resource on how to develop all types of surveys. Provides a very practical step-by-step approach to the design of questionnaires, including the use of cognitive interviewing.
- S. Presser, J. Rothgeb, M. Couper, J. Lessler, E. Martin, J. Martin and E. Singer, *Methods for Testing and Evaluating Survey Questionnaires* (New York: Wiley-Blackwell, 2004)
  Provides an excellent account of the methods associated with the design and testing of questionnaires. Includes a full section on cognitive interviewing.
- B. Willis, *Cognitive Interviewing: A Tool for Improving Questionnaire Design* (New York: Sage, 2005)
  Provides a good overview of the theory that underpins cognitive interviewing as well as practical examples of how to undertake cognitive interviewing in real world research.

Examples of the use of cognitive interviewing in health care research

The following papers provide excellent examples of how cognitive interviewing has been used in health care research.

- C. Christodoulou, D. Junghaenel, D. DeWalt, N. Rothrock and A. Stone, Cognitive interviewing in the evaluation of fatigue items: Results from the patient-reported outcomes measurement information system (PROMIS), *Quality of Life Research*, 17(10) (2008), 1239–46

- P. Housen, G. Shannon, B. Simon, M. Edelen, M. Cadogan, L. Sohn, M. Jones, J. Buchanan and D. Saliba, What the resident meant to say: Use of cognitive interviewing techniques to develop questionnaires for nursing home residents, *The Gerontologist*, 48(2) (2008), 158–69
- F. Murtagh, J. Addington-Hall and I. Higginson, The value of cognitive interviewing techniques in palliative care research, *Palliative Medicine*, 21(2) (2007), 87–93

Useful websites

- Willis has provided an excellent resource for carrying out the cognitive interview technique – http://fog.its.uiowa.edu/~c07b209/interview.pdf

References

Adair, C., Holland, A., Patterson, M., Mason, K., Goering, P. and Hwang, S. (2011) Cognitive interviewing methods for questionnaire pre-testing in homeless persons with mental disorders, *Journal of Urban Health: Bulletin of the New York Academy of Medicine*, 89(1): 36–52.

Ahmed, N., Bestall, J., Payne, S., Noble, B. and Ahmedzai, S. (2009) The use of cognitive interviewing methodology in the design and testing of a screening tool for supportive and palliative care needs, *Supportive Care in Cancer*, 17(6): 665–73.

Beatty, P. (2004) The dynamics of cognitive interviewing, in S. Presser, J. Rothberg, M. Couper, J. Lessler, E. Martin, J. Martin and E. Singer (eds) *Methods for Testing and Evaluating Survey Questionnaires*. New Jersey: Wiley, pp. 45–65.

Brown, G., Hawkes, N. and Tata, P. (2008) Construct validity and vulnerability to anxiety: A cognitive interviewing study of the revised Anxiety Sensitivity Index, *Journal of Anxiety Disorders*, 23(7), 942–9.

Christodoulou, C., Junghaenel, D., DeWalt, D., Rothrock, N. and Stone, A. (2008) Cognitive interviewing in the evaluation of fatigue items: Results from the patient-reported outcomes measurement information system (PROMIS), *Quality of Life Research*, 17(10): 1239–46.

Conrad, F. and Blair, J. (2004) Data quality in cognitive interviews: The case of verbal reports, in S. Presser, J. Rothberg, M. Couper, J. Lessler, E. Martin, J. Martin and E. Singer (eds) *Methods for Testing and Evaluating Survey Questionnaires*. New Jersey: Wiley, pp. 67–87.

Conrad F., Blair J. and Tracy E. (1999) Verbal reports are data! A theoretical approach to cognitive interviews, in *Proceedings of the Federal Committee on Statistical Methodology Research Conference*, Tuesday B Sessions, Arlington, VA, pp. 11–20.

Dillman, D. (2000) *Mail and Internet Surveys: The Tailored Design Method*, 2nd edn. New York: Wiley.

de Leeuw, E., Borgers, N. and Smits, A. (2004) Pretesting questionnaires for children and adults, in S. Presser, J. Rothberg, M. Couper, J. Lessler, E. Martin, J. Martin and E. Singer (eds) *Methods for Testing and Evaluating Survey Questionnaires*. New Jersey: Wiley, pp. 409–29.

Drennan, J. (2003) Cognitive interviewing: Verbal data in the design and pre-testing of questionnaires, *Journal of Advanced Nursing*, 42(1): 57–63.

Ericsson, K. A., and Simon, H. A. (1980) Verbal reports as data, *Psychological Review*, 87(3): 215–50.

Ericsson, A. and Simon, H. (1993) *Protocol Analysis: Verbal Reports as Data*, 2nd edn. Cambridge, MA: MIT Press.

Irwin, D., Varni, J., Yeatts, K. and DeWalt, D. (2009) Cognitive interviewing methodology in the development of a pediatric item bank: A patient reported outcomes measurement information system (PROMIS) study, *Health and Quality of Life Outcomes*, 7(3): 1–10.

Lessler, J. and Forsythe, B. (1996) A coding system for appraising questionnaires, in N. Schwartz and S. Sudman (eds) *Answering Questions: Methodology for Determining Cognitive and Communicative Processes in Survey Research*, San Francisco: Jossey-Bass, pp. 259–92.

Matter, R., Kline, S., Cook, K. and Amtmann, D. (2009) Measuring pain in the context of homelessness, *Quality of Life Research*, 18(7): 863–72.

Miller, K., Mont, D., Maitland, A., Altman, B. and Madans, J. (2011) Results of a cross-national structured cognitive interviewing protocol to test measures of disability, *Quality and Quantity*, 45(4): 801–15.

Murtagh, F., Addington-Hall, J. and Higginson, I. (2007) The value of cognitive interviewing techniques in palliative care research, *Palliative Medicine*, 21(2): 87–93.

Naughton, C., Drennan, J., Lyons, I., Lafferty, A., Treacy, M., Phelan, A., O'Loughlin, A. and Delaney, L. (2012) Elder abuse and neglect in Ireland: Results from a national prevalence survey, *Age and Ageing*, 41(1): 98–103.

Presser, S., Couper, M., Lessler, J., Martin, E., Martin, J., Rothgeb, J. and Singer, E. (2004) Methods for testing and evaluating survey questions, *Public Opinion Quarterly*, 68(1): 109–130.

Schuwirth, L., Verheggen, M., van der Vleuten, C., Boshuizen, H. and Dinant, G. (2001) Do short cases elicit different thinking processes than factual knowledge questions do? *Medical Education*, 35(4): 348–56.

Snijkers, G. (2002) Cognitive laboratory experiences: On pre-testing computerised questionnaires and data quality. Unpublished PhD thesis, Utrecht University and Statistics Netherlands, Heerlen.

Taylor, C. (2000) Clinical problem solving in nursing: Insights from the literature, *Journal of Advanced Nursing*, 31(4): 842–9.

Tourangeau, R. (1984) Cognitive sciences and survey methods, in T. Jabine, M. Straf, J. Tanur and R. Tourangeau (eds) *Cognitive Aspects of Survey Methodology: Building a Bridge Between Disciplines*. Washington, DC: National Academy Press, pp. 73–100.

Willis, G. (1999) Cognitive interviewing, a 'how to guide': Reducing survey error through research on the cognitive and design processes in surveys. Short course presented at the 1999 meeting of the American Statistical Association, Research Triangle Institute.

Willis, G. (2004) Cognitive interviewing revisited: a useful technique, in theory?, in S. Presser, J. Rothberg, M. Couper, J. Lessler, E. Martin, J. Martin and E. Singer (eds) *Methods for Testing and Evaluating Survey Questionnaires*. New Jersey: Wiley, pp. 23–43.

Willis, G. (2005) *Cognitive Interviewing: A Tool for Improving Questionnaire Design*. New York: Sage.

Wu, H. and McSweeney, M. (2004) Assessing fatigue in persons with cancer: An instrument development and testing study, *Cancer*, 101(7): 1685–95.

15 Questionnaires and instruments for health care research

Elaine Lehane and Eileen Savage

Chapter topics

- Measurement in health care research
- Types of health care measures
- Conceptual considerations for measurement
- Psychometrics properties

- Methodological aspects for measurement
- Practicalities of using established instruments
- Critical appraisal of instruments

Introduction

This chapter presents an overview of the purpose and importance of using accurate quantitative measurement in using questionnaires and instruments for health care research. Different types of measures are detailed. Key questions that need to be asked when selecting or developing a questionnaire or instrument are considered. Conceptual, psychometric and methodological considerations for their development and evaluation are examined. The practicalities associated with using questionnaires or instruments are explored. Finally, two instruments are presented to illustrate, first, an example of instrument development (Beliefs about Medication Compliance Scale) and, second, the use of an instrument across a range of health-related quality of life studies (Short Form 36 Health Survey). It is not the purpose of this chapter to explore theories underpinning measurement or to provide a step-by-step guide to item development. For information on these issues, the reader is referred to *An Introduction to Psychometric Theory* (Raykov and Marcoulides 2011), *Measurement in Nursing and Health Research* (Waltz et al. 2010), and *Scale Development: Theory and Applications* (DeVellis 2012). Measurement issues in qualitative research are not addressed in this chapter, an area which is considered by Waltz et al. (2010) in *Measurement in Nursing and Health Research*.

Types and uses of measurement instruments in health care research

In simple terms, measurement is a process of quantifying a phenomenon by assigning numbers to it. Measurement is a fundamental activity in health care practice and research. In everyday clinical practice health care professionals are charged with measurement, especially in relation to health assessment and health outcomes of individuals in their care. For example, an individual admitted to an emergency department following a head injury will typically have initial and continuous measurement of vital signs (respiratory rate, heart rate, temperature and blood pressure). In addition, measurement of the individual's state of consciousness can be expected using a neurological scale such as the Glasgow Coma Scale. For each of these observations, specific clinical tools or instruments are used for measurement. Accurate measurement is important for judging the clinical health status of the individual and informing decisions around treatment and care options.

In the context of research, measurements also exist for the purpose of accurately quantifying a phenomenon under study. Although quantifying phenomena by assigning numbers to them is fundamental to research measurement, many phenomena in health care research are abstract concepts such as quality of life, patient adherence, medication compliance, social support or self-management. Abstract concepts for research are known as theoretical constructs. For the purpose of measurement, these theoretical constructs need to be operationalized into defined variables, following which newly developed or existing instruments are used to quantify the variables and relationships if applicable (de Vaus 2002). For example, health-related quality of life may be operationalized into variables of social, physical and emotional well-being. A related measurement would therefore measure these variables in terms of quality of life scores for each dimension. According to Cano and Hobart (2011), research instruments that measure target variables of the phenomena of interest are the cornerstones of measurement in health care research.

Questionnaires or instruments are tools used to collect information relevant to the questions or aims and objectives of a study. They comprise a collection of items grouped together as scales to reveal levels of theoretical variables not readily assessed by direct means (DeVellis 2012). Although the term *questionnaire* is most commonly associated with measurement in health care research, questionnaires typically include rating scales, and therefore are instruments of measurement. Other terms also associated with instruments of measurement include inventories, checklists, surveys and schedules. It is the focus on scales, however, that is important in terms of measuring theoretical variables.

Selecting a measurement

The growth of rating scales for any given concept (for example, quality of life, medication compliance) over the past two decades can leave researchers somewhat confused about which measurement to select for their studies. Although it may be necessary to develop a new measure for a study, a researcher's starting point should always be to consider existing scales that seem relevant to the research area. Kimberlin and Winterstein (2008: 2280) draw attention to a select number of questions when considering existing measures:

- Do instruments already exist that measure a construct in the same way or in a very similar way to the one you wish to measure?
- How well do the constructs in the instruments you have identified match the construct you have conceptually defined for your study?
- Is the evidence of reliability and validity well established?

- In previous research, was there variability in scores with no floor or ceiling effects?
- If the measure is to be used to evaluate health outcomes, effects of interventions, or changes over time, are there studies that establish the instrument's responsiveness to change in the construct of interest?

Taken together, the above questions concern theoretical, psychometric and methodological issues that need to be considered by researchers in their use of measurement in their studies. Health care stakeholders need assurances that credible, quality data can be collected from instruments measuring subjective health outcomes. The application of rigorous development criteria to instruments used by researchers and health care practitioners is therefore essential.

Conceptual considerations for measurement

Key measurement texts in health and social sciences (McDowell 2006; Streiner and Norman 2008; Waltz et al. 2010; DeVellis 2012) collectively recommend that instrument development proceeds from theory. Similarly, review articles focused on developing appraisal criteria for selecting the most appropriate and robust measurement instruments include theoretical input as an essential criterion (Scientific Advisory Committee of the Medical Outcomes Trust 2002; Rothman et al. 2007; Valderas et al. 2008; Feldman-Stewart and Brundage 2009). Atheoretical or empirically developed instruments also have a place in social and health sciences research; however, these are becoming increasingly limited to areas where measurement has a practical purpose such as ascertaining patient discharge criteria in terms of age, gender or socio-economic status, or where an inductive approach to enquiry is required, that is, developing a theory or model (McDowell 2006; DeVellis 2012).

Why is there such an emphasis on the development of theoretically based measures? Phenomena of interest to professionals in the health and social sciences are often quite complex, abstract and not directly observable, making them difficult to measure. Coping, quality of life, psychological distress, adherence and social support are but a few examples of concepts which we are concerned with but which cannot be as easily measured or observed as more elemental data such as blood pressure or respiratory rate. If we take the example of adherence, specifically long-term adherence to anti-hypertensive medications, we would find after reviewing the literature that there are over 200 variables cited as influencing non-adherence in chronic conditions (Dunbar-Jacob and Mortimer-Stephens 2001). Taking 200 different variables and constructing a coherent, meaningful and valid instrument to measure this concept would be an arduous, if not impossible, undertaking. This task, however, would be made considerably easier, more rigorous and ultimately more accurate with theoretical input. For instance, the Medication Adherence Model (MAM) (Johnson 2002) points to three key areas responsible for long-term adherence to prescribed medications:

- high levels of *purposeful action* (the degree to which individuals intentionally decide to take medications based on perceived need, effectiveness and safety)

- *patterned behaviour* (the degree to which individuals initiate and establish a ritual, habit or pattern of taking medications through regularity of lifestyle or access, routine and remembering)
- *feedback* (the degree to which information, facts, prompts or events reinforce the need to maintain or modify medication taking).

A model such as the Medication Adherence Model helps to clarify what needs to be measured by 'unpacking' or reducing the abstract concept of adherence into its various components and dimensions of adherence behaviour. These components can then be measured using a set of questions or items on a rating scale or questionnaire. This unpacking or reduction of abstract concepts into measurable items is known as operationalization of concepts for measurement (DeVellis 2012). For example, if we take the component of *purposeful action* from the Medication Adherence Model above, the relevant dimensions of this would include perceived need, perceived effectiveness and perceived safety. Each of these dimensions would then require a set of items or questions on a measurement scale. This unpacking and focused approach effectively limits the number of questions or items that can be generated from a vast pool of potential questions available on a given topic (e.g. adherence), leading to a more systematic and sophisticated process of item generation for measurement.

A word of caution in relation to the use of theory as a guiding framework for instrument development must be noted. Just as a theory or model can lead to conceptual clarity and therefore a well-defined measurement process, inadequate theoretical input in the form of a misguided or ill-defined conceptual framework can sabotage the measurement process. Here, item generation, grouping and scoring, as well as analysis and interpretation of scores, all of which are interrelated, would be adversely affected and therefore the evaluation or measurement of the phenomenon under study would be compromised (Rothman et al. 2007). When developing or appraising an instrument, therefore, careful consideration must be given to the conceptual approach taken. In this regard, key questions need to be asked. Is the theory well established? In other words, are the underlying philosophical assumptions, concepts and dimensions explicit and empirically tested? To what extent do the instrument items collectively represent the dimensions or components of what is being conveyed by the theoretical framework (Prior et al. 2011)? Again, refer to the example above on the Medication Adherence Model. Seeking answers to these questions and clearly linking theory to instrument development is fundamental to ensuring that credible data can be collected from measures used in the social and health sciences.

Psychometric considerations for measurement – the fundamentals

Psychometrics defined

Psychometrics can be simply defined as the study of methods for measuring social and psychological variables (Hobart and Cano 2009; DeVellis 2012). As previously mentioned, many phenomena in health and social sciences cannot be measured easily as they are not directly observable. Such phenomena must be *made* measurable even though the variable is not directly quantifiable – it can be estimated indirectly from items that are written to access it. Psychometric methods are therefore concerned with the construction of instruments which make the variable of interest operational from a measurement perspective. Psychometric analyses, in turn, seek to establish the *extent* to which this quantitative conceptualization of a phenomenon has been operationalized successfully (Hobart and Cano 2009).

To have a robust appreciation of psychometrics and its relationship to instrument development, an understanding of the various measurement frameworks (also termed methods, models or theories) and the concept of measurement error must be acquired. While it is not possible to cover the full breadth and depth of literature necessary for such an understanding in this chapter (the key measurement texts provide excellent accounts in these areas), brief mention will be made here.

Measurement frameworks

Measurement frameworks specify measurement rules that guide how an instrument will be constructed, and provide definitive assumptions and conditions as to how the instrument can be analysed and how such analyses can be interpreted. A number of frameworks exist, but they can be broadly divided into *traditional* and *modern* categories. Traditional frameworks, which to date have been used most frequently by developers in the health and social sciences, are based on the assumptions underlying classical test theory, which include parallel and domain sampling models and, by extension of classical test theory, generalizability theory. Modern frameworks refer mainly to Item Response Theory (IRT) and associated Rasch Measurement. The use of modern frameworks by developers is gaining momentum due to the fact that they try to address the often quoted limitations of traditional methods, but, more importantly, access to software that can compute the complex calculations required has improved (Hobart and Cano 2009).

Measurement error

Measurement error is a further central concern in psychometrics. When constructing any instrument, error to some extent will be introduced, whether it is through the accuracy of the items written, the scaling measurement level used or the scoring system chosen. Such error impacts on the developed items' ability to accurately represent the variable of interest. Two types of error exist: random and systematic. In brief, random error is caused by *chance* factors that hamper accurate measurement. Such sources of error are unsystematic in nature and affect the consistency or reliability with which the instrument measures the variable (Waltz et al. 2010). For example, music playing in a waiting room on one of the data-collection days might distract patients from completing the instrument accurately, resulting in a different set of instrument scores than on the other three days that the measure was used to collect data. Systematic error is caused by sources within the measuring instrument, measurement process or subject. An example of this may be the inclusion of items that inadvertently tap into a different variable (e.g. pain) from the one that you set out to measure (e.g. fatigue). This affects the instrument's ability to accurately measure the concept of interest – in the above case fatigue – and therefore the validity of the measure is compromised. Waltz et al. (2010) provide further practical illustrations and unambiguous explanations of both types of error, which the reader may find useful. While it is inevitable that error will be present, such error and its resulting impact on data quality can be reduced by a rigorous approach to measurement. The extent of success in decreasing the amount of error may be gauged by two psychometric properties: reliability and validity.

At the outset it must be emphasized that evidence for an instrument's reliability and validity falls along a continuum rather than being considered a dichotomous index. For this reason, claiming that an instrument is completely 'reliable' or 'valid' is inappropriate (Frost et al. 2007; Streiner and Norman 2008). Rather, psychometric testing may provide evidence for instrument reliability and validity when it is used with a specific population for a specific purpose under certain conditions. The more evidence that is accrued, therefore, over time that the instrument is reliably measuring what it is supposed to be measuring, the more confidence one can have in the accuracy of derived data (Frost et al. 2007; Streiner and Norman 2008; Waltz et al. 2010).

Reliability

Reliability is defined as the extent to which a measure yields the same number or score each time it is administered, or the degree to which an instrument is free from random error (Frost et al. 2007). Classical approaches for examining reliability include: 1) internal consistency reliability, typically using Cronbach's coefficient alpha (α); and 2) reproducibility (e.g. test–retest or inter-observer (interviewer) reliability). Internal consistency reliability provides information about the associations among different items in an instrument (Frost et al. 2007), and essentially refers to the degree to which the subparts of an instrument are all measuring the same attribute. The coefficient alpha is a reliability index that estimates the internal consistency or homogeneity of a measure (DeVellis 2012). Reproducibility data look at inter-rater agreement at one point in time and the stability (test–retest reliability) of an instrument over time (at least two time points). Intraclass correlation coefficients are now regarded as the most appropriate choice of calculation for this aspect of reliability (Streiner and Norman 2008). In modern measurement framework applications, reliability – or in this case termed the *degree of precision* of measurement – is expressed in terms of error variance, standard error of measurement (SEM) (the square root of the error variance), or test information (reciprocal of the error variance). Error variance (or any other measure of precision) takes on different values at different points along the scale (Frost et al. 2007; Hobart and Cano 2009). See Chapter 16 for additional information on reliability.

Validity

Validity refers to the extent to which an instrument measures what it is intended to measure, and not something else (Frost et al. 2007). Validity is considered a unified or unitary concept, in that all evidence accumulated from different validation processes supports the interpretation of the measure's test scores and performance (American Educational Research Association 1999). There are a number of validation processes, the most common of which are content, criterion and construct validation.

Content validation is a fundamental step in developing new, high-quality instruments, and refers to the extent to which an instrument contains the relevant and important aspects of the concept it intends to measure (Rothman et al. 2009). A panel of experts (both lay and professional) on the content of interest is assembled and the items are judged by these experts for their relevance and clarity in representing the concept underlying a measure (Waltz et al. 2010).

Criterion validation involves determining the relationship between an instrument and some criterion or 'gold standard' (Polit and Beck 2004; DeVellis 2012). Once a criterion is selected, a correlation coefficient is computed between scores on the instrument and the criterion. The magnitude of the coefficient is a direct estimate of how valid the instrument is according to this validation method. Validation by means of the criterion-related approach in health care research can be difficult given the lack of 'gold-standard' criteria for social and psychological variables.

Construct validation is concerned with the theoretical underpinnings of a construct and seeks to determine the extent to which the instrument measures the abstract concept of interest (Polit and Beck 2004). Establishing construct validity is a challenging and ongoing developmental task that requires the gradual accumulation of evidence which illustrates that the instrument scores relate to observable behaviours in the ways that were predicted by the guiding theoretical framework and hypotheses generated by developers (DeVellis 2012). Common methods to obtain construct-related validity data include examining the logical relations that should exist with other measures and/or patterns of scores for groups known to differ on relevant variables, and factor analyses (exploratory and confirmatory) which can determine the underlying structure of an instrument when little is known or to test hypotheses in the theoretical structure. Chapter 16 provides further in-depth detail about the different types of validity and reliability tests that are available to researchers and how they should be used in health care research.

Psychometrics, while complex, is essential for determining the credibility of data collected from instruments used in research and practice. Depending on data quality, this in turn can influence decision making in relation to patient care as well as health and social policy (Hobart and Cano 2009).

Methodological considerations for measurement

Methodological decisions about item-generation techniques, scaling/scoring procedures, instrument administration methods and respondent burden require careful deliberation for the development of accurate and robust measurement.

Item generation

Successful item generation can only take place if the developers have a thorough familiarity with the relevant work in the area of study (Pollard et al. 2007). Optimal item generation therefore entails gathering information from a *number* of different sources (Shikiar and Rentz 2004). Appropriate methods include literature reviews (including instrument appraisals), patient interviews and expert panels. In particular, patient elicitation techniques (for instance, focus groups, structured interviews, open interviews) are essential to the development of an initial item list. Such an approach to item generation aids researchers in identifying the salient aspects of the variable in question from patients' perspectives, which in turn helps in the refinement of the guiding theoretical framework and lends enhanced credibility and content validity to measurements (de Vaus 2002; Frost et al. 2007).

Scaling and scoring

For decisions on instrument scaling and scoring, a range of procedures are available to developers, with the final choice being determined by the intended use of the instrument and the nature of the variable being measured (Turner et al. 2007; DeVellis 2012). Standard scaling procedures exist, and are a theoretically sound method of developing and scoring measures by applying a standard approach to attributing numerical values to item responses (Pollard et al. 2007). Such scaling procedures begin by collecting a large number of items, and then use prescribed methods to reduce the number of items, attach a response format, and score the final scale (Pollard et al. 2007). The most common standard scaling procedures in health care instruments are based on assumptions from classical measurement theory, which have been derived from the scaling of attitudes (Thurstone 1929; Likert 1932; Guttman 1944). These methods ensure that the scoring, scaling and response format for items are consistent. For example, Likert scaling is widely used in instruments measuring beliefs, opinions and attitudes in diverse health and social care applications (DeVellis 2012). In a Likert scale, the item is presented as a declarative statement followed by response options that indicate varying degrees of agreement or disagreement. When the Likert scaling technique is used, *all* items should conform to Likert response formats and use an additive scoring method – that is, the scores on the items are either summed or averaged to yield an individual score for each participant.

When making a decision as to the best scaling procedure to opt for, scale variability and the respondent's ability to discriminate response options meaningfully are two important considerations (DeVellis 2012). Scale variability is significant because if a scale fails to discriminate differences in the underlying attribute, its correlations with other measures will be restricted and its utility therefore limited (Streiner and Norman 2008; DeVellis 2012). In terms of response discrimination, fewer response categories can result in a loss of discrimination, while a larger number of categories can result in respondent fatigue, frustration and confusion. Furthermore, an even number (e.g. four) response option format forces a respondent to make a commitment in terms of agreeing or disagreeing with a declarative statement, whereas an odd number (e.g. five) response option format allows equivocation (e.g. 'neither agree nor disagree') or uncertainty (e.g. 'not sure'). Neither response format is considered to be superior, and decisions regarding this choice are influenced by the purpose and content of the scale. Developers also need to consider the quality and ordering of the response options and ensure that there is as little ambiguity as possible in both the language and spatial arrangement of the response descriptors (DeVellis 2012).

Administration

A further methodological issue requiring attention by developers relates to how the instrument will be administered. Depending on the method chosen, whether it be face-to-face interview, telephone, mail or computer-assisted, this can impact on the type of question that can be asked, and therefore how effectively it can be answered (Streiner and Norman 2008). Each method has distinct advantages and disadvantages, and to make an informed decision as to the most appropriate administration mode judicious consideration must be given to the target population, the situation (home or outpatient department) of administration, the resources required (e.g. computer software, administrator training) and, most important of all, respondent burden (Scientific Advisory Committee of the Medical Outcomes Trust 2002).

Respondent burden

Respondent burden is a fundamental issue in instrument development which is often overlooked by developers, to their detriment. Respondent burden can be defined as the time, effort and other demands placed on those to whom the instrument is administered (Scientific Advisory Committee of the Medical Outcomes Trust 2002). Three main issues must be taken into account: 1) length of time needed by patients to complete the instrument; 2) ease of response in terms of the reading and comprehension level required; and 3) patient acceptability in relation to whether the instrument 'makes sense' in terms of what information is sought. In addition, acceptability also encompasses whether or not completion of the measure places respondents under undue physical or emotional strain (Pollard et al. 2007). From a common sense perspective, reducing respondent burden enhances patient comfort and convenience, which in turn can increase participation rates and reduce levels of missing data. Pretesting the instrument and conducting a pilot study are therefore essential steps to take in the development process to ensure respondent burden is kept to a minimum.

Practicalities of using instruments

In addition to addressing questions about theoretical, psychometric and methodological issues concerning measurement instruments, there are also practicality questions to be addressed. The following questions posed by Kimberlin and Winterstein (2008: 2280, 2282) are useful in thinking about practicalities:

- Is the instrument in the public domain?
- How expensive is it to use the instrument?
- How will the instrument be administered?
- Will the instrument be acceptable to subjects?

If an instrument is available in the public domain (for instance, published in the literature, available on the web), it is necessary to note whether permission from the author and publisher is needed to use it in your study. Permission from the author will certainly be needed if the instrument is not in the public domain. The instrument may also be copyrighted, in which case you may be required to pay a fee to use it. Additional fees may be required for scoring the instrument (Kimberlin and Winterstein 2008). In relation to copyright, Jacobson (2004) advises that researchers should never use an instrument if permission from the original author or legal designee cannot be obtained. For instruments assumed to be in the public domain, these should only be used in cases where a notice concerning public availability is clearly evident in the instrument or related article (Jacobson 2004).

Undoubtedly, there will be costs associated with using instruments (apart from purchasing the instrument, if required). Sample size will have cost implications: the larger the size, the more copies of the instrument will be needed. Administering instruments over the telephone or in face-to-face interviews will be more costly than mail administration (Kimberlin and Winterstein 2008). For ease of administration, consideration may be given to administering instruments by web surveys. For example, *SurveyMonkey* offers various plans ranging from 'Basic', with limited design features (e.g. permits only a small number of questions and respondents), through to 'Platinum', which contains more sophisticated design features. The Basic design plan is free, whereas the cost of other plans increases with greater sophistication in terms of features available. From the outset, the costs of using instruments need to be factored into the overall costs of conducting a study. There is a range of options available for administering instruments, for example telephone interviews, face to face, mail and online. The pragmatics of instrument administration have direct methodological implications because, as noted in the previous section, decisions about which method to use are often linked to considerations around maximizing response rates, obtaining quality, and obtaining complete datasets. Therefore it is important to reiterate that you should always keep in mind that the method of administering an instrument is critical to any study, because it influences the number, length and quality of responses.

An instrument should be acceptable to potential respondents. For this, Kimberlin and Winterstein (2008) draw attention to the reading level required of potential respondents to complete the instrument. Additional considerations include the level of burden imposed on potential respondents in terms of the amount of time it is likely to take to complete the instrument, as well as how complex it might be to complete.

Review of measurement instruments

In this section two measures are examined to illustrate an example of instrument development (Beliefs about Medication Compliance Scale) and the use of an instrument across a range of health-related quality of life studies (Short Form 36 Health Survey).

Example 1 Beliefs about Medication Compliance Scale (BMCS) (Bennett et al. 1997)

Scale description

Bennett et al. (1997) developed a 12-item, five-point Likert scaled (1 = *strongly disagree*, 5 = *strongly agree*), cardiac-specific instrument, the purpose of which is to measure beliefs about medication compliance in patients with heart failure. The items are focused on diuretic therapy compliance because the side effects of diuretic therapy are commonly reported by patients as problematic and interfering with daily living (Bennett et al. 2005). On the original scale, six items assess perceived benefits of medication compliance and six items assess barriers to medication compliance. A 'benefits' score and 'barriers' score are obtained by summing the responses to the items on each subscale. Higher scores on the benefits subscale indicate more perceptions of benefits, whereas higher scores on the barriers subscale indicate a greater number of perceived barriers.

Conceptual, psychometric and methodological considerations

The items for the BMCS were influenced by the 'benefits' and 'barriers' constructs in the Health Belief Model. In addition, a literature review of past studies of perceived benefits and barriers in this population of patients was performed, and data from six interviews with patients diagnosed with heart failure were used for item generation. Content validity of the scale was conducted with two nurses with expertise in caring for patients with heart failure. The experts were requested to review items for clarity and consistency in line with the conceptual definitions of perceived benefits and barriers. The content validity index was 0.81, which was determined to be an acceptable level of agreement. Initial confirmatory factor analysis with a sample of 98 patients demonstrated tentative support for construct validity of the BMCS, which yielded the predicted two subscales, interpretable as perceived benefits and barriers to compliance with medications, especially diuretics. Both subscales demonstrated acceptable internal consistencies, which were estimated by Cronbach's alpha (0.87 (benefits) 0.91 (barriers)). Test–retest reliability estimates were not reported during initial testing. A further validation study was reported by Bennett et al. (2001) with a larger (n = 196) and more heterogeneous sample of patients diagnosed with heart failure. Again, confirmatory factor analysis provided tentative support for the original two-factor structure, with the benefits and barriers subscales explaining 43 per cent and 41 per cent of the total variance in the factor analysis. Internal consistency estimates in this study ranged from 0.63 to 0.71 for the benefits subscale and 0.65 to 0.71 for the barriers subscale. Some of the reliability estimates were lower than 0.70, which the developers attributed to the heterogeneous nature of the items, the patients' illness level, the literacy level of patients, or the relatively low numbers of items on the scales (Bennett et al. 1997, 2001). In terms of test–retest reliability, estimated intraclass correlation coefficients were calculated. The intraclass correlation coefficients of the benefits scale for baseline to time point 1 (8 weeks) and time point 2 (52 weeks) ranged from 0.23 to 0.47 respectively. For the barriers subscale the intraclass correlation coefficients were all greater than 0.40. While other researchers have also used the instrument in this population (van der Wal et al. 2006, 2007), further psychometric information was not reported.

In relation to methodological considerations, information regarding the time it would take for patients to complete the scale was not reported. However, all items are short and concise, ensuring a minimum burden for respondents. The reading level of the BMCS is grade six, which is considered acceptable reading levels for self-administered instruments.

Scale appraisal and research application

The instrument development process can be commended in terms of its use of a theoretical framework, patient input, disease specificity and patient acceptability. Initial and follow-on psychometric validation of the scale, while promising, requires continued systematic testing. Overall, the instrument is of value to researchers and health care professionals working with patients on diuretic therapy for the treatment of heart failure.

Example 2   Quality of life – Short Form 36 Health Survey (SF-36)

Quality of life (QOL), particularly health-related quality of life (HRQOL), is one of the most measured concepts in health care research. Yet the concept of QOL is continuously debated in the literature, with little consensus on a gold standard for measurement methodology (Varrichio 2006). Among the challenges of measurement are that QOL remains conceptually ill-defined and multiple measurement instruments exist, potentially leading to confusion about which one to choose. Conceptual and methodological debates concerning QOL measurement can be read elsewhere (Moons et al. 2006; Varrichio 2006), and although not addressed in detail here, some issues around QOL measurement are considered when examining the SF-36 health survey instrument.

Description of SF-36

The SF-36 was originally developed over 20 years ago as a measure of health status, assessing functional status and well-being. It comprises 36 items across eight subscales of health states, which are: physical functioning; role limitations due to physical problems; social functioning; bodily pain; general mental health; role limitations due to emotional problems; vitality; general health perceptions. In addition, the SF-36 measures health transition using a single item. Two summary scores can also be gleaned from the SF-36: the physical component summary (PCS) and the mental component summary (MCS). The scores range between 0 and 100, with lower scores representing poorer health status. The scale can be administered by a trained interviewer by telephone, or can be self-administered (Ware and Sherbourne 1992). Drawing on population studies, the SF-36 is reported to be psychometrically reliable and valid, and able to detect differences between groups in terms of age (over 14 years), gender, socio-economic status, and clinical condition (Hemingway et al. 1997; Failde and Ramos 2000; Khader et al. 2011). Detailed accounts of the history and development of the SF-36, evaluations of its psychometric properties, and its revised version (SF-36v2) can be found elsewhere (Ware and Sherbourne 1992; McHorney et al. 1993; Ware et al. 1993, 2000).

Application of SF-36 in previous research

Although originally developed as a measure of health status, the SF-36[1] is now one of the most widely used generic (that is, not disease-specific) measures of HRQOL in health care research, and has been translated for use in over 50 countries (Contopoulos-Ioannidis et al. 2009). Drawing on our earlier emphasis on the need to use theoretically based measures, the SF-36 may be considered a conceptual fit for a study on HRQOL if this construct is defined broadly in terms of functional abilities, mental health status and personal sense of general well-being. This broad definition of HRQOL has been conceptualized in the contexts of 'normal life' roles and abilities (Moons et al. 2006), or 'achievements' (Dijkers 2005). This contrasts with other conceptualizations of QOL such as 'satisfaction with life' in terms of enjoyment and contentment with life, or 'utility' in terms of preferences for particular health states (Moons et al. 2006). Therefore, the SF-36 would not be conceptually suitable for a study aiming to measure HRQOL in terms of satisfaction with health status or preferences for health states. In using the SF-36 to study HRQOL, few researchers have made explicit their theoretical underpinnings, although it can be gleaned from studies that this measure is commonly used to establish functioning status and general well-being as a consequence of disease (for example, Picavet and Hoeymans 2004; Puhan et al. 2008; van der Heijde et al. 2009).

With regard to reporting on the psychometric properties (reliability and validity) of the SF-36 to measure HRQOL across a range of illnesses or populations, researchers tend to report mostly on reliability with reference to internal consistency (freedom from random error) of the subscales. Although the internal consistency (estimated with Cronbach α coefficient) of the SF-36 subscales is commonly reported to be good, scores can vary across studies. For example, in a Swiss population with asthma, Puhan et al. (2008) found the internal consistency for all its subscales to exceed 0.70, which has not been the case for a Dutch (Picavet and Hoeymans 2004) or Thai (Lim et al. 2008) version of the SF-36, which yielded scores of 0.67 and 0.55 respectively for the social functioning subscale. A coefficient score of 0.70 is recommended to deem a scale reliable (de Vaus 2002). With reference to various translations of the SF-36, Lim et al. (2008) noted difficulties associated with translating items on the social functioning subscale of the SF-36 because of cultural differences regarding this concept.

With regard to validity, it is important to keep in mind that instruments considered valid in one study situation may not be valid in another situation. The tendency by some researchers to use previously published data on the SF-36 as an indication of validity is inappropriate because, as noted by Picavet and Hoeymans (2004), population means vary by country, culture and language, thereby reducing the validity of international comparisons. The validity of the SF-36 for use in some populations has also been questioned. For example, Fitzpatrick (2007) noted that the SF-36 is an inappropriate measure for use in

---

[1]A newer version of the SF-36, the SF-36v2, was published in 1996, reflecting refinements in item wording and format, and an increase in the range of scores covered. Although the title SF-36 was used in all studies reviewed for this chapter, it is likely that the revised SF-36v2 survey was actually used, since the original version is no longer available for purchase.

older adults because their principal concerns may not correspond with the SF-36 emphasis on functional activities. It is also now increasingly common for researchers to use disease-specific HRQOL measures in conjunction with generic measures such as SF-36 because disease-specific scales are considered more sensitive to assessing changes in a given population than in a general population (Corica et al. 2006). However, this may not always be the case, as shown by Puhan et al. (2008), who compared the validity of a disease-specific and generic HRQOL measure in people with asthma from the general population. Both instruments were found to have good internal consistency and the SF-36 showed better discrimination between different aspects of HRQOL. The researchers concluded that the SF-36 may be a more valid measure of HRQOL than the disease-specific measure when applied to people with asthma from the general population.

The SF-36 measures HRQOL using Likert scaling, which as noted earlier is the type of scale widely used to measure beliefs and attitudes. It is relatively quick to complete, taking approximately ten minutes. Respondent fatigue is therefore unlikely. In this regard the instrument is likely to be acceptable to potential respondents, which in turn has implications for increasing response rates and decreasing the amount of missing data. Evidence from a range of HRQOL studies involving the SF-36 suggest that as little as 3 per cent of data are missing, and this is only for some items on the scale (see, for example, Lim et al. 2008; Puhan et al. 2008). As previously noted, the acceptability of a measure also concerns physical or emotional issues associated with its completion. Dijkers (2005) draws attention to the potential of the SF-36 to be insulting to individuals with spinal injury, with specific reference to one question on this instrument: 'Does your health now limit you in . . . walking more than a mile?' Dijkers noted that some researchers have replaced the word 'walking' with 'going', and while this change in terminology is less offensive to individuals with spinal injury who cannot walk, this modification to the instrument changes the conceptual basis of the SF-36 and destroys comparability with data for the population at large.

The SF-36 survey can be administered in paper, electronic and web formats. The instrument can be purchased from QualityMetric Incorporated (http://www.qualitymetric.com), which is a company based in the USA that provides health status and outcome measurement products and services to researchers, and academic and health care organizations. Details about obtaining a licence to use the SF-36 are available at http://www.sf-36.org/wantsf.aspx. The user manual for the instrument is also available. Information on costs associated with purchasing a licence to use the SF-36 and the manual are not readily available on the QualityMetric website; however, a Survey Information Request Form is available for this purpose.

Conclusion

In this chapter, the importance of measurement in using questionnaires and instruments for health care research was addressed. The need for accurate measurement of health care concepts was highlighted. Anything less hinders data confidence, leading to ambiguous research findings and conclusions. However, accurate measurement of health care concepts is complex, requiring careful consideration of conceptual, methodological and psychometric issues. Developing a new instrument for your research may be necessary if no suitable measure already exists. However, it is always advisable to source an instrument that has already been developed to measure your research area of interest, which could be modified if necessary, provided that the fundamental principles of measurement are adhered to. We hope that the conceptual, psychometric and methodological issues discussed in this chapter will provide an insight into the depth of knowledge and dedication required for developing a research instrument. It is a demanding process, but one that can be rewarding if conducted in a rigorous manner.

Key concepts

- Measurement in health care research involves accurate quantification of the phenomenon under study.
- Although various types of research instruments exist (e.g. questionnaires, checklists, inventories), it is the inclusion of rating scales that is important for measuring theoretical or conceptual variables.
- Theory makes an important contribution to measurement because it helps to operationalize abstract concepts into concrete groups of items representing various dimensions of the concept being studied.
- The psychometric properties (reliability and validity) of measurement must be viewed as falling along a continuum rather than as a dichotomous index.
- Methodological decisions about item generation technique, scaling/scoring procedures, instrument administration methods, and respondent burden require careful deliberation for the development of accurate and robust measurement.

Key readings on measurement instruments for health care research

- R. DeVellis, *Scale Development: Theory and Applications*, 3rd edn (London: Sage, 2012)
  This textbook provides a concise, step-by-step guide to developing a health and social science measure.
- C. Waltz, O. Strickland and E. Lenz, *Measurement in Nursing and Health Research*, 4th edn (New York: Springer Publishing Company, 2010)
  An excellent resource for a comprehensive understanding of conceptual, methodological and psychometric considerations in developing measurements relevant to health care research.
- J. Hobart and S. Cano, Improving the evaluation of therapeutic intervention in multiple sclerosis: The role of new psychometric methods, *Health Technology Assessment*, 13(12) (2009), 1–200
  A detailed monograph which provides a contemporary account of methodological debates concerning psychometric approaches to health measurement.
- R. Turner, A. Quittner, B. Parasuraman, J. Kallich and C. Cleeland, Patient-reported outcomes: Instrument development and selection issues, *Value in Health*, 10(Supp. 2) (2007), S86–93
  A straightforward but thorough review paper that focuses on instrument development and selection issues which require consideration by health care practitioners and researchers.

Examples of the use of questionnaires and instruments in health care research

The following papers provide examples of issues relevant to the use of measurement instruments in health care research.

- Y. Achhab, C. Nejjari, M. Chickri and B. Lyoussi, Disease-specific health-related quality of life instruments among adults diabetic: A systematic review, *Diabetes Research and Clinical Practice*, 80(2) (2008), 171–84
- C. Barnes and E. Adamson-Macedo, Perceived Maternal Parenting Self-Efficacy (PMP S-E) tool: Development and validation with mothers of hospitalized preterm neonates, *Journal of Advanced Nursing*, 60(5) (2007), 550–60
- C. Garcia, Conceptualization and measurement of coping during adolescence: A review of the literature, *Journal of Nursing Scholarship*, 42(2) (2010), 166–85
- J. Rolley, P. Davidson, A. Ong, B. Everett and Y. Salamanson, Medication adherence self-report instruments: Implications for practice and research, *Journal of Cardiovascular Nursing*, 23(6) (2008), 497–505

Useful websites

- HaPI: Health and Psychosocial Instruments – http://www.ebscohost.com/academic/health-and-psychosocial-instruments-hapi
  The HaPI database identifies measurement tools relevant for investigations and explorations in the fields of medicine, nursing, public health, psychology, social work, communication, sociology, and organizational behaviour/human resources. HaPI is available through personal or university subscriptions, from Ovid Technologies or EBSCOhost.
- PROMs: Patient Reported Outcomes Measurement Group, Oxford University – http://phi.uhce.ox.ac.uk/
  The resources, which include a bibliographic database on patient-reported outcome measures, systematic reviews of PROMS relevant to specific diseases and populations, and links to related websites, are available free on this website.

References

American Educational Research Association APA, National Research Council on Measurement in Education (1999) *Standards for Educational and Psychological Testing*. Washington, DC: AERA.

Bennett, S.J., Milgrom, L.B., Champion, V. and Huster, G.A. (1997) Beliefs about medication and dietary compliance in people with heart failure: An instrument development study, *Heart and Lung*, 26(4): 273–9.

Bennett, S.J., Perkins, S.M., Lane, K.A., Forthofer, M.A., Brater, D.C. and Murray, M.D. (2001) Reliability and validity of the compliance belief scales among patients with heart failure, *Heart and Lung*, 30(3): 177–85.

Bennett, S.J., Lane, K.A., Welch, J., Perkins, S.M., Brater, D.C. and Murray, M.D. (2005) Medication and dietary compliance beliefs in heart failure, *Western Journal of Nursing Research*, 27(8): 977–93.

Cano, S. and Hobart, J. (2011) The problem with health measurement, *Patient Preference and Adherence*, 5: 279–90.

Contopoulos-Ioannidis, D.G., Karvouni, A., Kouri, I. and Ioannidis, J.P.A. (2009) Reporting and interpretation of SF-36 outcomes in randomised trials: Systematic review, *British Medical Journal*, 338(a3006), doi:10.1136/bmj.a3006.

Corica, F., Corsonello, A., Apolone, G., Lucchetti, M., Melchiolda, N., Marchesini, G. and Quo-vadis Study Group (2006) Construct validity of the Short Form-36 health survey and its relationship with BMI in obese outpatients, *Obesity*, 14(8): 1429–37.

de Vaus, D. (2002) *Surveys in Social Research*, 5th edn. New South Wales, Australia: Allen & Unwin.

DeVellis, R. (2012) *Scale Development: Theory and Applications*, 3rd edn. London: Sage.

Dijkers, M. P. (2005) Quality of life of individuals with spinal cord injury: A review of conceptualization, measurement, and research findings, *Journal of Rehabilitation Research & Development*, 42(3): 87–110.

Dunbar-Jacob, J. and Mortimer-Stephens, M.K. (2001) Treatment adherence in chronic disease, *Journal of Clinical Epidemiology*, 54(Supp. 1): S57–60.

Failde, I. and Ramos, I. (2000) Validity and reliability of the SF-36 health survey questionnaire in patients with coronary artery disease, *Journal of Clinical Epidemiology*, 53(4): 359–65.

Feldman-Stewart, D. and Brundage, A. (2009) A conceptual framework for patient–provider communication: A tool in the PRO research tool box, *Quality of Life Research*, 18(1): 109–14.

Fitzpatrick, R. (2007) Measurement issues in health-related quality of life: Challenges for health psychology, *Psychology & Health*, 15(1): 99–108.

Frost, M.H., Reeve, B.B., Liepa, A.M., Stauffer, J.W., Hays, R.D. and Mayo/FDA Patient-Reported Outcomes Consensus Meeting Group (2007) What is sufficient evidence for the reliability and validity of patient-reported outcome measures?, *Value in Health*, 10(Supp. 2): S94–105.

Guttman, L. (1944) A basis for scaling qualitative data, *American Sociological Review*, 9(2): 139–50.

Hemingway, H., Stafford, M., Stansfeld, S., Shipley, M. and Marmot, M. (1997) Is the SF-36 a valid measure of change in population health? Results from Whitehall II study, *British Medical Journal*, 315(7118): 1273–9.

Hobart, J. and Cano, S. (2009) Improving the evaluation of therapeutic intervention in multiple sclerosis: The role of new psychometric methods, *Health Technology Assessment*, 13(12): 1–200.

Jacobson, S. (2004) Evaluating instruments for use in clinical nursing research, in M. Frank-Stromborg and S.J. Olsen (eds) *Instruments for Use in Clinical Health-Care Research*. London: Jones & Bartlett International, pp. 3–19.

Johnson, M.J. (2002) The Medication Adherence Model: A guide for assessing medication taking, *Research and Theory for Nursing Practice*, 16(3): 179–92.

Khader, S., Hourani, L. and Al-Akour, N. (2011) Normative data and psychometric properties of Short Form 36 Health Survey (SF-36, version 1.0) in the population of north Jordan, *Eastern Mediterranean Health Journal*, 17(5): 368–74.

Kimberlin, C.L. and Winterstein, A. G. (2008) Validity and reliability of measurements instruments used in research, *American Journal of Health System Pharmacists*, 65(23): 2276–84.

Likert, R. (1932) *A Technique for the Measurement of Attitudes (Archives of Psychology)*. New York: Columbia University.

Lim, L.-Y., Seubsman, S. and Sleigh, A. (2008) Thai SF-36 health survey: Tests of data quality, scaling assumptions, reliability and validity in healthy men and women, *Health and Quality of Life Outcome*, 6(52), doi:10.1186/1477-7525-6-52.

McDowell, I. (2006) *Measuring Health: A Guide to Rating Scales and Questionnaires*. 3rd edn. Oxford: Oxford University Press.

McHorney, C., Ware, J.E. and Raczek, A.E. (1993) The MOS 36-item short-form health survey (SF-36®): II. Psychometric and clinical tests of validity in measuring physical and mental health constructs, *Medical Care*, 31(3): 247–63.

Moons, P., Budts, W. and De Geest, S. (2006) Critique on the conceptualisation of quality of life: A review and evaluation of different conceptual approaches, *International Journal of Nursing Studies*, 43(7): 891–901.

Picavet, H.S.J. and Hoeymans, N. (2004) Health related quality of life in multiple musculoskeletal diseases: DF-36 and EQ-5D in the DMC3 study, *Annals of the Rheumatic Diseases*, 63(6): 723–9.

Polit, D. and Beck, C. (2004) *Nursing Research: Principles and Methods*. Philadelphia: Lippincott Williams & Wilkins.

Pollard, B., Johnston, M. and Dixon, D. (2007) Theoretical framework and methodological development of common subjective health outcome measures in osteoarthritis: A critical review, *Health and Quality of Life Outcomes*, 5(14), doi:10.1186/1477-7525-5-14.

Prior, M., Hamzah, J., Francis, J., Ramsay, C., Castillo, M., Campbell, S., Azuara-Blanco, A. and Burr, J. (2011) Pre-validation methods for developing a patient reported outcome instrument, *BMC Medical Research Methodology*, 11(112), doi:10.1186/1471-2288-11-112.

Puhan, M.A., Gaspoz, J.M., Bridevaux, P.O., Schindler, C., Ackermann-Liebrich, U., Rochat, T. and Gerbase, M.W. (2008) Comparing a disease-specific and a generic health-related quality of life instrument in subjects with asthma from the general population, *Health and Quality of Life Outcomes*, 6(15), doi:10.1186/1477-7525-6-15.

Raykov, T. and Marcoulides, G. (2011) *An Introduction to Psychometric Theory*. New York: Routledge Academic.

Rothman, M., Beltran, P., Cappelleri, J., Lipscomb, J. and Teschendorf, B. (2007) Patient-reported outcomes: Conceptual issues, *Value in Health*, 10(Supp. 2): S66–75.

Rothman, M., Burke, L., Erickson, P., Kline Leidy, N., Patrick, D. and Petrie, C. (2009) Use of existing patient-reported outcome (PRO) instruments and their modification: The ISPOR good research practices for evaluating and documenting content validity for the use of existing instruments and their modification – PRO Task Force report, *Value in Health*, 12(8): 1075–83.

Scientific Advisory Committee of the Medical Outcomes Trust (2002) Assessing health status and quality-of life instruments: Attributes and review criteria, *Quality of Life Research*, 11(3): 193–205.

Shikiar, R. and Rentz, A.M. (2004) Satisfaction with medication: An overview of conceptual, methodologic, and regulatory issues, *Value in Health*, 7(2): 204–15.

Streiner, D. and Norman, G. (2008) *Health Measurement Scales: A Practical Guide to Their Development and Use*, 4th edn. Oxford: Oxford University Press.

Thurstone, L.L. (1929) The measurement of psychological value, in T. Smith and W. Wright (eds) *Essays in Philosophy by Seventeen Doctors of Philosophy of the University of Chicago*. Chicago: Open Court, pp. 157–74.

Turner, R., Quittner, A., Parasuraman, B., Kallich, J. and Cleeland, C. (2007) Patient-reported outcomes: Instrument development and selection issues, *Value in Health*, 10(Supp. 2): S86–93.

Valderas, J., Ferrer, M., Mendívil, J., Garin, O., Rajmil, L., Herdman, M. and Alonso, J. (2008) Development of EMPRO: A tool for the standardized assessment of patient-reported outcome measures, *Value in Health*, 11(4): 700–8.

van der Heijde, D.M., Revicki, D.A., Gooch, K.L., Wong, R.L., Kupper, H., Harnam, N., Thompson, C. and Sieper, J. (2009) Physical function, disease activity, and health-related quality-of-life outcomes after 3 years of adalimumab treatment in patients with ankylosing spondylitis, *Arthritis Research and Therapy*, 11(4), doi:10.1186/ar2790.

van der Wal, M.H., Jaarsma, T., Moser, D.K., Veeger, N.J., van Gilst, W.H. and Van Veldhuisen, D.J. (2006) Compliance in heart failure patients: The importance of knowledge and beliefs, *European Heart Journal*, 27(4): 434–40.

van der Wal, M. H., Jaarsma, T., Moser, D.K., van Gilst, W.H. and van Veldhuisen, D.J. (2007) Unraveling the mechanisms for heart failure patients' beliefs about compliance, *Heart and Lung*, 36(4): 253–61.

Varricchio, C.G. (2006) Measurement issues in quality-of-life assessments, *Oncology Nursing Forum*, 33(Supp. 1): 13021.

Waltz, C., Strickland, O. and Lenz, E. (2010) *Measurement in Nursing and Health Research*, 4th edn. New York: Springer Publishing Company.

Ware, J.E. and Sherbourne, C.D. (1992) The MOS 36-item short-form health survey (SF-36), *Medical Care*, 30(6): 473–83.

Ware, J.E., Snow, K.K., Kosinski, M. and Gandek, B. (1993) *SF-36® Health Survey Manual and Interpretation Guide*. Boston, MA: New England Medical Center, The Health Institute.

Ware, J.E., Kosinski, M. and Dewey, J.E. (2000) *How to Score Version Two of the SF-36 Health Survey*. Lincoln, RI: QualityMetric.

16   Issues and debates in validity and reliability

Roger Watson

Introduction

The purpose of this chapter is to explore issues around the reliability and validity of measures used in health care; these measures could be clinical, educational or for research. Broadly speaking, this chapter is concerned with psychometrics and I will begin by exploring what psychometrics is about and why it applies directly to the issues of measurement in nursing. This is followed by a discussion of the concept of measurement and why it is fundamental to understanding psychometrics. Various definitions and types of reliability are discussed; in addition, methods used in research to ascertain the reliability and validity of instruments are also outlined. The chapter concludes with a brief discussion of other approaches used in the testing of instruments, including sensitivity, specificity, receiver operating characteristics and item response theory.

Psychometrics

Psychometrics is concerned with theories and practices in measuring psychological parameters; it has its roots, as the name suggest, in psychology but is widely applied in the social sciences. Psychologists are concerned with measuring things that are in the mind and these include mental ability, personality and memory as well as psychologically distressing phenomena such as depression, anxiety and stress. We all have a working knowledge of these issues and some understanding that they can be measured. However, unlike the entities that we measure – or more often estimate – on a daily basis (height, weight, distance and volume), we cannot see, feel or visualize psychological phenomena. In other words, they are hidden from us and therefore are referred to as being 'latent'.

A simple example of the application of psychometrics is the measurement of mental ability. We know mental ability differs between individuals; the reasons are open to debate involving, as they do, elements of both nature (genetics) and nurture (environment) and they also involve circumstances. However, at school, for the person within the normal range of mental ability – and that describes the majority of us within one standard deviation of the mean for mental ability – there were always, consistently, those who outperformed us and those who underperformed us. We saw this in common tests and examinations. We were not able to visualize an entity called mental ability (we often called it 'brains', 'cleverness', 'smartness' etc.) but we knew it was there – it was latent, but made manifest (no longer hidden) by virtue of performance. Taking this a step forward into psychology, there are a great many tests and questionnaires that have been developed specifically to measure mental ability in a more abstract way – often referred to as 'IQ' (intelligence quotient) tests – so our everyday example has a direct psychometric equivalent as psychologists strive to explain what mental ability is and why it differs between people.

Measurement

The concept of measurement has been referred to several times above and it is clearly fundamental to psychometrics; in fact, psychometrics and measurement are virtually synonymous. However, psychometrics refers exclusively to latent traits whereas measurement is more general, including the measurement of physical entities and ascribing a value, such as metres, kilograms or litres, to them. According to one theory of measurement (Stevens 1946; Watson et al. 2005), measurement is made on four different scales: nominal, ordinal, interval and ratio. Nominal measurement is merely labelling, e.g. 'male' or 'female', and not really measurement. Ordinal measurement merely ascribes order to entities: for example, a group of three people could be ordered on the basis of height, e.g. smallest, medium and tallest. With ordinal measures the distance between the points on the scale are not equal, unlike interval and ratio measures.

Interval and ratio measures are more familiar to us. For example, height and weight are ratio level measures and are described as such because they have a genuine zero point. On the other hand, interval level measures have arbitrary zero points – a classic example is the measurement of temperature in either Celsius or Fahrenheit. Clearly, interval and ratio level measurements are preferable levels of measurement as we can do more with them; they can be added, subtracted and multiplied, for example. However, what is gained in utility with higher-order levels of measurement is achieved at the introduction of measurement error – the difference between the real value and the one you estimate – which ordinal and nominal levels of measurement are less prone to. In psychometrics, the scales we use are often scored at the item level using ordinal level measurement but the aggregated scores on instruments composed of these items are usually treated as interval level measures.

Reliability and validity

The effort to derive instruments to measure latent variables such as quality of life, stress, anxiety, depression and coping lies at the heart of psychometrics and this relies on the concepts of reliability and validity. Reliability and validity are very specific concepts in psychometrics and they will be defined and explained below. It should become self-evident why they are crucial concepts: they are what add meaning and purpose to the measurement instruments we use and, using the example of mental ability, what use would such a test have if it meant nothing and could not be used?

Reliability

Reliability in psychometrics is simply the extent to which something gives the same measurement each time it is used, in other words, how free from error the measure is. For example, if a 10 cm ruler was actually 11 cm long it would be reliable and would give the same measurement each time it was used to measure something. However, the measurement would not be correct. This leads in logically to the definition of validity and an examination of the relationship between reliability and validity.

Validity

Validity refers to the extent to which something measures what it is supposed to measure. Therefore, referring to the case of the ruler above, one that claimed to be 10 cm long but was, in fact, 11 cm would be invalid – it would not be measuring what it was supposed to measure. To be valid, the ruler would have to measure the correct length and that would be obtained from an agreed standard unit of length.

In describing something very obvious to you, such as the necessity for an every-day measure such as length to be measured in agreed units and how you could be misled by something that was not graduated in these units raises two very important points about reliability and validity. First, validity is predicated on reliability; in other words, as you saw above, it is possible for an instrument to be perfectly reliable but to be invalid. Therefore, while reliability is absolutely necessary in measurement, it is insufficient on its own without validity. In other words, for something to be valid it simply has to be reliable and something that is truly valid simply has, logically, to be reliable.

Second was the idea of some agreed external standard whereby validity could be measured. This is relatively easy with physical measures such as length and weight because such agreed external standards do exist; they are kept by government agencies so that weights and measures can be checked periodically and the instruments used to do this are calibrated against the standard measures. However, in the case of psychometrics, which – as explained above – deals with measuring latent phenomena, how is this possible? Where are the standard measures for mental ability, depression and quality of life, for example? How clever does someone have to be to be considered clever? How depressed does someone have to be to be considered depressed, and so on? If reliability and validity are the essence of psychometrics, these questions are the essence of the challenge of psychometrics.

The 'gold standard'

A concept that is referred to often in all fields of measurement, including psychometrics, is the 'gold standard', and this arises from the fact that some currencies used to be compared with an arbitrary amount of the precious metal gold. The idea was that, within a country, the basic unit of currency or some multiple of it would always buy that arbitrary but fixed amount of gold. In this way, the value of the currency could be compared with that standard across the world to see how much it was worth in relative terms. The gold standard in economics was abandoned decades ago, but the idea persists.

With reference to psychometrics, in most cases, when using instruments to measure psychological and even clinical phenomena, there is no 'gold standard' against which to compare the measurements we make with questionnaires and observation schedules. This raises a significant question: how do we ever know that we are measuring something that we cannot see if we have nothing with which to compare it? The answer is not simple, but lies in the array of methods available to psychometricians and it is these methods that will form the bulk of the remainder of this chapter.

Reliability and validity: methodology

How do we take the abstract notions that we often refer to, such as 'patient satis-faction', 'quality of life' and 'self-efficacy', and take them to a point where we can measure them?

Theory

All measurement starts with theory. Whether that theory is inductive or deductive is irrelevant but it is pointless to pursue the measurement of a vague notion without having a clear theoretical perspective of what it is that you are trying to measure. This has to be the first step as it is, ultimately, against this theory and predictions about it that you will be able to gauge the success of your measurement instrument. Theory will also guide the content of the instrument, that is, what you ask in the instrument either directly or by observation.

For example, you may have developed the theory that people have different qual-ities of life, and to explore this theory you decide that you need to measure it. You will have some idea of the things that you think contribute to quality of life, such as security, health, income and friendship, and this will allow you to develop questions around these phenomena. Once you have developed your questionnaire, according to your theory, people who score higher on the items on your questionnaire will have a higher quality of life and vice versa, and you could also predict that people with different levels of quality of life have other characteristics that are related to quality of life such as illness and visits to hospital, availability of work and so on. An example of a theoretical construct that has been used to develop a commonly used instrument in social research is Bandura's (1977) theory of self-efficacy whereby people feel con-fident that they will succeed in certain situations. Self-efficacy was first described by Bandura, who proceeded to develop several self-efficacy scales related to a range of situations such as exercise, eating habits and pain.

In the course of developing a measurement instrument the endeavour may seem to become like an end in itself. However, that should not be the case; the process should begin with a theoretical perspective on some aspect of the human condition and that theory should enable you to develop the instrument and, subsequently, test it.

Operationalization

Operationalization means being able to put abstract ideas into actions that can be specifically enquired about, observed and then rated. This is fundamental to questionnaire design but, in the context of reliability and validity, is no less important as your instrument will only be as reliable and valid as the specific questions you ask.

Therefore, formulating the items for your instrument is important and this is directly related to one form of validity, the content validity, of your instrument. We will return later to looking at formal methods for assessing content validity. The steps involved in arriving at the right set of items begin with establishing the 'nomological network'[1] around the concepts you wish to measure, and this means drawing up a pool of candidate items that could be included and then deciding which ones should be included. There are several ways this can be done but one is by 'brainstorming' the relevant issues – either alone or with a team – to draw up a long list. This process could be done more formally using focus groups, Delphi techniques[2] or nominal group techniques[3] (see Chapter 3) and also using qualitative research methods. There are no rules, as such. It is important, simply, that you try to find as many relevant items as possible but, in the end, include as few items as possible; that is only those items you need and no more. The idea here is to keep the instrument as short and simple as possible. Again, there are no set rules for reducing the items in the instrument down to those that are absolutely necessary, but a group of relevant experts can be used, comprising those who might require the instrument and those with whom it might be used: for example, clinicians and patients. You can draw up a draft of the questionnaire, having made some preliminary decisions about what is important to include, and then ask an expert group to rate each of the items for importance or to spot any redundancy among the questions; redundancy refers to those questions asking essentially the same thing. Sometimes you may want to include similar items to check that people are answering consistently, but those aspects of questionnaire design are beyond the scope of this chapter.

Authenticity and directness

Ultimately, you are trying to achieve an appropriate balance between two antagonistic concepts, which stem from the design of educational tests: 'authenticity' and 'directness' (Messick 1994). Authenticity refers to the extent to which the items in

[1]A nomological network is a representation of the concepts (constructs) of interest in a study, their observable manifestations, and the interrelationships among and between these (http://en.wikipedia.org/wiki/Nomological_network).

[2]The Delphi method is a structured communication technique, originally developed as a systematic, interactive forecasting method (http://en.wikipedia.org/wiki/Forecasting), which relies on a panel of experts (http://en.wikipedia.org/wiki/Delphi_method).

[3]The nominal group technique (NGT) is a decision-making method for use among groups of many sizes, who want to make their decision quickly, as by a vote, but want everyone's opinions taken into account (as opposed to traditional voting, where only the largest group is considered) (http://en.wikipedia.org/wiki/Nominal_group_technique).

your instrument cover all of the concepts you are interested in, and directness means the extent to which the instrument only asks about the concepts in which you are interested. You will be able to see, of course, that – despite the antagonistic nature of these concepts – they are both required and both necessary. It is easier to achieve authenticity by including as many relevant items as possible in the instrument, all of which may be direct. However, as soon as questions become marginal to the issue under investigation then you begin to lose directness. Authenticity is a threat to how completely you investigate the phenomenon of interest and directness threatens the utility of the questionnaire by making it too long and possibly distracting for the respondent. There are no specific formal methods for establishing either of these parameters; largely, it is a matter of judgement but some of the formal methods described below can contribute.

Reliability and validity: methods

It is conventional to consider methods for establishing reliability and validity separately and to consider reliability first. However, despite the predication of validity on reliability, some validity methods precede those for testing reliability and there is a process of iteration between the two. The categorization and description, therefore, of methods for establishing reliability and validity are based on what they aim to do rather than on a hierarchy of these methods. With one exception, all of the methods in this area are statistical and, mainly, they are based on the statistical technique of correlation. While many readers will have at least a rudimentary understanding of correlation I will ensure that all readers have the same understanding by explaining it here in relatively non-mathematical terms.

Correlation

Correlation is a measure of the extent to which two or more variables vary together (Watson et al. 2005). Variables – for example age, distress, mental ability, anxiety – are so called because they can vary or differ between people, across time and under different circumstances. For example, people differ in their age and this variable may be of interest in terms of whether it is related to other variables such as mental ability. Likewise, distress may change under the influence of circumstances or as other variables such as counselling are applied and, again, this could be of interest. This difference in variables is described in statistical terms as 'variance' and this can be calculated mathematically. However, variance is expressed in arbitrary units and, with some further mathematics (dividing variance by the standard deviation), the correlation – which is expressed in units between 0 and 1 that can be understood – is obtained. Correlation can be positive (both variables vary in the same direction), or it can be negative (one variable increases while the other decreases). For example, you could expect a positive correlation between the amount of rainfall and the rate of growth in grass and you could expect a negative correlation between the level of analgesic and a measure of pain. It is noteworthy that correlation does not necessarily mean causation; in other words, it does not tell us the direction of causation or that two variables are necessarily directly linked. For example, while we can be sure, as we understand the biology, that increasing rain leads to more growth in grass and we could be sure that the growth in the grass is not causing the rain to fall, we cannot be sure that some other cause (called a confounder) is not leading to both. Correlation becomes especially difficult to interpret when it comes to measures in social sciences such as correlating social class and mental ability: if we find that people with higher mental ability tend to be in a higher social class then we cannot know if people are more clever as a result of their social circumstances or if they are in a particular social class because they are more clever. However, the correlation and causation argument is not really relevant to the use of correlation in psychometrics as we are not trying to establish causation, merely that a relationship exists between two variables; the relationship between the two variables is, patently, the people using the instrument that you are testing.

Interpretation of correlation

Correlation is the square root of the variance shared between two variables; therefore, the square of the correlation gives the variance. For example, if the correlation between two variables is 0.5 then the variance explained between the variables is 0.25; if the correlation is 0.7 – which is considered good – the variance explained is 0.49, that is less that 50 per cent of the variance. The level of variance considered to be acceptable in psychometric tests is, to some extent, a matter of judgement. As with all statistical tests, it is also possible to test for the probability of a correlation. However, large correlations are usually significant and even small correlations with large samples are usually significant, so some caution and interpretation are required, often with the help of a statistician. As a 'rule of thumb', Pearson's correlations (a measure of a linear relationship between two variables) are usually considered small, medium or large (Table 16.1). In estimating reliability, correlation is used to compare measures made either at the same time by more than one person or at different times by the same people. If a measure is reliable then where more than one person makes measures at the same time then their two sets of measures should correlate; likewise for the same people making the same measure at two times. In estimating validity, correlation is used to compare two or more measures of the same phenomenon, using different instruments. For example, where measures are valid they should correlate with other similar measures.

Note of caution

Before proceeding to describe the actual methods used to investigate reliability and validity it is worth noting that this is not an easy area to study. Researchers, especially

Table 16.1   Effect size, correlation and variance

Size of effect	r	% variance
Small	0.1	1
Medium	0.3	9
Large	0.5	25

PhD students, frequently report confusion over the different methods and this is due to considerable inconsistency in the way the methods are reported in textbooks and, increasingly, on the internet. I will not review the inconsistency that is evident, even on a superficial review of the methods, but instead will try to provide a straightforward division of methods and clear descriptions of what each does and why it is important. From your perspective, as someone learning about research methods and possibly applying them for the first time, what is important is that you understand why you are carrying out a psychometric evaluation of an instrument and what each of the tests you apply actually shows you, regardless of how the test is described or labelled in any of the textbooks you read or websites you visit.

Methods for establishing reliability

A range of methods exist for establishing reliability (Bannigan and Watson 2009) and these can be classified under tests to establish:

- internal consistency
- stability
- equivalence

Internal consistency

Sometimes internal consistency is classified under equivalence methods and is sometimes referred to as a non-repeat method of establishing reliability. Nevertheless, it is significantly different from either of these types of methods and is often considered on its own, as I do here. Internal consistency is the extent to which all of the items in an instrument are correlated or measuring the same phenomenon. However, there are different ways of establishing this and all are based, essentially, on 'split-half' techniques whereby the data are, literally, split in half and the two halves correlated with each other. A dataset can be split in many directions and the most common method is Cronbach's alpha, which is described as the mean of all the split-half methods. As with all correlation-based methods, the value of Cronbach's alpha can range from 0 to 1 with 0 meaning there is no internal consistency (this is very unusual as there is always some correlation between items, some of this occurring by chance) and 1 meaning that there is perfect internal consistency. Values of Cronbach's alpha greater than 0.7 are considered acceptable and values greater than 0.8 are considered to indicate good internal consistency. It is not uncommon to obtain values of Cronbach's alpha exceeding 0.9 and, while this seems like a very good result, it could indicate redundancy in the questionnaire; in other words, all of the items are essentially measuring the same thing. Therefore, fewer questions or even one question may be all that is required. Statistical packages enable the investigator to identify items that are a threat to internal consistency and remove them serially to see if the value of Cronbach's alpha is increased to an acceptable level.

There are detractors from the concept of internal consistency using methods like Cronbach's alpha on the basis that they exaggerate the extent to which reliability in a set of items exists (Schmitt 1996; Sijtsma 2009). Also, Cronbach's alpha is dependent on the number of items in the instrument, with larger numbers of items tending to produce larger values of Cronbach's alpha. Therefore, it is very unusual for instruments with very large numbers of items not to be internally consistent on the basis of Cronbach's alpha, meaning that it requires considerable caution in its interpretation. Cronbach's alpha is often used as an adjunct to factor analysis and this technique will be described later under methods aimed at studying validity.

Stability

Stability methods are used to examine the extent to which a test gives the same measurement on two or more administrations (Bannigan and Watson 2009). The methods used are:

- test–retest
- intra-rater reliability

Test–retest and intra-rater reliability, although related, are different techniques.

Test–retest reliability

Test–retest reliability is a method of establishing reliability in self-administered questionnaires (those that are given to people to complete themselves), and is a general term under which intra-rater reliability – to be described below – is included. However, intra-rater reliability, as the name suggests, is specifically for observational instruments.

The basic method in test–retest reliability is to administer the test to the same group of respondents on two occasions which are separated by enough time to minimize the risk that the respondents will recall their first set of answers but not so long that the respondents have, themselves, changed such that this would alter their responses to the test. In this case, 'test' is simply another word for instrument and belies the origin of this method in educational research. For example, to see if an educational test was reliable it could be administered to a group of students on one occasion and then on another, later, occasion. If the test is unreliable, that is, the responses to it are completely different between the two times, it is not a good measure of the aspect of education that is being studied, and these principles apply to any self-administered instrument. If the test is not reliable from this perspective then it cannot possibly be used to measure the construct of interest and will, by definition, be invalid.

The decision about how long you should leave between tests depends, largely, on the test. For example, in our educational example above, you could administer the test at least a week or maybe a month apart, assuming that the respondents had not undertaken any education specific to the content. In psychology, some traits such as personality and mental ability are relatively stable and there is no need for the test times to be very close. However, when we are measuring states such as depression or rapidly changing clinical states then the times cannot be too long, as the state may have changed spontaneously or under the influence of treatment.

Intra-rater reliability

Intra-rater reliability is a unique case of test–retest reliability applied to rating scales and is specifically designed to test whether the same person, or people, obtain the same rating on two occasions (Bannigan and Watson 2009). For example, this has been applied to a rating scale to assess the feeding difficulty of older people with dementia. As with test–retest, the time between ratings needs to be optimal to prevent a rating being done purely from memory of the previous one and not so far apart that the people being rated have changed. There is no specified period but, as with test–retest, it depends on the phenomenon being rated; often one day is too short and a month is too long in clinical practice but this is just a 'rule of thumb' approach. In rapidly changing situations the time between ratings may need to be quite short, from between less than a day to a few days. The concept of intra-rater reliability is easy enough to grasp but it is, practically, very difficult to carry out. The basic premises are that the same situation must be rated on both occasions; usually this will be the same patient or participant in a research study. In addition, the same people must carry out the rating on both occasions. Again, this is easy to grasp but the practical problems include the loss of participants and also the loss of raters; in clinical practice in the real world, rather than in a tightly controlled research situation, this can be very hard to achieve.

Equivalence

Equivalence investigates the extent to which people agree in their use of an instrument and this can be evaluated by giving the same test to more than one person to use and seeing how much they agree (inter-rater reliability) and also by administering equivalent but alternative forms of an instrument and seeking agreement between them. I will only consider inter-rater reliability as the use of alternative forms of a test is problematic and is also easily confused with concurrent validity which will be discussed below.

Inter-rater reliability

Inter-rater reliability provides insight into how well more than one person (rater) agrees with another or others in the use of a rating instrument (Bannigan and Watson 2009). Clearly, as the name suggests, this kind of reliability only applies to rating scales and not to self-administered tests (where alternative forms could be used). The aim of inter-rater reliability is to obtain instruments that will provide the same measurement regardless of who is using them; clearly, if two people use the same instrument to rate the same situation and obtain different results then – all other things such as appropriate knowledge and training for both people being equal – the instrument cannot be reliable and, thereby, cannot be valid.

Precisely how to conduct inter-rater reliability is not always clear and there are various ways it can be achieved. For example, independent pairs of raters could be asked to rate the same thing (person or situation) using your instrument or they could be asked to rate several people or situations, ideally one per pair of raters. In both of the above situations the two ratings from each pair are compared by correlation. Alternatively, a group of raters could be asked to rate the same thing and all of the possible pairs of ratings in the group could, again, be compared by correlation. Before you set up an inter-rater reliability test you need to set up your protocol very carefully and instruct your raters very clearly. The analysis will depend on how you have designed your test.

Intraclass correlation

As mentioned above, many of the tests used in psychometrics use correlation analysis and, while there is a range of correlation tests available, the recommended methods now are those falling under a group of methods called intraclass correlation (Rankin and Stokes 1998). Intraclass correlation methods are favoured over other forms of correlation (e.g. Pearson's correlation) as they tend to be more flexible, conservative, and take into account different types of correlation graphs. They are flexible in that they can be used for any number of raters rating any number of situations or people, and the order in which the ratings are done is immaterial. They are conservative in that they tend not to overestimate the correlation between raters or ratings and they take into account, for example, if the line of correlation does not pass through the origin – where the x-axis and the y-axis are both zero – of the graph.

There is a range of intraclass correlation models available and intraclass correlation is available in common statistical packages such as SPSS. The tests are described as either one-way or two-way depending on whether the correlation to be calculated is between two or more pairs, respectively, and the model can have fixed or random effects depending on how the test has been set up – but random effects is usually best as this is less restrictive. There seems to be no agreement on what an acceptable level of intraclass correlation is, but one that was not statistically significant would not be acceptable and anything below 0.7 could be considered to be low; again, expert advice may be required in the interpretation of intraclass correlations.

Validity

As with tests of reliability, there is an array of tests of validity, and the distinctions between some of these are quite subtle and often confused. As explained, the literature in the area does not always help as sometimes slightly contradictory definitions are provided. For the purposes of this chapter I am going to consider validity under the following broad headings (DeVon et al. 2007):

- translational validity
- criterion validity

Construct validity

Before proceeding, however, I will consider the concept of construct validity, which refers to the overall concept or construct that you are purporting to measure using your instrument and how much you can generalize from the measurements you make to inferences about the construct in general. Strictly speaking, since the construct you are attempting to measure is latent, construct validity is unattainable; you can never really know how close you are to measuring it even if the instrument you develop gives results very close to a gold standard measure. The gold standard measure will also be an approximation. Some people claim that nothing can be measured or that measuring latent constructs is a waste of time and use the above argument about lack of precision to support their position. However, it is precisely the latent nature of many phenomena in social research that leads us to develop instruments, and the application of psychometrics is precisely to ensure that these are as accurate and meaningful (i.e. reliable and valid) as we can possibly make them.

Translational validity

Translational validity, which is concerned with the practical utility of an instrument, covers three methods (DeVon et al. 2007):

- face validity
- content validity
- factorial validity

Face validity

Face validity is controversial and some dismiss it as not truly being a form of validity; it lacks precise definition and is impossible to quantify. Therefore, it can be dealt with quickly. My understanding of this form of validity is just that an instrument looks as if it makes sense and that it can be completed and understood by participants. Beyond that, there is little else to say about face validity.

Content validity

Content validity is certainly a measure of validity in the true sense, and in some respects the most important aspects of validity in that it is the link between the items in the instrument and the construct that is being measured. Without content validity there can be no approach to construct validity; in addition, it is also possible to quantify content validity.

However, despite the predication of validity on reliability, content validity is the first step in designing an instrument and needs to take place prior to establishing reliability or any of the other types of validity. The approaches to content validity have been described earlier and the use of experts who can be used to generate items and for formal content validation; however, it is better not to use the same set of experts for both. The number of experts to use often depends on availability rather than statistical power calculations, but 10–20 should be sufficient; for these you should produce a version of the instrument that asks them to rate the importance of all of the items for inclusion in the questionnaire. In this way you are trying to get insight into the relevance of each item to the overall construct being measured – this is why these should be experts who understand the phenomenon. The rating for the items can be simply 'yes' or 'no' to inclusion or you could ask for a Likert-type response. The proportion of agreement between the raters can be expressed as a content validity index (CVI) where a CVI = 0.9 indicates good agreement between raters (Lynn 1986; Polit et al. 2007). Once the experts have rated the items you can quantify the responses and then decide on the basis of these responses which items to include and which to exclude; this can be done using formal criteria. Once you have arrived at your final set of items the questionnaire should be prepared in as close to its final form as possible and then piloted with a small group of people – again 10–20 – who meet the criteria of the intended respondents and any final problems with comprehensibility and legibility resolved.

Factorial validity

Factorial validity is sometimes called structural validity as it is concerned with the underlying structure to, or the relationship between, the items in the questionnaire; this is called the factor structure. This is sometimes treated separately from face and content validity but it is concerned with translational validity as it is about how sensible either the overall grouping of the items is, or the association of subgroups (factors) in the instrument. Until it is mathematically analysed, this structure is hidden or 'latent', a term we met earlier with reference to latent traits.

The method used to analyse a set of items for factor structure is called factor analysis and this is one of several methods of multivariate statistical analysis. Factor analysis is, essentially, a correlational technique in that it looks for correlations between items in an instrument. However, where the correlational methods described above usually only consider the correlation between two sets of scores, factor analysis can analyse the correlation between hundreds of items and thousands of people. The only limit, usually, is sample size, which is related to the ratio between the number of items in your instrument and the number of people responding. The minimum ratio of items to people is 1:5. The basic requirement is that you have more people than items, and ratios of 1:10 are considered best (Kline 1994). Therefore, you can see that the more items in your instrument the more respondents you will require; one good reason for keeping instruments as short as possible.

Factor analysis is very complex and it is not to be undertaken lightly; expert advice may be required to run it and interpret the analysis. There is excellent published advice available for conducting factor analysis (Ferguson and Cox 1993; Watson and Thompson 2006) and you should at least have a working knowledge of it before using it. There are two broad approaches to factor analysis:

- exploratory factor analysis
- confirmatory factor analysis

For the purposes of this chapter it is worth knowing that factor analysis may be used to explore the underlying structure of an instrument and also, where an underlying structure is suspected or has previously been demonstrated, this structure can also be hypothesized and confirmed. There are several types of exploratory factor analysis, but what is most commonly used is a technique closely related to factor analysis called principal components analysis. Confirmatory factor analysis is carried out using structural equation modelling techniques (Byrne 2001).

Factors and internal consistency

Internal consistency was referred to earlier in the context of reliability testing and, while some doubts are raised about the use of internal consistency, the use of factor analysis is often combined with analysis of internal consistency. The larger the number of items in an instrument the higher the internal consistency; therefore, the use of factor analysis is essential to ensure that high levels of internal consistency in an instrument do not mislead the investigator into thinking that all of the purported underlying dimensions of the instrument are internally consistent.

Criterion validity

Criterion validity can be considered under the following types of validity (DeVon et al. 2007):

- concurrent validity
- predictive validity
- convergent validity
- discriminant validity

Concurrent validity

Concurrent validity is a measure of the extent to which a measurement with the instrument being developed correlates with an established measure of the same phenomenon, at the same time. The measurement instrument used to compare your instrument may well be considered to be a gold standard measure. For example, if you were developing an instrument to measure psychological morbidity then a version of the *General Health Questionnaire* could be the instrument of choice. Clearly, the issue of concurrent validity raises the question of whether or not a new instrument is required; this should have been considered long before you begin to develop a new one, and the reasons for developing a new instrument may be to have one that is more appropriate for a specific population such as children or people with a specific disorder. All that is required for concurrent validity is that your instrument correlates with the gold standard; the correlation will not be perfect and concurrent validity alone is not sufficient to establish validity.

Predictive validity

Predictive validity is a measure of the extent to which a measurement made with your instrument correlates with a different but related measure at a future point in time. For example, a measure of psychological morbidity could be hypothesized to correlate with a measure of depression in future.

Convergent validity

Convergent validity (and its converse, discriminant validity) is described in two ways. Convergent validity refers, on the one hand, to the extent to which an instrument correlated contemporaneously with another related measure (for example psychological morbidity and depression or quality of life). Convergent validity also refers to the extent to which items or dimensions within an instrument correlate with one another.

Discriminant validity

Discriminant validity refers to the extent to which either two measures that would not be expected to correlate do not correlate or to lack of correlation between unrelated items and dimensions within an instrument. Discriminant validity is also referred to in the context of an instrument being able to discriminate between people, for example those with and without a diagnosis.

Which statistical tests are best for estimating validity?

A range of statistical tests may be used to estimate validity but basically they rely mainly on tests of correlation or tests of difference. In addition, factor analysis was mentioned above – essentially a test of intercorrelation – which is used to examine underlying dimensions, and in the context of instrument development it is worth mentioning receiver operating characteristics (ROCs).

The most commonly applied test of correlation is Pearson's r which assumes that the data are parametric, that is normally distributed; if this is in doubt then an alternative non-parametric test – Spearman's *rho* – may be used (Watson et al. 2005). These are very commonly applied tests of correlation which have 'stood the test of time' and are perfectly adequate for most purposes. The usual advice about any situations where you are in doubt is to consult a statistician at the stage when you are designing your study. For a consideration of the relative sizes of correlation see the earlier section on the use of correlation measures; normally, it is wise only to accept a large correlation as acceptable in tests of validity but it is not uncommon to see lower levels reported. If correlations are reported properly then, with your own knowledge of what correlation means, you can make your own judgement about the strength of a relationship and the likely validity. To some extent, the expected correlation between two instruments in a test of validity will depend on the instrument selected against which to test your developing instrument; for example, if the new instrument was a modification or a derivation of an existing instrument and purported to measure the same construct then you would expect the correlation to be high. However, if there was not a closely related instrument or you had to use one that measured another construct that could be expected to be correlated, then you would expect the correlation to be moderate or low.

Tests of difference

Where your test of validity depends on measuring a difference between people – discriminant validity – then you are concerned with tests of difference and the appropriate test is a t-test whereby the mean scores of the two groups of people you wish to discriminate can be compared (Watson et al. 2005). Therefore, if your instrument was designed to measure a diagnosis you would administer it to two groups of people: those with the diagnosis and those without. You would expect the mean scores of the two groups to be statistically significantly different. All of these tests depend on sample size, and this is especially the case with the t-test, where your sample size depends on the likely difference between the groups – the effect size. The smaller the effect size the larger the number of people in the groups is required to be and, while there are online calculators and other published advice available, you are often best to consult a statistician about sample size calculations.

Sensitivity and specificity

The concepts of sensitivity and specificity are worth considering and can be used to test how good a diagnostic instrument which provides a score is at discriminating between cases and non-cases – i.e. between those with the diagnosis and those without the diagnosis, where a definitive diagnosis can be determined. Sensitivity refers to the ability of an instrument to detect a case if it is real and specificity refers to the ability of an instrument only to detect those cases and not to provide 'false positive' results. In the case of sensitivity and specificity, the results of the instrument have to be dichotomized to give a 'yes' or a 'no' answer and these are compared in a contingency table with the 'yes' and 'no' of the true diagnosis. The results of the contingency table are used to work out the probability of obtaining a proper diagnosis (sensitivity) and the probability of avoiding false positives (the specificity). In theory, as these are probabilities, the sensitivity and specificity can both range from 0 to 1 but are rarely either. Clearly, an instrument that gives both high sensitivity and high specificity is desirable but there is a 'trade-off' between these: as sensitivity increases, the likelihood of specificity decreases.

Receiver operating characteristics

Receiver operating characteristics is a way of combining sensitivity and specificity of a measurement instrument against a dichotomous outcome whereby the best possible combination of the two can be used and, thereby, the level of measurement on the instrument that provides the best outcome in terms of detecting real cases (sensitivity) and avoiding false positives (specificity). Receiver operating characteristics is based on early radio technology whereby, before more sophisticated technology was available both to send and receive signals, the radio had to be set to maximize the chances of picking up the desired signal but to minimize the chances of picking up the wrong signal. In the use of instruments for diagnostic purposes the receiver operating characteristics are obtained by plotting the sensitivity against one minus the specificity, and the area under the curve is used, first, to indicate if the receiver operating characteristics are appropriate. If the area under the curve is 1 then the instrument has perfect sensitivity and specificity; if the area under the curve is 0 then the instrument has neither sensitivity nor specificity; and if the area under the curve is 0.5 then the sensitivity is equal to the specificity and therefore you are likely to make as many false positives as correct diagnoses. The minimum acceptable area under the curve is considered to be 0.7.

Item response theory

Item response theory covers a range of methods that, rather than the methods based on correlation and internal consistency described above (sometimes referred to as classical test theory), analyse the behaviour of and relationship between items (Watson et al. 2011). Item response theory is used in the development of questionnaires to select subsets of items from large item sets that are consistently related to each other in a hierarchy, i.e. items are scored by people in a specific order with some being more readily endorsed than others. These methods are becoming more commonly applied as instrument developers increasingly appreciate the value of hierarchical scales where the score on the scale is related to a specific set of items rather than to a combination of items. Scales developed using item response theory are more meaningful than simply summing scores on sets of items, and the reliability of these scales can be tested using a non-repeat method. Their validity can also be tested as described above by correlating them with existing scales.

Conclusion

This chapter has provided an overview of the concepts of reliability and validity and the main methods associated with their determination. Reliability and validity are not ends in themselves and the development of instruments should be driven by theory and the need to measure, properly, human attributes and behaviours.

Key concepts

- Reliability is absolutely necessary in quantitative social research, but not sufficient.
- Validity is predicated on reliability and is the real point of psychometrics.
- Reliability and validity are both crucial in understanding psychometrics.
- Reliability and validity can be estimated using statistical methods.

Key readings in reliability and validity

- K. Bannigan and R. Watson, Reliability and validity in a nutshell, *Journal of Clinical Nursing*, 18(23) (2009), 3237–43
  A very practical and readable recent paper on the issues of reliability and validity.
- H.A. DeVon, M.E. Block, P. Moyle-Wright, B.M. Ernst, S.J. Hayden, D.J. Lazzara, S.M. Savoy and E. Kostas-Polston, A psychometric toolbox for testing validity and reliability, *Journal of Nursing Scholarship*, 39(2) (2007), 155–64
  A very clear account of how to apply reliability and validity in instrument development.
- C.J. Jackson and A. Furnham, *Designing and Analysing Questionnaires and Surveys* (London: Whurr, 2000)
  A comprehensive and easy-to-read guide to questionnaire development including reliability and validity.
- J. Kottner, L. Audigé, S. Brorson, A. Donner, B.J. Gajewski, A. Hróbjartsson, C. Roberts, M. Shoukri and D. L. Streiner, Guidelines for reporting reliability and agreement studies (GRRAS) were proposed, *International Journal of Nursing Studies*, 48(6) (2011), 661–71
  A guide to reporting studies where reliability is measured.

Examples of the use of reliability and validity in health care research

The following papers provide an excellent example of how reliability and validity have been used in health care research.

- A. Carvajal, C. Centeno, R. Watson and E. Bruera, A comprehensive study of psychometric properties of the Edmonton Symptom Assessment System (ESAS) in Spanish advanced cancer patients, *European Journal of Cancer*, 47(12) (2011), 1863–72
- Y.-H. Chen, L.-C. Lin and R. Watson, Evaluation of the psychometric properties and the clinical feasibility of a Chinese version of the Doloplus-2 scale among cognitively impaired older people with communication difficulty, *International Journal of Nursing Studies*, 47(1) (2010), 78–88
- L.-C. Lin, R. Watson, Y.-C. Lee, Y.-C. Chou and S.-C. Wu, Edinburgh Feeding Evaluation in Dementia (EdFED) scale: Cross-cultural validation of the Chinese version, *Journal of Advanced Nursing*, 62(1) (2008), 116–23

References

Bandura, A. (1977) Self-efficacy: Toward a unifying theory of behavioral change, *Psychological Review*, 84(2): 191–215.

Bannigan, K. and Watson, R. (2009) Reliability and validity in a nutshell, *Journal of Clinical Nursing*, 18(23): 3237–43.

Byrne, B.M. (2001) Structural equation modelling with AMOS. London: Lawrence Erlbaum Associates.

Ferguson, E., Cox, T. (1993) Exploratory factor analysis: A users' guide, *International Journal of Selection and Assessment*, 1(2): 84–94.

DeVon, H.A., Block, M.E., Moyle-Wright, P., Ernst, D.M., Hayden, S.J., Lazzara, D.J., Savoy, S.M. and Kostas-Polston, E. (2007) A psychometric toolbox for testing validity and reliability, *Journal of Nursing Scholarship*, 39(2): 155–64.

Kline, P. (1994) *An Easy Guide to Factor Analysis*. London: Routledge.

Lynn, M.R. (1986) Determination and quantification of content validity, *Nursing Research*, 35(6): 382–5.

Messick, S. (1994) The interplay of evidence and consequences in the validation of performance assessments, *Educational Researcher*, 23(2): 13–23.

Polit, F.D., Beck, C.T. and Owen, S.V. (2007) Is the CVI an acceptable indicator of content validity? Appraisal and recommendations, *Research in Nursing & Health*, 30(4), 459–67.

Rankin, G. and Stokes, M. (1998) Reliability of assessment tools in rehabilitation: An illustration of appropriate statistical analyses, *Clinical Rehabilitation*, 12: 187–99.

Schmitt, N. (1996) Uses and abuses of coefficient alpha, *Psychological Assessment*, 8(4): 350–3.

Sijtsma, L. (2009) On the use, misuse, and the very limited usefulness of Cronbach's alpha, *Psychometrika*, 74(1): 107–20.

Stevens, S.S. (1946) On the theory of scales and measurement, *Science*, 103(2684): 677–80.

Watson, R. and Thompson, D.R. (2006) Use of factor analysis in *Journal of Advanced Nursing*: A literature review, *Journal of Advanced Nursing*, 55(3): 330–41.

Watson, R., Atkinson, I. and Egerton, P. (2005) *Successful Statistics for Nursing and Healthcare*. Basingstoke: Palgrave.

Watson, R., van der Ark, L.A., Lin, L.-C., Fieo, R., Deary, I.J. and Meijer, R.R. (2011) Item response theory: How Mokken scaling can be used in clinical practice, *Journal of Clinical Nursing*, 21(19–20): 2736–46, doi: 10.1111/j.1365-2702.2011.03892.x.

PART 5

Analysing and presenting data

17   Understanding probability

Siobhan Corrigan

Introduction

Is it possible to predict all events completely accurately? Or is there always some level of uncertainty or unexpected events that may impact the final outcome? Uncertainty is both 'irreducible' and inescapable in health care: no intervention ever leads with complete certainty to a given clinical outcome, no diagnosis is ever completely established, and no prognosis is ever completely accurate (Thompson 2009). For example, clinicians will never have *all* of the reliable and valid clinical information needed to achieve 100 per cent diagnostic certainty. However, building on their clinical intuition and experiences, they attempt to make decisions on the basis of probability. How often have we heard clinicians state something along the following lines: 'the patient will probably return from surgery and be back in the ward within three hours'; 'there is a 50–55 per cent chance that surgery will be required'. Therefore the concept of probability is used in everyday activities and conversations, although not in a very precise manner. These qualitative expressions of uncertainty, although relatively easy to use, are prone to misunderstanding. When asked to quantify their uncertainty in response to hearing words such as 'rare' or 'likely', patients and professionals – even when given access to the same information – often give widely variable estimates of what the phrase means to them (Thompson 2009).

In the study of statistics and research methods, probability plays a systematic and specific role in making evidence-based decisions.

What is probability?

There are many definitions of probability, and put simply it can be defined as a mathematical-based framework for understanding, describing and providing accurate estimates for the likelihood that a specific event will occur. Therefore it is one of the key basic building blocks in drawing inferences and generalizing findings from sample research data to the wider population. Thus, probability establishes a connection between samples and populations, and inferential statistics rely on this connection when sample data are used as the basis for making conclusions about populations (Gravetter and Forzano 2012).

Understanding probability should not be perceived as something very complicated or intimidating, as probability is a common element in our everyday lives. Every time we buy a lottery ticket or roll a die we are involved in the world of probabilities. It is a huge topic and this chapter does not attempt to examine all aspects of probability and probability calculations. The logic of this chapter is to cover the key concepts and approaches to probability as a first step and how that is then applied to research and random sampling, highlighting the importance of producing a sample that represents the population and enables the researcher to use powerful statistical techniques and generalize findings to the wider population.

Basic terminology

A specific terminology has developed around the terms used in probability, so before examining probability it is important to review the basic terminology as these terms will be used throughout this chapter. Table 17.1 provides an overview of some of the key terms.

The basic probability concept of any event can vary from 0 to 1. If an event is certain to occur, it has a probability of 1; while, if it is certain the event will not occur, it has a probability of 0. Therefore probability of any event E, P(E), must be greater than or equal to 0 and less than or equal to 1. That is $0 \leq P(E) \leq 1$.

The sum of the probabilities of all outcomes must be equal to 1. That is, if the sample space is:

$$S = \{e_1, e_2 \ldots e_n\}, \text{ then } P(e_1) + P(e_2) + P(e_n) = 1$$

The classical approach

The easiest way to appreciate probability is to follow the more classical approach. In this, any event is considered as the one that actually happens from among all the possible outcomes which might have happened – therefore the exact number of outcomes is required. One of the most common ways to demonstrate this is to use the example of tossing a coin. For example, when a coin is tossed there are only two possible outcomes – a head or a tail. These two events are mutually exclusive; you cannot get both (Watson et al. 2006). Therefore in calculating probability the following occurs:

$$P(event) = \frac{number\ of\ ways\ event\ occurs}{total\ number\ of\ possible\ outcomes}$$

Table 17.1   Overview of basic terminology

Term used	Definition
Event	The basic bit of data is called an event. When referring to the probability of something, the something is called an event (e.g. when flipping a coin, the event is the outcome of that flip).
Independent events	Two events when the occurrence or non-occurrence of one has no effect on the occurrence or non-occurrence of the other.
Mutually exclusive	Two events are mutually exclusive if the occurrence of one event precludes the occurrence of the other.
Exhaustive	A set of events is exhaustive if it includes all possible outcomes.
Population	The large group of interest to the researcher is called the population. Typically, populations are huge, containing far too many individuals to measure and systematically study, therefore the entire population does not participate in the research.
Sample	A sample is a selected small collection of individuals or units, and can represent the overall intended population of the research study.
Target population	A target population refers to the specific sample of individuals or cases that the researcher wants to study.
Sampling ratio	The ratio of the size of the sample to the size of the target populations is the sampling ratio. For example, the population has 50,000 people; draw a sample of 150 from it – thus the sampling ratio is 150/50,000 = 0.003, or 0.3 per cent. If the population is 500 and the sample 100, then the sampling ratio is 100/500 = 0.20, or 20 per cent (Neuman 2007).
Random variable	A variable whose value is determined by the outcome of a random experiment.
Discrete random variable	Discrete random variables are obtained by counting, and have values for which there are no in-between values. These values are typically the integers 0, 1, 2, etc.
Continuous random variable	A random variable where the data can take infinitely many values. For example, a random variable measuring the time taken for something to be done is continuous since there are an infinite number of possible times that it could take.

Consequently, the probability of tossing a head is:

$$P(1\ head) = \frac{number\ of\ ways\ 1\ head\ can\ occurs}{total\ number\ of\ possible\ outcomes} = \frac{1}{2}$$

The empirical approach

Another way in which probability can be understood and measured refers to the empirical approach, which determines probability value by observation and experimentation, and relates more to experience of real life. By repeated trials of 'experiments' over extended periods, we can get a 'feel' for the relative frequency of any given event occurring (Watson et al. 2006). Probabilities in these experiments are defined as the ratio of the frequency of the occurrence of an event to the number of trials in the experiment.

$$P(E) = \frac{number\ of\ times\ event\ E\ occurs}{total\ number\ of\ observed\ occurrences}$$

The probability obtained using the empirical approach is approximate because different runs of the probability experiment lead to different outcomes and, therefore, different estimates of P(E). Imagine flipping a coin 20 times and recording the number of heads and then using the results of the experiment to estimate the probability of obtaining a head. However, if the experiment is repeated, the results of the second run of the experiment may not necessarily yield the same results. Therefore we cannot say the probability equals the relative frequency; rather we say the probability is approximately the relative frequency. As the number of trials in a probability experiment are increased, the estimate becomes more accurate and the relative frequencies settle down to a consistent figure (this is also known as the law of large numbers). Therefore the empirical approach to determining probabilities relies on data from actual experiments and adequate sample sizes to determine approximate probabilities, instead of the assumption of equal likeliness.

Whichever method is used, the probability of any event is always calculated to be a positive number between 0 and 1. As in the tossing of the coin, we can leave it as a fraction '1/2', or we can convert it to decimal notation '0.5', or record it as a percentage '50 per cent'.

Rules of probability

Two important rules are central for understanding probability, and they are usually referred to as the *additive rule* and the *multiplicative rule*.

The additive rule

A formal definition of the additive rule – a statistical property that states the probability of one and/or two events occurring at the same time is equal to the probability of the first event occurring, plus the probability of the second event occurring, minus the probability that both events occur at the same time. For example, how can we determine the probability of drawing a king and/or a queen out of a deck of cards on only one draw? Using the addition rule for probabilities, we get the following:

P(King) = 4/52, P(Queen) = 4/52, and P(King and Queen) = 0

Since it is impossible to draw both a king and a queen on the same draw, we can conclude that the probability of drawing either a king or a queen from a deck of cards is 8/52, or about 15.4 per cent.

The multiplicative rule

The multiplicative rule is a result used to determine the probability that two events, A and B, both occur, and follows from the definition of conditional probability (see the next section). To calculate the probability of two or more independent events (for example, a head followed by another head in two independent tosses of the coin) simply multiply the independent probabilities together. Therefore the probability of getting two heads with two tosses of the coin is $1/2 \times 1/2 = 1/4$. The chance of a head or a tail with two tosses of the coin is 1/2 because there are two ways of obtaining this: head/tail or tail/heads (Mc Killup 2005).

If the events are not independent (for example, the first event being a number in the range of 1–3 inclusive when rolling a six-sided die and the second event being that this is an even number), the multiplication rule also applies, but this requires having to multiply the probability of one event by the conditional probability of the second. When rolling a die, the independent probability of a number from 1 to 3 is $3/6 = 1/2$, and the independent probability of any even number is also 1/2 (the even numbers are 2, 4 and 6, divided by the six possible outcomes). If, however, a rolled number from 1 to 3 comes up, the probability of that restricted set of outcomes being an even number is 1/3 (because 2 is the only even number possible in this set of outcomes). Therefore the probability of both related events is $1/2 \times 1/3 = 1/6$. This can also be looked at in another way – the chance of an even number when rolling a die is 1/2 (numbers 2, 4 or 6) and the probability of one of these numbers being in the range 1 to 3 is 1/3 (the number 2 out of these three outcomes). Therefore the probability of both is again $1/2 \times 1/3 = 1/6$ (Mc Killup 2005).

Conditional and joint probabilities

Two types of probabilities need to be highlighted in order to understand the role of probability: *conditional* and *joint* probabilities.

Conditional probability

The concept of conditional probability is one of the most important concepts in probability theory. It is extremely useful in problem solving. Conditional probabilities express the fact that probabilities alter when the available information alters. The concept of conditional probability is intuitive for most people. For example, most people reason as follows to find the probability of getting two aces when two cards are selected at random from an ordinary deck of cards. The probability of getting an ace on the first card is 4/52. Given that one ace is gone from the deck, the probability of getting an ace on the second card is 3/51. The desired probability is therefore $4/52 \times 3/51$ (Tijms 2004). The probability of contracting lung cancer if you smoke cigarettes is a conditional probability, as is the probability of coronary heart disease if you are excessively overweight and over 60 years old.

Joint probability

A joint probability is defined as the probability of the co-occurrence of two or more events at the same time, and can only be applied to situations where more than one observation can occur at the same time. For example, a joint probability cannot be calculated when tossing a coin on the same flip. However, the joint probability can be calculated on the probability of rolling a 2 and a 5 using two different dice. This type of probability depends on whether the experiment is done *with* or *without* replacement.

With replacement means that the object chosen on one stage is returned to the sample space before the next choice is made. Independent events are considered with replacement since they do not affect each other, interfere with each other, or cause each other. For example, tossing a head on the first toss of a coin does not affect the outcome of flipping the coin a second time. The probability that independent events A and B happen simultaneously is found by using the multiplication rule, or the product of the individual probabilities.

Without replacement uses the same idea, only we consider the change in the sample space if the first choice is not replaced. These can be considered dependent events, since changing the sample space changes the probability. We still use the multiplication rule, but the numerator and/or denominator decrease(s) for each of the stages.

Applying probabilities to data analyses: inferential statistics

Why is probability relevant to inferential statistics? Statistics are, in one sense, all about probabilities. Inferential statistics deal with establishing whether differences or associations exist between sets of data. The data come from the sample we use, and the sample is taken from a population. When testing a sample of individuals or events we are generally doing so to facilitate an understanding of the population and draw conclusions about the population from which the sample was drawn.

Therefore we need to think about whether the sample represents the population from which it has been taken. The larger the sample we take, the greater the probability that it is representative of the population. If we took the whole population for a study the probability would equal 1 since the sample = the population. A sample smaller than the whole population means that we cannot guarantee that it is similar to the population. There is a probability that it is not. We want to keep this probability of sampling error as small as possible, so researchers often set a limit of probability (p) of a sampling error at no more than 0.05. Some studies might be more stringent and set the chance of a sampling error at 0.01. And in some studies where little chance of error is critical (for instance testing new drugs) some researchers may even use a probability of error being very small indeed at 0.001, saying that the chance of an error is one in a thousand (http://www.nottingham.ac.uk/nursing/sonet/rlos/statistics/probability/5.html).

Whenever we use samples we are prone to sampling error. This means we do not know whether the patterns of results we find in our samples accurately reflect what is happening in the population or whether they are simply a result of sampling error (Dancey and Reidy 2007).

The unavoidable problem with using probability is that there is always a chance of making a wrong decision, with no way of telling when this has been done. Every time a statistical test is applied there is the risk of a *type 1* or *type 2 error*, and they are unavoidably associated with using probability to make a decision.

Type 1 errors

Say we want to see if a group of patients, who have been given a new drug, have recovered more quickly than a group of patients who received the standard drug. We can use a statistical test to see if there is a difference. Whatever test we use, we need to remember that the data we are analysing comes from groups that originally started off as similar to one another. If this were not the case we could not tell if the new drug had made the difference. So if we find a difference, it might be due to the trial, but there is a possibility that it is due to sampling error. Another way of thinking about sampling errors is that it is the error that gives rise to the difference between the sets of data. If the error were not present then there would not be a difference. The type 1 error (also known as a 'false positive' or 'alpha error') states that a difference is found when no difference exists. It is one of the reasons why researchers publish the results of their research. This then enables other researchers to repeat the study to see if they find similar results. If the results were originally due to an error (which has a small chance of happening, i.e. less than 1 in 20, or 0.05) then repeating the study may not be able to reproduce the result. An undetected type 1 error could have serious consequences in a clinical practice. The fluke recovery of a few patients might cause us to believe that an innovative treatment is effective, when in fact it is not; this could result in resources being wasted on worthless treatments (Watson et al. 2006).

Type 2 errors

There is also the possibility of a type of error known as a type 2 error (or 'false negative'). Such possibilities have a probability of occurrence. They arise when it is reasonable to expect a difference and the sampling has resulted in no difference being found. Think about a drug trial, and in this instance think about the possibility that people taking the new drug will each react differently to the drug. Not everybody will respond in exactly the same way to the drug. Some will show a big improvement and for some it will be very minor, if any, improvement. So there is a probability that the trial group is unrepresentative if the sample that forms this group includes participants who do not respond to the new drug. In the end, the type 2 error means we find no difference when one should be found. The probability of such an event can be determined. Researchers usually set the probability in this case at 0.2. That is, a one in five chance of a type 2 error (http://www.nottingham.ac.uk/nursing/sonet/rlos/statistics/probability/5.html). The clinical implication of a type 2 error might be that an ineffectual remedy continues to be applied, in the mistaken belief that it is more effective than a new development (Watson et al. 2006).

Sampling methods

Sampling methods fall into two basic categories: *probability sampling* and *non-probability sampling*.

Probability sampling

A probability sampling method is any method of sampling that utilizes some form of random selection. To have a random selection method, it is critical to set up some process or procedure that assures that the different units in a chosen population have equal probabilities of being chosen. For example, if each individual in a population of 100 people is likely to be selected, then the probability of selection is 1/100 for each person. Probability sampling has three important conditions:

1   The exact size of the population must be known and it must be possible to access all of the individuals in the population.
2   Each individual in the population must have a specified probability of selection.
3   When a group of individuals are all assigned the same probability, the selection process must be unbiased so that all group members have an equal chance of being selected. Selection must be a random process, which simply means that every possible outcome is equally likely. For example, each time a coin is tossed, the two possible outcomes (heads and tails) are equally likely (Gravetter and Forzano 2012).

Probability sampling requires extensive knowledge of the population. Specifically, we must be able to list all of the individuals in the population. In most situations, this information is not available to the researcher. As a result, probability sampling is rarely used for research in the social and behavioural sciences. Nonetheless, this kind of sampling provides a good foundation for introducing the concept of representativeness and demonstrating how different sampling techniques can be used to help ensure a representative sample (Gravetter and Forzano 2012). Table 17.2 provides a summary of the key probability sampling methods.

It is also possible to combine two or more sampling strategies to select participants. For example, a health board may first divide the population into the two biggest teaching hospitals in a particular part of the country, which involves stratified sampling. From the two different teaching hospitals, the health board may then only select second year medical students, which involves cluster sampling. Selection strategies are combined to optimize the chances that a sample is representative of a widely dispersed or broad-based population, such as in a wide market survey or a political poll.

Non-probability sampling

The difference between non-probability and probability sampling is that non-probability sampling does not involve random selection and probability sampling does. Does that mean that non-probability samples are not representative of the population? Not necessarily. But it does mean that non-probability samples cannot depend on the rationale of probability theory. At least with a probabilistic sample we know the odds or probability that we have represented the population well. We are able to estimate confidence intervals for the statistic. With non-probability samples, we may or may not represent the population well, and it will often be hard for us to

Table 17.2 Summary of probability sampling methods

Type of sampling	Overview	Application
Simple random sampling	The most basic type of probability sampling. The simple random process ensures that each individual has an equal and independent chance of selection. The two principal methods of random sampling are: *sampling with replacement* – this method requires that an individual selected for the sample be recorded as a sample member and then returned (replaced) to the sample before the next selection is made; and *sampling without replacement* – each selected element is removed from the population before the next selection is made.	The popularity of simple random sampling is due to the fact that most statistical techniques assume this mode of sampling (Knapp 1985). While statistically the most expedient, simple random sampling is not always feasible as researchers must have a listing of every element in the population. The selection process is fair and unbiased, and when the population is of a limited nature (e.g. patient records) the task of enumerating the population becomes manageable.
Systematic sampling	Starts by listing all the elements of the population, then randomly picks a starting point on the list (e.g. selecting every fifth born baby in a given hospital in a given month).	An easy method for obtaining an essential random sample, but even with the random start, the possibility of obtaining a biased or non-representative sample exists.
Stratified random sampling	A sample can be obtained from dividing the overall population into subpopulations (e.g. males/females; different income levels). Stratified random sampling is very useful when a researcher wants to describe or compare and contrast segments of the population. To do this, each segment must contain enough elements to adequately represent the subpopulation.	The overall sample is not representative of the population. The chance of obtaining a non-typical sample is reduced.

(continued)

Table 17.2 (*Continued*)

Type of sampling	Overview	Application
Proportionate stratified sampling	A sample is obtained by subdividing the population into strata and then randomly selecting from each stratum a number of participants so that the proportions in the sample correspond to the proportions in the population.	Guarantees that the composition of the sample (in terms of the identified strata) will be perfectly representative of the composition of the population, but some strata may have limited representation in the sample. Can create a lot of extra work and requires a lot of preliminary measurement before the study begins, and it can discard many of the sampled individuals.
Cluster sampling	In cluster sampling, a cluster (i.e. a group of population elements) constitutes the sampling unit, instead of a single element of the population.	Can be used when well-defined clusters exist in a population of interest. It has two advantages – it is quick and easy to obtain a large sample, and measurement of individuals can be done in groups. Its disadvantage is that it can raise concerns about the independence of individual scores. It may not reflect the diversity of the community. Other elements in the same cluster may share similar characteristics. Provides less information per observation than a stratified random sample of the same size (redundant information: similar information from the others in the cluster). Standard errors of the estimates are high, compared to other sampling designs with the same sample size.

know how well we've done so. In general, researchers prefer probabilistic or random sampling methods over non-probabilistic ones, and consider them to be more accurate and rigorous. However, in applied social research there may be circumstances where it is not feasible, practical or theoretically sensible to do random sampling (http://www.socialresearchmethods.net/kb/sampnon.php).

Non-probability samples are limited with regard to generalization. Because they do not truly represent a population, we cannot make valid inferences about the larger group from which they are drawn. Validity can be increased by approximating random selection as much as possible, and making every attempt to avoid introducing bias into the sample selection.

Table 17.3 Summary of non-probability sampling methods

Type of sampling	Description	Application
Convenience sampling Nagpal et al. (2012): Failures in communication and information transfer across the surgical care pathway: Interview survey	Participants are selected on the basis of their availability, ease of access and willingness to participate. This sampling is probably used more than any other kind of sampling. Most researchers use two strategies to help alleviate the drawbacks of this type of sampling – try to ensure that their samples are reasonably representative and not strongly biased, and provide a clear description of how the sample was obtained and specific information on the participants.	Considered to be a weak form of sampling because no attempt is made to know the population or to use random processes in selection. Biased sample, but quick and easy way of obtaining a large sample.
Quota sampling Morrow et al. (2007): The utility of non-proportional quota sampling for recruiting at-risk women for microbicide research	Quota sampling is the non-probability version of stratified sampling. The population is divided into homogeneous subpopulations and samples from these subgroups are selected based on predefined characteristics, traits or focused phenomena.	Samples may be biased as not everyone gets a chance to be selected.
Volunteer sampling Barbour (1999): The case for combining qualitative and quantitative approaches in health services research	Researchers simply ask for participation in the research or may interview or send questionnaires to a randomly selected group.	Those individuals who choose to respond represent a voluntary rather than a truly random sample of individuals – the sample could be biased. This applies to both a survey and randomly selected individuals.
Purposive sampling Benzer et al. (2011): The relationship between organizational climate and quality of chronic disease management	The researcher deliberately selects the units to be included in the study. The sampling units are selected because they are representative of the wider population. When the desired population for the study is rare or very difficult to locate and recruit for a study, purposive sampling may be the only option.	The major problem with purposive sampling is that the type of people who are available for study may be different from those in the population who can't be located, and this might introduce a source of bias.

Here, we consider a range of non-probabilistic alternatives. Among the widely used non-probability sampling methods are convenience, quota, purposive and volunteer sampling. Table 17.3 provides a summary of some of the key non-probability sampling techniques. This table also includes a specific reference that demonstrates or discusses each of the non-probability sampling techniques from applied health research.

In undertaking any research study, the sample selected is critical to the overall research process.

An interesting research question is only the start of the process, but it is in the confidence of the sample that research can make inferences regarding the findings and differences found from the analysis. In reviewing other studies or developing your own study, pay careful attention to how the sample was drawn. If the sample is biased, then are the results valid? You set forth before the start of any study to lay out specific rules for selection of your sample so that you can limit the amount of bias in your sample so that generalizations can be made (Landreneau 2004).

Conclusion

Probability is one of the key basic building blocks in drawing inferences and generalizing findings from sample research data to the wider population. Determining the statistical significance of a research result means knowing what probability means; and individualizing the results of research studies to patients requires knowledge of probability and how it works (Thompson 2009). Like any approach, there are rules and structures to be learned, and the key objective of this chapter was to focus on the key concepts and approaches to understanding probability and the role it plays in describing and providing accurate estimates for the likelihood that a specific event will occur.

Key concepts

- The probability of any event E, P(E), must be greater than or equal to 0 and less than or equal to 1, and probabilities can be represented in terms of odds (e.g. 1 in 5), decimals (0.2) or percentages (20 per cent).
- There are two key approaches to assigning probabilities:
  - Classical probability is predicated on the assumption that the outcomes of an experiment are equally likely to happen. It utilizes rules and laws, and we can apply classical probability when the events have the same chance of occurring (called equally likely events), and the set of events are mutually exclusive and collectively exhaustive. It involves an experiment.
  - The empirical-based approach is based on cumulated historical experimental data to determine approximate probabilities instead of the assumption of equal likeliness.

- There are many rules associated with solving probability problems. This chapter dealt with the additive rule and multiplicative rule.
- Joint probability refers to the likelihood of two events occurring together and at the same point in time.
- Conditional probability is the probability that one event will occur given that some other event has occurred. The probability that a person will contact AIDS given that he or she is an intravenous drug user is a conditional probability (Howell 2013).
- Whenever we use samples we are prone to sampling error. This means we do not know whether the patterns of results we find in our samples accurately reflect what is happening in the population or whether they are simply a result of sampling error (Dancey and Reidy 2007). Every time you do a statistical test you run the risk of a type 1 or type 2 error, and they are unavoidably associated with using probability to help you make a decision.
  - A type 1 error (also known as a false positive or alpha error) happens when you reject the null hypothesis even if it is true – that a difference is found when no difference exists.
  - A type 2 error (also known as a false negative) happens when you accept the null hypothesis when you should in fact reject it. This means we find no difference when one should be found.
- There are a number of common strategies for obtaining adequate samples, and the two basic categories of sampling techniques are probability and non-probability sampling:
  - In probability sampling, the odds of selecting a particular individual or event are known and can be calculated. Types of probability sampling include simple random sampling, systematic sampling, stratified sampling, proportionate stratified sampling and cluster sampling.
  - In non-probability sampling, the probability of selecting a particular individual or event is not known because the researchers do not know the population size or the members of the population. Types of non-probability sampling include convenience sampling, quota sampling, volunteer and purposive sampling. Each sampling method has advantages and limitations, and differs in terms of the representativeness of the sample obtained.
- Mastering the language of probability is the key to thinking creatively about uncertainty in decision making.
- Without learning the rules, health care professionals are artificially limiting the size of their problem-solving toolkit for clinical practice. Without competence in this basic building block for giving 'due weight' to research evidence, clinicians will always fall back on the intuitive, the familiar, and the experiential—all of which have some severe limitations (Thompson and Dowding 2009).
- This chapter has provided the initial steps in introducing some of the concepts that are key for reasoning probabilistically; only by acknowledging uncertainty, making it transparent, and factoring it into our decisions can we move towards truly shared decision making with both patients and researchers.

Key readings in probability

- H. Tijms, *Understanding Probability*, 3rd edn (Cambridge: Cambridge University Press, 2012)

  This book provides a fairly straightforward guide to learning and applying basic probability principles. Also the key concepts and ideas from probability theory are treated in a very clear way.

- C. Barboianu, *Understanding and Calculating the Odds: Probability Theory Basics and Calculus Guide for Beginners, with Applications in Games of Chance and Everyday Life.* (Romania: INFAROM Publishing, 2006)

  This book covers the fundamentals of probability very well, and is easy to read with a good variety of problems and excellent examples and algorithms for solving.

- Probability and statistics e-book: http://wiki.stat.ucla.edu/socr/index.php/Probability _and_statistics_EBook

  This is an internet-based 'probability and statistics e-book'. There are three novel features of this specific 'statistics e-book'. It is community-built, completely open access (in terms of use and contributions), and blends information technology, scientific techniques and modern pedagogical concepts.

Examples of the use of probability in health care research

- L. Field, R. Pruchno, J. Bewley, E. Lemay and N. Levinsky, Using probability vs. non-probability sampling to identify hard-to-access participants for health-related research, *Journal of Ageing Health*, 18(4) (2002), 565–83
- T.M. Gale, C.T. Hawley and T. Sivakumaran, Do mental health professionals really understand probability? Implications for risk assessment and evidence-based practice, *Journal of Mental Health*, 12(4) (2003), 417–30
- R. Fuller, N. Dudley and J. Blacktop, How informed is consent? Understanding of pictorial and verbal probability information by medical inpatients, *Postgraduate Medical Journal,* 18(923) (2003), 543–4
- M. Marshall, Sampling for Qualitative Research, *Family Practice*, 13(6) (1996), 522–6
- C. Pope, P. van Royen and R. Baker, Qualitative methods in research on health-care quality, *Quality Safety Health Care*, 11(2) (2002), 148–52
- C. Thompson, Probability: The language of uncertainty, *Evidence Based Nursing*, 12(3) (2009), 67–70

Useful websites

- http://www.natco1.org/research/research_guidelines.htm
- http://www.socialresearchmethods.net/kb/sampnon.php
- http://www.nottingham.ac.uk/nursing/sonet/rlos/statistics/probability/5.html
- http://www.nottingham.ac.uk/nmp/sonet/rlos/statistics/probability/index.html

- http://www.iwh.on.ca/at-work/62/what-researchers-mean-by-probability
- http://www.umanitoba.ca/faculties/medicine/units/pediatrics/sections/neonatology/media/DiagnosticTest2.pdf
- http://www.nursingplanet.com/Nursing_Research/basic_statistical_concepts_nurses1.html

References

Barbour, R.S. (1999) The case for combining qualitative and quantitative approaches in health services research, *Journal of Health Service Research Policy*, 4(1): 39–43.

Benzer, J.K., Young, G., Stolzmann, K., Osatuke, K., Meterko, M., Caso, A., White, B. and Mohr, C. (2011) The relationship between organizational climate and quality of chronic disease management, *Health Service Research*, 46(3): 671–711.

Dancey, C.P. and Reidy, J. (2007) *Statistics Without Maths for Psychology*, 4th edn. Harlow: Pearson Education.

Gravetter, F.J. and Forzano, L.B. (2012) *Research Methods for the Behavioural Sciences*, International edn, 4th edn. Canada: Wadsworth, CENGAGE Learning.

Howell, D.H. (2013) *Statistical Methods for Psychology*. Belmont, CA: Wadsworth, CENGAGE Learning.

Knapp, R.G. (1985) *Basic Statistics for Nurses*, 2nd edn. Albany, NY: Delmar Publishing.

Landreneau, K. J. (2004) Sampling strategies. Available at http://www.natco1.org/research/files/SamplingStrategies.pdf [Accessed 16 February 2012].

Mc Killup, S. (2005) *Statistics Explained*. Cambridge: Cambridge University Press.

Morrow, K., Vargas, S., Rosen, R., Christen, A., Salamon, L., Shulman, L., Barroso, C. and Fava, J. (2007) The utility of non-proportional quota sampling for recruiting at-risk women for microbicide research, *AIDS & Behavior*, 11(4): 586–95.

Nagpal, K., Arora, S., Vats, A., Wong, H.W., Sevdalis, N., Vincent, C., and Moorthy, K. (2012) Failures in communication and information transfer across the surgical care pathway: Interview study, *British Medical Journal Quality & Safety*, 21(10): 843–9.

Neuman, W.L. (2007) *Basics of Social Research: Qualitative & Quantitative Approaches*. New York: Pearson Education.

Tijms, H. (2004) *Understanding Probability: Chance Rules in Everyday Life*. Cambridge: Cambridge University Press.

Thompson, C. (2009) Probability: The language of uncertainty, *Evidence Based Nursing*, 12(3): 67–70.

Thompson, C. and Dowding, D. (2009) *Essential Clinical Decision Making for Nurses*. London: Elsevier Science.

Watson, R., Atkinson, I. and Egerton, P. (2006) *Successful Statistics for Nursing & Healthcare*. New York: Palgrave Macmillan.

18 Analysing data from small and large samples and non-normal and normal distributions

Catherine Comiskey and Orla Dempsey

Chapter topics

- Nominal and ordinal data
- Discrete data
- Continuous data

- Hypothesis testing
- Parametric and non-parametric tests
- Non-normal data

Introduction

Quite often in phase one clinical trials, in smaller-scale studies or studies dealing with sensitive topics the number of cases is necessarily small, and the resulting data may need to be analysed using specific techniques. In addition, even data arising from a large study may have some key variables with a non-normal distribution. In this chapter these issues are addressed, methods of analyses for regular and small datasets are presented and additional approaches for dealing with non-normal data are also provided. Finally we demonstrate, using real-life research examples, how meaningful results can be obtained once these challenges are overcome.

Regardless of the scale of a study it is important to first have a clear and focused overarching research question. Secondly, one must recognize the types of data the study has generated to answer that question, and finally one must be clear on the nature of the study design. Once these are clear in the researcher's mind then the answer to the question, 'what statistical test do I use?' will be a matter of working through these three questions. The key aim of this chapter is to lead the reader through these steps by describing the different data types and introducing a range of methods for analysing the data types from both large- and small-scale studies.

Types of data

Before addressing types of data, an explanation of some basic terminology is required. The facts and figures collected, summarized, analysed and interpreted in a study are known as the *data*. The data collected in a particular study are known as a *dataset*. A set of data contains *elements* or *cases*, which are the entities on which the data are collected; they may be individuals with a particular infection, animals with a particular disease, or things such as medical devices. A characteristic of interest for an element, such as age, gender or marital status, is known as a *variable*. An *observation* is the set of measurements collected for a particular element or case.

Example

A hospital patient database contains information on every patient attending the hospital. The patient is the element or case. For each element or case, the data contain variables such as date of birth, gender, condition, type of treatment, number of times hospitalized, severity of symptoms.

Data can be classified as either *categorical* or *numerical* variables.

Categorical variables

Categorical variables describe a set of observations which can be assigned to non-overlapping categories. There are two types of categorical variables: *nominal* and *ordinal* data.

Nominal data

A nominal variable is categorical data which has no natural order or rank. Examples of nominal variables are gender, marital status and employment status. The observations in a nominal dataset can be counted, however this type of data cannot be ordered or measured.

Ordinal data

A categorical variable which has a natural order is known as an ordinal variable. Examples of ordinal variables are level of education, state of health and deprivation score. The observations in an ordinal dataset can be ranked and assigned a ranking scale. This type of data can be counted and ordered but not measured.

Example

A group of patients are asked to rank their knowledge of their medical condition, type 1 diabetes; the options available were 'no knowledge', 'limited knowledge', 'good knowledge' or 'very good knowledge'.

Numerical data

A dataset which records measurements of the amount of something on a numerical scale is numerical data. Numerical variables can be measured and analysed using statistical measures and techniques. There are two types of numerical variables: *discrete* and *continuous* variables.

Discrete data

Discrete data count how many, and the answers are usually whole numbers. Discrete variables have a finite number of values. Examples: the number of patients with arthritis attending a clinic, or the number of health centres in a region.

Continuous or scale data

Continuous data measure how much, and the answers are not necessarily whole numbers. Continuous variables have an infinite number of values within a given range. Examples: level of psychological concerns associated with cancer, the Lerman Cancer Worry Scale (Lerman et al. 1991).

The type of data available, whether it is categorical or numerical, determines the type of statistics that must be used to answer the predetermined research question. Numerical data are generally more detailed, allowing more powerful statistical analysis to be conducted. The following sections outline some of the different statistical tests available for analysing the data.

Testing for significance and understanding hypothesis testing

In the previous sections the different types of data were explained and described. Before these data can be analysed and results interpreted, an understanding of the nature of hypothesis testing is required. Hypothesis testing is also often referred to as significance testing or testing for significance (Page et al. 1995). While the nature of the statistical test used may change depending on the different types of data and the size of the sample, the nature and the steps involved in a hypothesis test never change. Once the researcher has a clear and basic understanding of the steps involved in hypothesis testing and their rationale for undertaking a test, they will find that they can understand and interpret the results of their statistical tests more easily. Often the researcher knows some of these steps intuitively but has never made the connection between this intuitive understanding and the statistics behind them. Regardless of the type of data or the statistic used, the steps involved in a hypothesis test include the following.

Identify and state the null hypothesis: This is a statement of the form: 'There is no difference between the mean value of the study sample and the population mean'; 'There is no difference between the mean value of sample one and sample two'; 'There is no difference between the sample mean before and after some intervention'; 'There is no difference between the sample proportion and the proportion in the population'; 'There is no association between variable one and variable two'; and so on. The common word in each of these null hypotheses is 'no'. The *null* hypothesis, as the term suggests, always assumes *no* relationship, *no* change, *no* difference, *no* association and so forth.

Identify and state the alternative hypothesis: If the null hypothesis states that there is no difference or relationship, then the alternative hypothesis always states that there is a difference or relationship between your sample statistic and the population, or your sample and another sample. For example, the alternative hypothesis may state: 'There is a difference between the mean value of the study sample and the population mean'. An alternative hypothesis which states that there is a difference is called a two-sided or two-tailed hypothesis test. If the alternative hypothesis was more specific, and stated: 'The sample mean is less than the population mean', or if it stated: 'The sample mean is greater than the population mean', then it is said that a one-sided or one-tailed hypothesis test is required. The choice of whether to use a two-tailed or one-tailed hypothesis test is up to the researcher, and will depend on the application. If the researcher is unsure, then a two-tailed test is usually chosen.

Compute the test statistic and the related p-value: The type of statistic to compute will depend on the type of data and the study design. If the data are categorical, the test statistic may be a chi-square, denoted by χ^2. If the sample size is small it may be a Fisher's exact statistic. If the data are continuous and the mean value is to be tested, then the test statistic may be a t-value. If a non-parametric test is to be used the test statistic may be a Mann Whitney U value, and so forth. Once the test statistic is decided then the probability, p, of getting that statistic, given your data, is computed. This is usually computed by a statistical software package but can be computed by hand.

Make a decision to reject or not to reject the null hypothesis: The fourth step in hypothesis testing is to make the decision whether or not to reject the null hypothesis. The decision is easy to make once the p-value is calculated. In general, the null hypothesis is rejected if the p-value is less than or equal to 5 per cent: $p \leq 0.05$. The value 0.05 is called the α (alpha) value, and it is the probability of making a type 1 error: that is, the probability of rejecting the null hypothesis when in fact the null hypothesis is true. In some cases, for example in clinical trials, the alpha value is set at 1 per cent or $\alpha = 0.01$. In other cases, for example in pilot studies testing interventions, the alpha value is set at 10 per cent or $\alpha = 0.10$. If the researcher is unsure of the alpha value, the standard approach is to choose 5 per cent, $\alpha = 0.05$ (Scot and Mazhindu 2009).

State the conclusion: Once the decision to reject or not reject the null hypothesis is taken, the researcher must state the implications of that decision – that is, the result of the hypothesis test must be concluded. This is in effect the answer to the test and in applied research this is the most interesting and meaningful step. The conclusion will follow on from the original hypothesis. For example, if the null hypothesis is not rejected the conclusion may take the form: 'There is no difference between the mean value of sample one and the mean value of sample two'. If the null hypothesis is rejected and a two-tailed test was conducted, the conclusion will take the form: 'There is a difference between the mean value of sample one and the mean value of sample two'. If a one-tailed test was conducted and the null hypothesis was rejected, then the conclusion may take the form: 'The mean value of sample one is less than the mean value of sample two', and so forth.

A two-minute video summary of the steps in a hypothesis can be found on YouTube at http://www.youtube.com/watch?v=_oYnItIapTk

Analysing categorical data

Earlier, the different types of data that might be generated in a research study were explained and the steps taken when performing hypothesis or significance tests (regardless of the type of data) were described. In this section these two topics are brought together to demonstrate the types of statistics that need to be used for analysing both nominal and ordinal categorical data. For nominal and ordinal categorical data the chi-square test, the Fisher's exact test for small samples, and the McNemar and Cochran's Q test for two or more related samples are explained. For ordinal data with three or more related samples the Friedman test and correlation statistics are described (Plichta and Kelvin 2013).

Two-way contingency tables and chi-square tests

With both nominal and ordinal categorical data, researchers are often interested to know if there is an association between two variables or if the two variables are independent of one another. For example, one may wish to know if there is an association between level of nurse education and level of the quality of patient care, or if they are independent of one another. Similarly, a researcher may wish to know if there is an association between gender and parenting style or between age group and income group. To test for independence of two categorical variables the simplest test to use is a chi-square test. For each chi-square test the null hypothesis is given by a statement of the form, *there is no association between variable one and variable two* (that is, variables one and two are independent of one another). The alternative hypothesis test is therefore stated as, *there is an association between variable one and variable two* (that is, variables one and two are dependent on one another). Note how the alternative hypothesis suggests a two-tailed test, as the researcher is only interested in whether or not there is an association rather than any less than or greater than relationship between the two variables. A full example of the chi-square test is provided below.

Example

A professor of paediatrics wishes to know if there is an association between the side a mother holds her baby on and the hand the mother writes with. A sample of 287 mothers were interviewed and the results are presented in Table 18.1. Test the association at the 1 per cent level of significance.

Table 18.1 Numbers of mothers who hold their baby on a particular side and the mother's handedness

		Side		
		Left	*Right*	*Totals*
	Left	25	7	32
Hand	Right	212	43	255
	Totals	237	50	287

The null hypothesis is: 'There is no association between the side a mother holds her baby on and handedness' (the two variables are independent).

The alternative hypothesis is: 'There is an association' (the two variables are dependent).

The chi-square statistic is: $\chi^2 = 0.50$.

The probability of getting this chi-square value given the two variables are independent is found to be $p > 0.01$.

As the p-value is greater than the alpha, $p \geq 0.01$, the paediatrician decides not to reject the null hypothesis. The paediatrician concludes that the side a mother holds her baby on is not associated with handedness (that is, the side a mother holds her baby on is independent of handedness).

The value of the chi-square statistic is found using a common statistical software package such as SPSS (Field 2009) but it can be computed by hand for tables with two rows and two columns. The formulae for computation are available in any undergraduate statistics textbook.

Violations of the chi-square test and Fisher's exact test for small samples

The chi-square value is based on the differences between the observed values in Table 18.1 and the values the researcher would expect to see in the table if the variables were independent. The chi-square test is not reliable if two or more of the expected values are less than 5. If this occurs the statistical package will often still compute the chi-square and the p-value, but the software may issue a warning. This situation can occur when the researcher is working with a small sample size, when the researcher has a large study but is looking at the occurrence of rare events, or when the researcher again has a large study but wishes to study smaller groups within the large sample. When two or more of the expected values are less than 5 then it is said that an assumption of the chi-square test is violated, and Fisher's exact test may be used.

Example of Fisher's exact test

Two schools decided to test the implementation of a Healthy Schools programme. One school was randomly chosen to be the school to receive the intervention and the other school was the control. Researchers wished to see if the health of the children in the two schools differed in any way prior to the implementation of the intervention, as if they did differ this might influence the interpretation of the results following the intervention. Children in the age range 8 to 12 years old were asked how often they drank alcohol, and the results are presented in Table 18.2. The school nurse wished to see if the frequency of alcohol consumption was independent of the type of school.

The null hypothesis is: 'There is no association between the frequency of alcohol use and the type of school (intervention or control)' (the two variables are independent).

Table 18.2 How often do children in intervention and comparison schools drink alcohol?

	Intervention (I) Comparison (C)	Self-report children aged 8 to 12 years		Total
		I	*C*	
How often do you drink alcohol?	**Never**	79.8% 142	61.3% 38	180
	One or two times ever	15.7% 28	30.6% 19	47
	Sometimes (on special occasions)	2.8% 5	1.6% 1	6
	Once or twice a week	0.6% 1	0.0% 0	1
	I don't know	1.1% 2	6.5% 4	6
Total		178	62	240

The alternative hypothesis is: 'There is an association' (the two variables are dependent).

The Fisher's exact statistic is: Fisher's exact = 12.214.

The probability of getting this value given the two variables are independent is: $p = 0.007$.

The p-value is less than the alpha, $p \leq 0.05$.

The school nurse decides to reject the null hypothesis. The school nurse concludes that there is an association between the frequency of alcohol use and the type of school (intervention or control) and the two variables are dependent – that is to say there is an association between frequency of alcohol use and type of school.

From Table 18.2 it can be observed that the pattern of use between the two types of school does appear to differ. Just under 80 per cent of children in the intervention school and just over 60 per cent of comparison school children indicated they never drank alcohol. In comparison, a little over 3 per cent of intervention school children and less than 2 per cent of comparison school children indicated they drank alcohol either 'sometimes' or 'once/twice a week'.

The value of the Fisher's exact statistic may be found using a common statistical software package such as SPSS (Field 2009). While it, too, can be computed by hand and the formulae for computation are available in any undergraduate statistics textbook (Field 2009), unlike the chi-square statistic its computation requires considerable work.

Table 18.3   Data required for a McNemar test

		Results at time point 1	
		No (absent)	Yes (present)
Result at time point 2	No (absent)	n_{11}	n_{12}
	Yes (present)	n_{21}	n_{22}

Binary data, two related samples and the McNemar test

In the previous example the two schools were not necessarily related. Often a researcher is following a group of study participants over a period of time, and may wish to see if a result observed at one time point is independent of a result observed at a second time point. This situation occurs quite often in outcome studies where participants are observed before and after treatment. In these situations researchers may use the McNemar test. In general, data on frequencies of the form specified in Table 18.3 are required.

In practice, however, all of the data in Table 18.3 is not reported. A practical example of a McNemar test is provided below and in Table 18.4.

Example of a McNemar test

A policymaker responsible for financing methadone treatment services for heroin users wishes to measure the proportion abstinent from heroin one year after treatment. The percentage abstinent at intake and at one year following treatment is measured with a cohort of 82 clients in receipt of methadone. The results are presented in Table 18.4.

The null hypothesis is: 'The proportion abstinent is independent of treatment' (there is no association between abstinence and treatment).

The alternative hypothesis is: 'The proportion abstinent is dependent on treatment'.

The test statistic is the McNemar test and the p-value is less than the alpha value of 1 per cent, $p < 0.01$. Therefore, the policymaker decides to reject the null hypothesis. The policymaker concludes that the proportion abstinent does depend on methadone treatment.

Table 18.4   Proportions abstinent from heroin use at intake to and one year after methadone treatment

	Intake to treatment % (n/N)	One year following treatment intake % (n/N)	Test of significance
% abstinent	6 (5/82)	33 (27/82)	McNemar $p < 0.01$

Binary data, three related samples and Cochran's Q test

When comparing data of the same nature as described above but across three time points Cochran's Q test may be applied. This is simply an extension of the McNamara testing procedure. In the event of a significant or close to significant result in Cochran's Q test the researcher may then decide to do a further analysis of all pairwise comparisons between the time points.

Ordinal data, three related samples and Friedman's test

In circumstances where data are ordinal and comparisons are to be made across more than two time points the Friedman's test may be used. This procedure considers the score given by a participant to a particular question at each time point under consideration. These scores are then ranked across time points. This is performed for each participant contributing a score to each time point and the ranks are summed over each time point for all of the participants. If the time points have summed ranks that do not differ largely then there will not be a significant time effect. On the other hand, if the summed ranks differ greatly across the time points this will result in a significant test statistic. Examples of the Friedman test are provided in Plichta and Kelvin (2013).

Numerical or ordinal data and appropriate correlation tests

Correlation is a statistical technique that measures the extent of a relationship between two variables. For example, in a study involving children a researcher might suspect that there is a relationship between a child's weight and their height. As height increases weight might be expected to increase also and a positive correlation may exist. Alternatively, a researcher working with an ageing population may suspect that as age increases bone density decreases and a negative correlation between these two variables is suspected. The simplest way to check if a relationship exists between two variables is to plot or graph one set of values against the other. If from the graph the researcher believes that a relationship exists then the strength and the direction of this relationship can be statistically tested by computing an appropriate correlation coefficient.

It should be noted that correlations are most appropriate for numerical data. They can be computed for ordinal data but cannot be computed for purely categorical data such as gender, ethnicity etc. When working with numerical data correlations produce precise numbers; when working with ordinal data correlations provide general indications, as ranks are not precise numbers equal distances apart. For example, when coding responses to the question 'how is your health?', one researcher may code the responses poor, average and excellent as 0, 1, 2 and another may code them as 0, 1, 3 as that researcher may believe excellent health to be far greater than average health.

The main result in a correlation test is the derivation of the correlation coefficient. This value can vary from a minimum of -1 to a maximum of $+1$. Values close to $+1$ indicate a strong correlation between the two variables. Positive values indicate that as one variable increases so too does the second; negative values indicate that as one variable increases the other decreases.

Pearson's correlation coefficient, denoted by rho or ρ for a population and r for sample data, should be computed for numerical data. A value close to +1 or –1 indicates a positive or negative linear relationship and graphing the two variables against one another should illustrate this linear relationship.

Spearman's rank correlation, also denoted for a population by the Greek letter rho or ρ, and Kendal's correlation, denoted by the Greek letter tau or τ, do not indicate a linear relationship but rather provide a measure of the association between two ranked or ordinal variables. Kendal's tau is more appropriate for square tables where the number of rows equals the number of columns. With sample data, to distinguish between Pearson's and Spearman's correlation a subscript is often used, hence r_s denotes Spearman's correlation. An example is provided below.

Example

In a national evaluation of advanced nursing roles in a range of hospitals, patients were asked a series of questions about the quality of the communication they had with their nurse. Responses to two questions are provided in Table 18.5. Researchers believe that the responses to these two questions are related and compute Spearman's correlation coefficient and a hypothesis test to check their assumption.

The null hypothesis is: 'There is no association between the responses to the two questions'. Spearman's sample correlation coefficient $r_s = 0$.

The alternative hypothesis is: 'There is an association between the responses to the two questions'. Spearman's correlation coefficient $r_s \neq 0$ (a two-tailed hypothesis).

Using a statistical software package it is found that the sample Spearman's rho $r_s = 0.240$ and the p-value is given as $p \leq 0.001$. Therefore the researchers decide to reject the null hypothesis at the $\alpha = 0.001$ level. The researchers conclude that there is an association (positive correlation) between the responses to the two questions.

Table 18.5 Questions asked of service users in an evaluation of advanced nursing roles

	When you had important questions to ask did you get answers you could understand?		Overall, did you feel you were treated with respect and dignity while you were in the hospital or service?	
	%	n	%	N
Yes, always	86.6	129	88.6	132
Yes, sometimes	9.4	14	10.7	16
No	1.3	2	0.7	1
I had no need to ask	2.7	4	0	0

Analysing numerical or scale data

The normal distribution and determining if data are normally distributed

Before starting statistical analysis on data it is essential to determine if the data are normally distributed. The most important distribution when describing continuous random variables is the normal probability distribution as it will determine the type of inferential procedure required when analysing the data – whether parametric or non-parametric statistical tests are appropriate.

Plotting the data

Often in health care research it is useful to illustrate the dataset to gain an initial understanding of the dataset. Plotting is the graphical technique used to illustrate the dataset. A graphical representation of the data can be used to demonstrate a relationship between one or more variables, for example the relationship between age and height or the relationship between smoking mothers and the birth weights of their infants. A scatter plot to demonstrate the relationship between the age and height of babies is provided in Figure 18.1.

Normally distributed data

Quite often in research, when plotting data from a large sample observations seem to follow a bell-shaped pattern (see http://www.netmba.com/statistics/distribution/normal/ for further information). As this pattern occurs quite regularly it is known as the normal distribution. Normal distributions are symmetrical bell-shaped curves with the greatest frequency of scores in the middle and lower frequency of scores at either extremity. There are many different normal distributions which can be determined by the mean μ and standard deviation σ of the sample. A normal distribution is centred around the mean μ and the spread of the curve is determined by the standard deviation σ.

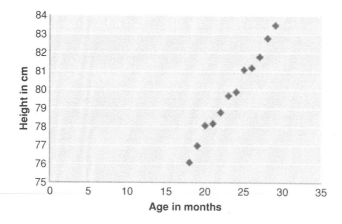

Figure 18.1   Scatter plot of age in months and heights in cm of a random sample of babies.

Characteristics of the normal distribution

- The highest point of the normal curve is at the centre, which is the mean μ.
- The distribution is symmetrical about the vertical line $x = \mu$, the left half of the curve is the mirror image of the right half, and the measure of skewness is 0.
- The standard deviation σ determines the spread of the curve; a large standard deviation will result in a wider, flatter curve and a small standard deviation will result in a narrow, more peaked curve.

As with all probability density functions, the total area under the normal distribution curve is 1.

Tests for normality, kurtosis and skewness

Plotting one's data on a histogram and comparing it to a normal probability density curve is an informal approach researchers sometimes take to ascertain if their data follow a normal distribution. The statistical package Minitab can be used to determine whether data follow a normal distribution using this graphical approach (see http://www.minitab.com).

The kurtosis is the measure of how peaked or flat the data are compared to the normal distribution curve. The kurtosis of the standard normal distribution curve is 3; data with kurtosis of more than 3 tend to be peaked near the mean, and those with low kurtosis tend to have a flat top near the mean. With some statistical software packages kurtosis can be computed in an alternative way, and in these cases the usual value of kurtosis is 0. With the alternative definition, positive kurtosis indicates a peaked distribution and negative kurtosis indicates a flat distribution.

The skewness of the data measures how symmetrical the data are; the normal distribution is a bell-shaped statistical curve and therefore the skewness of the normal distribution is 0. If the data follow a normal distribution they will have skewness close to 0. Data which are skewed to the left will have a negative value for skewness while data with positive values indicates data are skewed to the right. As a guide, a skewness value more than twice its standard error is taken to indicate a departure from symmetry. The skewness and kurtosis of data can be tested using the statistical package SPSS (Field 2009).

Z-tests for large samples

Data which are normally distributed, centred on zero, $\mu = 0$ and with a standard deviation of 1, $\sigma = 1$ are said to have standard normal distribution. The standard normal distribution is denoted by the letter Z. To determine the probability of an area under a normal curve the standard normal curve and the z tables are required (Peck and Devore 2011).

Firstly it must be determined whether a one-tailed or two-tailed test is required. If the data do not follow a standard normal distribution with $\mu = 0$ and $\sigma = 1$ then they must be converted from the approximate normal distribution to the standard distribution using the formula:

$$Z = \frac{X - \mu}{\sigma}$$

Once the Z value is calculated, use the Z tables to find the area under the standard normal curve to the left of the Z value.

Example

The length of pregnancy from conception to birth in an obstetrics and gynaecology clinic varies according to a distribution that is approximately normal with a mean of 266 days and a standard deviation of 16 days.

a   Determine the probability that a randomly selected woman will have a pregnancy of more than 278 days from conception to birth.

b   What percentage of women will have a pregnancy lasting between 258 and 278 days from conception to birth?

Part a:

Step 1: Determine the probability that the randomly selected woman's pregnancy will last more than 278 days, therefore a one-tailed Z-test is required.

Step 2: Convert to a standard normal distribution. The mean length of pregnancy $\mu = 266$. Let X be the length of the pregnancy, 278 days, and the standard deviation $\sigma = 16$, then:

$$P(X > 278) = P\left(Z > \frac{278 - 266}{16} = 0.75 \right)$$

Step 3: Determine the probability of $Z > 0.75$ using the cumulative probability table for the normal distribution:

$$P(Z > 0.75) = 1 - P(Z < 0.75)$$
$$= 1 - 0.7734$$
$$= 0.2266$$

There is a 23 per cent chance that the randomly selected woman will have a pregnancy lasting more than 278 days.

Part b:

Step 1: Determine the probability that the randomly selected woman's pregnancy will last between 258 and 278 days, therefore a two-tailed z-test is required.

Step 2: Let X be the length of pregnancy, the proportion of women with $258 \leq X \leq 278$ must be determined. Firstly convert to a standard normal distribution:

$$P(258 \leq X \leq 278) = P\left(\frac{258 - 266}{16} \leq Z \leq \frac{278 - 266}{16} \right)$$

$$= -0.5 \leq Z \leq 0.75$$

Step 3: As the standard normal distribution curve is symmetrical, the left side is the mirror image of the right side. Determine the probability of $Z > 0.5$ and $Z > 0.75$ using the cumulative probability table for the standard normal distribution:

$$P(-0.5 \leq Z \leq 0.75) = (1 - P(Z < 0.5)) + (1 - P(Z < 0.75))$$

$$= (1 - 0.6915) + (1 - 0.7734)$$

$$= 0.3085 + 0.2266$$

$$= 0.5351$$

The proportion of women having a pregnancy lasting between 258 and 278 days from conception to birth is 54 per cent.

A researcher will often have to make a decision regarding their research question based on the outcome of the statistical procedure they conduct, which may result in choosing a course of action associated with the null hypothesis or the alternative hypothesis. The approach outlined in hypothesis testing for conducting a hypothesis test regardless of the type of data or statistic used is demonstrated when testing the mean of some normal population below.

Example

An ambulance service claims that, on average, it takes no more than 8.9 minutes to reach its destination in emergency calls. To test this claim, a random sample of 50 emergency calls gave a sample mean of 9.3 minutes with a standard deviation of 1.9 minutes. Using this example, test at the 5 per cent significance level if the ambulance service's claim is true.

The null hypothesis is that: 'There is no difference in the time it takes an ambulance to reach its destination in an emergency'. $H_0: \mu = 8.9$.

The alternative hypothesis is that: 'It takes an ambulance more than 8.9 minutes to reach its destination in an emergency' (one-tailed test). $H_A: \mu > 8.9$.

x: time to reach destination. The sample size n = 50, the sample mean $\bar{x} = 9.3$ and the sample standard deviation $s = \hat{\sigma} = 1.9$ are substituted into the formula for the sample statistic:

$$Z = \left(\frac{\bar{x} - \mu_0}{\hat{\sigma} / \sqrt{n}} \right)$$

$$Z = \left(\frac{9.3 - 8.9}{1.9 / \sqrt{50}} \right)$$

$$Z = 1.49$$

$$P(Z > 1.49) = 1 - P(Z \leq 1.49)$$

$$= 1 - 0.9319$$

$$= 0.0681$$

The p-value of 0.0681 is greater than the α, p > 0.05, therefore do not reject the null hypothesis at the 5 per cent significance level. Conclude that the mean time to reach the destination is 8.9 minutes as claimed by the ambulance service.

t-tests for small samples

It is often the case in health care research that health care professionals will conduct studies which deal with a sensitive issue or a largely hidden population. As a result, the sample size will be small. Regardless of the scale of the study, there are important research questions that can and must be addressed once the appropriate statistical test is chosen. For small samples of n < 30 it is no longer acceptable to regard the standard deviation s as an accurate estimate for σ as it was in the section on Z-tests for large populations. If the sample size is small and the population X is considered approximately normal with mean μ and standard deviation σ then

$$t = \frac{(\bar{x} - \mu)}{(\hat{\sigma} / \sqrt{n})}$$

has the t-distribution.

Characteristics of the t-distribution

- There is no single t-distribution but rather a family of distributions which differ based on the number of degrees of freedom, d.f. = n − 1.
- Similar to the standard normal distribution, the t-distribution is centred on 0; however, the standard deviation is greater than 1.
- For d.f. = n − 1 (n ≥ 30) the t-distribution is approximately the standard normal distribution.

Example

The mean pulse rate for adult males is 72 beats per minute. A random sample of eight overweight males gave the following data in Table 18.6.

Do these findings suggest at the α = 0.05 level of significance that the mean pulse for overweight males is significantly greater than 72?

Table 18.6   Pulse rates for eight adult males

Person	1	2	3	4	5	6	7	8
Pulse rate	78	90	71	74	76	75	62	82

The null hypothesis states: 'There is no difference in the mean pulse rate', H_0: $\mu = 72$.

The alternative hypothesis states: 'The mean pulse rate for overweight males is greater than 72' (one-tailed test), H_A: $\mu > 72$.

The mean population pulse rate is $\mu = 72$, the sample mean $\bar{x} = 76$, the sample standard deviation $s = 8.1$ and sample size $n = 8$, then the test statistic t is:

$$t = \left(\frac{\bar{x} - \mu_0}{\hat{\sigma} / \sqrt{n}} \right)$$

$$= \left(\frac{76 - 72}{8.1 / \sqrt{8}} \right)$$

$$t = 1.39$$

From the t tables (Peck and Devore 2011), $t_{8-1} = 1.895$ is greater than 1.39, therefore we do not reject the null hypothesis at $\alpha = 0.05$. We therefore conclude that the mean pulse rate for overweight males is not significantly different from 72.

Compare means – t-test

It is quite often necessary in research to compare two groups, two different treatment types or even outcomes after an intervention. A researcher may be interested in comparing the health outcomes of drug users before and after treatment or the health outcomes of two groups of drug users in different treatment programmes. It is important to decide whether examining the difference in a group before and after an intervention or the difference between two independent groups is of interest.

If a researcher wishes to determine if there are statistically significant differences in the same group pre-intervention and post-intervention, for example the HbA1c levels in a group of patients with type 2 diabetes before and after introducing a new diet and exercise plan, a paired samples t-test must be conducted. In order to conduct a paired samples t-test a categorical variable with two groups, such as pre- and post-intervention groups, and a continuous variable such as the HbA1c level are required. The continuous variable HbA1c must be measured at two time points – pre- and post-diet and exercise intervention – to conduct a matched pairs t-test.

Example

The average weekly loss in work hours due to work-related accidents in ten health centres before and after a new health and safety programme was implemented is demonstrated in Table 18.7.

Test whether the health and safety programme is effective at the 5 per cent significance level.

Table 18.7   Average weekly work hours lost due to work-related accidents before
and after new health and safety programme

	Average time lost		
Health centre	Before	After	Difference
Centre A	45	36	9
Centre B	73	60	13
Centre C	46	44	2
Centre D	123	118	5
Centre E	33	35	−2
Centre F	57	51	6
Centre G	83	77	6
Centre H	34	29	5
Centre I	26	24	2
Centre J	17	11	6

The mean difference, $\mu_d = \mu_{pre} - \mu_{post}$

The null hypothesis states: 'There is no difference in the hours lost pre- and post-
intervention', H_0: $\mu_d = 0$.

The alternative hypothesis states: 'There is some difference in the hours lost post-
intervention', H_A: $\mu_d > 0$.

$$n = 10, \ \bar{x}_d = 5.2, \ \hat{\sigma}_d = 4.08, \ \text{d.f.} = n - 1 = 9$$

$$t = \frac{\bar{x}_d - \mu_d}{\hat{\sigma}_d / \sqrt{n}}$$

$$t = \frac{5.2 - 0}{4.08 / \sqrt{10}}$$

$$t = 4.03$$

$$t_{10-1} = 1.833$$

$t = 4.03 > t_9 = 1.833$ therefore reject the null hypothesis at the 5 per cent significance level and conclude that the health and safety programme is effective.

It may be the case that a researcher wishes to determine if there are statistically significant differences in the means from two different groups, for example the
self-esteem scores of males and females, then an independent samples t-test must be

conducted. To conduct an independent samples t-test a categorical variable such as gender and a continuous variable such as self-esteem score are required. The samples must be selected independently and can be of different sizes.

Example

The average number of patients which a random sample of general practitioners from two different clinics treat over a fixed period of time is presented in Table 18.8.

Is there a significant difference between the mean number of patients seen at the clinics?

Table 18.8 The average number of patients seen by GPs in clinic A and clinic B

Number of patients treated	
Clinic A	Clinic B
52	55
61	24
37	43
64	34
56	63
39	45
62	
47	
41	

X_1: the number of patients treated by a GP in clinic A
X_2: the number of patients treated by a GP in clinic B
The null hypothesis states: 'There is no difference between the mean number of patients seen at clinic A and at clinic B', H_0: $\mu_A = \mu_B$.
The alternative hypothesis states: 'There is some difference between the mean number of patients seen at clinic A and at clinic B', H_A: $\mu_A > \mu_B$.

$$n_A = 9,\ \bar{x}_A = 51,\ n_B = 6,\ \bar{x}_B = 44,\ \hat{\sigma}^2 = 142.8,\ \text{d.f.} = n_A + n_B - 2 = 9 + 6 - 2 = 13$$

$$t = \frac{\bar{x}_A - \bar{x}_B}{\sqrt{\hat{\sigma}^2(1/n_A + 1/n_B)}}$$

$$t = \frac{51 - 44}{\sqrt{142.8(1/9 + 1/6)}}$$

$$t = 1.11$$

$$t_{13} = 2.16$$

$t = 1.11 < t_{13} = 2.16$, therefore do not reject the null hypothesis at the 5 per cent significance level and conclude that there is no significant difference in the mean number of patients treated at the clinics.

Transforming non-normal data

In general, with large sample sizes data will be sufficiently close to a normal distribution to allow for the usual parametric tests to be conducted. However in some cases a situation may arise where this is not the case and the data must be transformed before any statistical tests are conducted. The three main ways to do this are the square root function, the natural log transform (denoted by ln) and the log to the base 10 transform. These transformations and many others are available on standard statistical packages. An example is provided below.

Example

A researcher working in a drug treatment centre measured the number of days clients had used heroin in the last three months, both at treatment intake to a methadone programme and one year following treatment intake. At one year follow-up the number of days clients had used heroin within the last 90 days is provided in Figure 18.2. The skewness value for these data was 1.895 and the kurtosis value was 2.260. For a normal distribution these values should be close to 0.

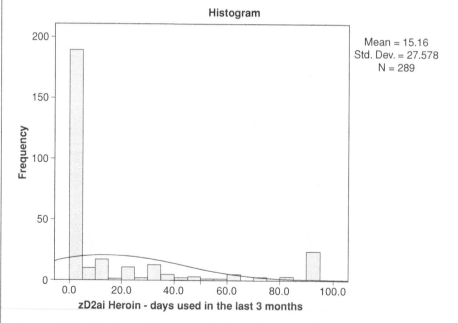

Figure 18.2 Number of clients who had used heroin on between 0 and 90 days in the last three months.

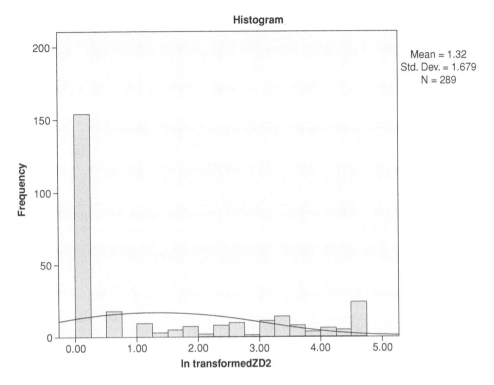

Figure 18.3 Plot illustrating the transformed data from Figure 18.2, that is the frequencies of the natural log of (days clients used heroin in last three months at one year follow-up + 1).

The researcher decided to transform the data using the natural log transformation, that is, the researcher first added the value 1 to each response and then obtained the natural log of that new number. The formula used was:

Days clients used heroin in last three months at one year follow-up = ln (days clients used heroin in last three months at one year follow-up + 1)

where ln denoted the natural log and +1 was added to each data point as the natural log of zero cannot be computed.

Frequencies for the data were plotted again and the new skewness value was 0.803 and kurtosis was −0.991. The revised plot of the new frequencies is provided in Figure 18.3.

Using non-parametric methods when transformations don't work

In the previous section the techniques for transforming non-normal data were outlined, however it is often the case that these transformations will not work and an alternative needs to be considered. If transformations are not appropriate, the use of non-parametric techniques to analyse the data can be considered. Non-parametric techniques are more robust tests which do not make assumptions about the underlying population of the distribution; these are often called distribution-free tests. These tests are appropriate when the sample size is very small or if the data violate one of the stringent assumptions of the parametric tests, such as normality.

The median and the Mann Whitney U-test for two independent samples

Often a researcher is interested in testing to see if there are differences between two independent groups. For example, the researcher may wish to know if there are differences in the health and well-being of patients with type 1 diabetes and type 2 diabetes. The Mann Whitney U-test is the non-parametric alternative to the independent samples t-test if the sample size is very small or the data violate the assumptions for an independent samples t-test. The Mann Whitney U-test compares the medians of the two groups. It is assumed that the group distributions have the same shape and possibly different medians. The observations across the two groups are ranked and then evaluated to determine if there are differences in the ranks across the two groups.

Example

Of the 17 babies born in a 24-hour period in a hospital, nine were born to non-smoking mothers and eight were born to smoking mothers. The birth weights of the infants are illustrated in Table 18.9.

Test at the 5 per cent significance level that the birth weight of babies born to non-smoking mothers is significantly greater than that for smoking mothers.

Table 18.9   Birth weights of babies born to smoking and non-smoking mothers

Birth weight (grams)			
Non-smoking mother	Rank	Smoking mother	Rank
3166	9	3204	10
2971	6	2809	3
3666	16	2771	2
3405	14	3133	8
2980	7	3476	15
3741	17	3222	12
2864	4	2732	1
3227	13	2934	5
3220	11		

The null hypothesis states: 'There is no difference in the medians of the two groups', $H_0: M_1 = M_2$.

The alternative hypothesis states: 'The median weight of infants born to non-smoking mothers is greater than that of babies born to smoking mothers', $H_A: M_1 > M_2$.

$$Z = -1.491$$
$$\text{p-value} = P(Z \leq -1.491)$$
$$= 0.0681$$

The p-value is greater than the 5 per cent significance level, therefore do not reject the null hypothesis and conclude that birth weights of babies born to non-smoking mothers are not significantly greater than those born to smoking mothers.

If testing for differences in three or more independent samples, the Kruskal-Wallis test must be used.

The median and the Wilcoxon test for two related or paired samples

The Wilcoxon Signed Rank Test is the non-parametric alternative to the paired samples t-test if the sample available is very small or if the data violate the assumptions for a paired samples t-test. The Wilcoxon Signed Rank is used when data for the sample are measured at two time points, for example before and after treatment. The test converts the scores to ranks and compares the medians at the two time points.

Example

The statistical knowledge of 29 student nurses was measured before and after attending a statistics for health care professionals course. Test at the 5 per cent significance level if there was a difference in their knowledge before and after the course.

The null hypothesis states: 'There is no difference in the nurses' knowledge before and after the course, $H_0: M_1 = M_2$.

The alternative hypothesis states: 'There is a difference in the nurses' knowledge before and after the course', $H_A: M_1 \neq M_2$.

$$Z = -2.115$$
$$\text{p-value} = 0.034$$

The p-value is less than the 5 per cent significance level, therefore reject the null hypothesis and conclude that there is a difference in the nurses' knowledge after attending a course in statistics for health care professionals.

The non-parametric tests mentioned in the previous sections can be conducted using the statistical package SPSS (Pallant 2010).

Conclusion

This chapter demonstrated how to approach the analysis of data arising not only from large-scale studies, but also smaller ones with fewer cases or participants as well as those with non-normally distributed data. In addition to the usual key statistical tests available for analysing data, other less well-known and less frequently used – but nonetheless, equally powerful – statistical tests were presented.

Key concepts

- Prior to deciding on the statistical test to use the data type must be identified.
- It is important to understand the nature of a hypothesis test and to understand that, while you may use different statistical formulae or tests, the steps in the hypothesis test do not change.
- The final steps in a hypothesis test stating the decision, conclusion and interpretation are of the greatest interest and have most relevance to the research question under study.

Key readings in analysing data from small and large samples

- J. Pallant, *SPSS Survival Manual: A Step by Step Guide to Data Analysis Using the SPSS Program*, 4th edn (Maidenhead: Open University Press, 2010)
  This is an invaluable hands-on book that describes the step-by-step process of conducting your hypothesis tests in the statistical package SPSS.
- S.B. Plichta and E. Kelvin, *Munro's Statistical Methods for Health Care Research*, 6th edn (London: Wolters Kluwer/Lippincott Williams & Wilkins, 2013)
  This book is useful for explaining the detailed statistics in a simple and clear way.

Examples of the use of analysis from small and large samples in health care research

- C.M. Comiskey, A 3 year national longitudinal study comparing drug treatment outcomes for opioid users with and without children in their custodial care at intake, *Journal of Substance Abuse Treatment*, 44(1) (2013), 90–6
- C. Begley, N. Elliott, J. Lalor, I. Coyne, A. Higgins and C. Comiskey, Differences between clinical specialist and advanced practitioner clinical practice, leadership, and research roles, responsibilities, and perceived outcomes (The SCAPE Study), *Journal of Advanced Nursing*, 69(6) (2012), 1323–37, doi:10.1111/j.1365-2648.2012.06124.x
- E. Hollywood, C.M. Comiskey, T. Begley, A. Snel, K. O'Sullivan, M. Quirke and C. Wynne, Measuring and modelling body mass index among a cohort of urban children living with disadvantage, *Journal of Advanced Nursing*, 69(4) (2013), 851–61, doi:10.1111/j.1365-2648.2012.06071.x

- J. Ballard, M. Mooney and O. Dempsey, Prevalence of frailty-related risk factors in older adults seen by community nurses, *Journal of Advanced Nursing*, 69(3) (2013), 675–84, doi:10.1111/j.1365-2648.2012.06054.x
- E. Smith, C.M., Comiskey A. Carroll and N. Ryall, A study of bone mineral density in lower limb amputees at a national prosthetics centre, *JPO Journal of Prosthetics & Orthotics*, 23(1) (2011), 14-20, doi:10.1097/JPO.0b013e318206dd72
- C.M. Comiskey and F. Larkan, A national cross-sectional survey of diagnosed sufferers of myalgic encephalomyelitis/chronic fatigue syndrome: Pathways to diagnosis, changes in quality of life and service priorities, *Irish Journal of Medical Science*, 179(4) (2010), 501–5

References

Field, A. (2009) *Discovering Statistics Using SPSS*, 3rd edn. London: Sage.

Lerman, C., Trock, B., Rimer, B.K., Jepson, C., Brody, D. and Boyce, A. (1991) Psychological side effects of breast cancer screening, *Health Psychology*, 10(4): 259–67.

Pallant, J. (2010) *SPSS Survival Manual: A Step by Step Guide to Data Analysis Using the SPSS Program*, 4th edn. Maidenhead: Open University Press.

Page, R.M., Cole, G.E. and Timmreck, T.C. (1995) *Basic Epidemiological Methods and Biostatistics: A Practical Guidebook*. London: Jones and Bartlett.

Peck, R. and Devore, J.L. (2011) *Statistics: The Exploration & Analysis of Data*, 7th edn. Boston, MA: Brooks/Cole.

Plichta, S.B. and Kelvin, E. (2013) *Munro's Statistical Methods for Health Care Research*, 6th edn. London: Wolters Kluwer/Lippincott Williams & Wilkins.

Scot, I. and Mazhindu, D. (2009) *Statistics for Healthcare Professionals an Introduction*. London: Sage.

19 Secondary data analysis

Deirdre Mongan

Chapter topics

- Advantages and disadvantages of secondary data analysis
- Locating datasets for secondary data analysis
- Ethical issues
- How to determine the feasibility and appropriateness of using a dataset for secondary data analysis
- Analysing secondary data
- Examples of secondary datasets and how they can be used for health care research

Introduction

Secondary data analysis can be described as the reanalysis of existing data or information that was either gathered by someone else or for some other purpose than the one currently being considered. The secondary analysis may explore a new research question or a different perspective on the original research question. It may literally be defined as 'second-hand' analysis. As studies often contain more data than are analysed by the original researchers, a variety of research projects can be undertaken using these existing data.

Secondary data analysis differs from primary data analysis in that primary data are collected by the researcher or research team who also analyse that data. With primary research, the researcher conceives of and designs the research study, collects the data from the research participants and analyses the data they have collected. While researchers may prefer to design and undertake their own research, this may actually be a waste of valuable time and resources, since it is not always necessary to undertake primary research in order to answer a unique research question.

Increasingly, there is a trend towards expedient and economical health research that can answer research questions in a timely manner and be relevant for policymakers. While collecting primary data is often the best way to obtain the information necessary to answer a particular research question, high-quality primary research can be expensive and time-consuming to conduct and may not always be feasible. If secondary data analysis is undertaken with due thoroughness and diligence it can provide a cost-effective alternative for understanding and answering research questions.

Secondary data are also helpful in designing subsequent primary research, and can provide a baseline with which to compare primary data-collection results. Therefore, it is always wise to begin any research activity with a review of the secondary data. The analysis of existing data can help to define a research question more clearly and can then lead to the generation of more hypotheses. Secondary analysis differs from systematic reviews and meta-analyses of studies, whose objective is to combine the results of several studies that address a set of related research hypotheses. Examples of secondary data sources include survey data and data found in administrative and clinical databases. In this chapter I describe the advantages and disadvantages of secondary data analysis, how to locate relevant datasets and how to assess the quality of and analyse secondary data.

Advantages of secondary data analysis

The primary advantage of secondary data analysis is its potential for cost effectiveness, in terms of both time and money. Where high-quality datasets are available for secondary data analysis, it is considerably cheaper and faster for researchers to use these existing data rather than collecting primary data. With secondary data analysis the researcher benefits from the time and effort involved in gathering the original primary data. This is particularly pertinent when the funds available for research are limited or uncertain. The costs associated with hiring and paying personnel with sufficient expertise are eliminated. With large-scale surveys, expertise is required for designing the research study, obtaining funding, designing and testing the questionnaire, sampling, data collection and data cleaning, and the costs associated with these can be considerable (Kiecolt and Nathan 1985).

Larger-scale national surveys are more likely to have highly experienced researchers working on them, which for the most part ensures high-quality data. The institutions involved are more likely than individual researchers to have the capacity for rigorous and complex sampling, obtaining large enough sampling sizes and reducing the likelihood of non-responses. The secondary data analyst benefits from a high level of expertise that may not be available to them were they to undertake their own primary research.

Conducting research can be time-intensive, and secondary data analysis often provides access to data which may have taken months or longer to collect. This can provide the researcher with an opportunity to go straight to the analysis stage and to devote more time to analysis than would be possible with primary research. This can also be of benefit to policymakers, who sometimes need research information in a short time frame to provide a basis for policy decisions.

Secondary data analysis can also generate new information that was not identified in the original study. Surveys generally contain data with potential for analysis beyond the specific research questions that they were designed to answer. Secondary data analysis allows the researcher to analyse variables in further detail than was originally reported or to undertake more sophisticated statistical analysis. It can therefore provide a cost-effective means to test specific hypotheses that have not been adequately examined and can help in the development of new research questions. The analysis of existing data can serve as a pilot study whose purpose is to define a research problem more clearly. By using information systems or longitudinal datasets it may be feasible to conduct trend analysis and monitor change over time. For example, using hospital discharges as a proxy for prevalence it may be possible to monitor trends in a particular medical condition over time (Nicoll and Beyea 1999).

Disadvantages of secondary data analysis

A major disadvantage of secondary data analysis is that the data were originally obtained by a different researcher and to answer a different question than the one currently under investigation. Consequently the secondary data analyst has no control over the quality of the data or the variables that are included in the dataset. The secondary data analyst has no control over the data-collection process and is also dependent on the original researcher's decisions regarding the population studied, sampling design, and the questionnaire used during data collection. The research procedures that were followed may not have been sufficiently documented to enable secondary analysts to appraise errors in the data. If errors were made in the original research they may no longer be visible, or it may not be possible to identify whether the errors occurred at the interviewing, data coding or data entry stages. Large-scale national studies tend to be well documented; however, even detailed documentation of procedures is often no substitute for the knowledge that is acquired when collecting data (Kiecolt and Nathan 1985).

Even if the dataset is of high quality it may not contain all the information of interest to the secondary data analyst. For example, the data may only include people aged 65 years or under although it would be preferable to study the whole adult population. Variables may be defined or categorized differently, age information may be presented as age groups rather than as a continuous variable, or it may not be possible to analyse the data by geographic region. Secondary data analysts therefore often have to 'make do' with variables that are not exactly those desired, and in order to undertake data analysis these variables may end up being manipulated and transformed in a way that might lessen the validity of the original research (Vartanian 2011).

Another disadvantage is that the data may be outdated. Given that the primary researcher expends so much time and effort in designing the research, collecting the data and organizing them so that they are ready to be analysed, it is understandable that he or she would be keen to be given the first opportunity to publish the results from the research – as reputations are made by publishing papers and reports from a body of data. It may therefore take some time for the dataset to become available to other researchers (Trzesniewski et al. 2011).

Locating datasets for secondary data analysis

While there is a vast quantity of secondary data that can be used in health research, the process of actually locating and accessing these data may not always be straightforward.

There are a number of examples of secondary datasets (Huston and Naylor 1996; McCaston 2005; Boslaugh 2007), which include:

- vital statistics – registers of deaths and births
- disease registries – cancer and cystic fibrosis
- national surveys – longitudinal and cross-sectional surveys
- administrative data – hospital discharge data

Locating existing data to answer a specific research question begins with the formulation of the question. It may be worthwhile for the researcher to conduct a thorough review of the literature to see if any previous research similar to that currently being undertaken has been done (Garmon 2007). This may help in compiling combinations of predictor and outcome variables that might help answer the research question. Once the question is set, then the population of interest needs to be specified. Do you wish to study children, elderly people, or people of all ages? Do you want to confine the analysis to a defined geographical region or do you want to study a national sample (Boslaugh 2007)?

When the researcher is satisfied with the research question, the next step is to locate databases and surveys that might include the variables of interest (Hearst et al. 2001). The researcher needs to determine which institutions conduct research or maintain information systems on the topic area of interest. Large national surveys are expensive and time-consuming to conduct and therefore they are usually done by government departments or commissioned out to large research institutions or universities. Government documents and official statistics may be a good starting place for gathering secondary data. Often these secondary data are stored in electronic databases that can be accessed and analysed. In addition, many research projects store their raw data in electronic form in computer archives so that others can also analyse the data.

The final step in this process involves choosing the best database for the research question. It may be useful to create a list of datasets that include information related to the research question and to document what other required information (age group studied, year of data collection) each dataset contains. Secondary analysis often involves combining information from multiple databases to examine research questions. For example, health data may be combined with census information to assess patterns in a certain disease by age and geographical region, so there may be a requirement to access more than one secondary data source (McCaston 2005).

Once the secondary data source is identified, it is often necessary to obtain permission from the data owner to use these data. If the data are confidential and contain information that could potentially identify individuals then the data owner may require the researcher and their host institution to sign a contract regarding its use. The researcher may also be asked to provide a justification as to why they need the data and how their analysis will provide benefits, and a comprehensive plan regarding how the data will be analysed.

Ethical issues

As with any research study, the researcher will have to consider whether there are any ethical issues associated with accessing and/or using the secondary data. The researcher should confirm that ethical approval was obtained for the original study and determine if there were any conditions regarding its use for subsequent studies. As a condition of funding, researchers are increasingly being required to undertake to place data in archives, and the possibility of the data being used for secondary analysis may already be covered in the original application for ethical approval. If this is the case then there should be no ethical issues regarding the use of the data (Huston and Naylor 1996; Safran et al. 2007).

As with any study, it is critical that the confidentiality of the information is respected and the use of personal identifiers such as dates of birth are minimized. Any identifiers that are necessary should be removed as soon as possible from the data file. If the data are anonymized and the original participants are not individually identifiable or recognizable in any way then there should be no need to require approval from a research ethics board (Economic and Social Research Council 2012). However, even when data have been anonymized there is still a risk that participants could become identifiable. For example, if deaths from rare causes are being reported by geographical region and age, it is possible that individuals may be identified. In these situations it is advisable not to report very low frequencies, such as those with five or fewer cases. Other housekeeping procedures that can help ensure confidentiality include guaranteeing that all files are password-protected and stored in a secure area in the host institution, on computers that have appropriate encryption. Only those researchers working on the secondary data analysis should have access to the files and there may be a requirement for the researcher to destroy the data at a given time after the analysis has been completed (Lowrance 2003).

How to determine the feasibility and suitability of using a dataset for secondary data analysis

Before undertaking secondary data analysis the researcher must determine firstly whether using secondary data is appropriate for answering the research question, and secondly if there is an appropriate fit between the secondary dataset and the research question. The researcher should become very familiar with the dataset before conducting any analysis, and considerable effort must be expended in identifying any limitations in the original study and in assessing the overall quality of the data (McCaston 2005). The following questions should be considered to determine whether secondary data analysis is the most appropriate means of answering the research question.

Is there sufficient information in relation to the secondary dataset?

While large-scale surveys will usually have enough accompanying documentation to assess the quality of the data, other datasets from smaller surveys or from health information systems may not have this level of documentation available. The researcher should access technical reports of surveys to gain information in relation to why the survey was conducted, what questionnaire was used, how the data were collected, how the data were cleaned and how the data were weighted. In the case of obtaining data from information systems, the system's protocol should be read to gain a better understanding of the methodology of the system itself, what quality control checks are in place, and what data are collected. For data relating to both surveys and information systems, other sources of information may include the website of the agency or institution responsible for collecting or hosting the data, research papers or reports based on the data, and personal communication with the relevant individuals involved (Garmon 2007).

If no documentation is available or if it gives a poor description of the dataset, then it is extremely difficult to come to any conclusions regarding its quality, and the researcher should consider using an alternative dataset. If a decision is made to use the data then any limitations associated with invalid or unreliable data should be clearly addressed in the research report. However, the use of poor-quality data can lead to inaccurate conclusions and can affect the reliability and the validity of the evidence that is generated. Therefore, if a researcher cannot guarantee that the dataset is of high quality, complete and representative, then serious consideration should be given to using the data, and if no other alternative dataset can be identified then it may actually be necessary to undertake primary research to answer the research question.

What was the original purpose for which the data were collected?

It is important to determine the original purpose of the data collection as this may have influenced what population was targeted and the questions that were asked of participants. Knowing the purpose of data collection will help to evaluate the quality of the data and discern the potential level of bias. The survey's source of funding should also be considered (Boslaugh 2007) – for example, if you are looking at attitudes to smoking or alcohol policies then it would be important to establish whether the tobacco or alcohol industries, who may have vested interests regarding the survey's results and outcomes, were involved in funding or designing the survey.

When were the data collected?

The researcher needs to know when the data were collected to determine whether they are current or out of date. A dataset that is released in 2012 may relate to data that were collected a few years previously, and some topic areas where there is continuing or rapid development may demand more current information. If you want to look at the impact of a policy change it is important that you have data relating to the time both before and after its introduction (Hanney et al. 2003).

How were the data collected?

It is useful to know how the data were collected – was it via face-to-face interviews, postal interviews, telephone interviews, or through data extraction from charts? If the data are from an information system, then the checks in place to ensure quality and completeness should be identified. If the data were collected through a survey, the researcher must ascertain what the response rate was, and how many attempts were made to interview non-respondents. A low response rate can be problematic as it can lead to non-response bias (which can be described as the bias that occurs when a significant number of people in the survey sample fail to respond and have relevant characteristics that differ from those who do respond). If the sample is biased and no longer random, then it lacks the potential to be representative of the larger population from which the sample was drawn, thereby limiting the survey's external validity and the secondary data analysis (Bowling 2002).

Does the dataset contain the variables of interest?

Researchers need to ensure that they are sampling from the appropriate populations in order to answer their research question. If they fail to get an appropriate sample, they will not be able to do the research they wish to do (Vartanian 2011). At this stage the researcher should have developed a conceptual model that will form the basis of the analysis and will have identified the dependent variable (outcome of interest) and the independent (predictor) variables. For example, if you wanted to study diabetes in a population, the dependent variable would be a diagnosis of diabetes (yes/no question), and the independent variables could include body mass index category, age and gender.

Codebooks are among the most important pieces of documentation for secondary data. In addition to describing the methodology, they generally provide a listing of all the variables in a dataset and should include the exact wording of each question and the options that the respondents were given when answering the questions. If the dataset does not contain the exact variable of interest then the researcher needs to consider whether there is an alternative variable that is conceptually comparable to the variable of interest that will answer the research question. It should be noted that sampling frames generally do not include people in institutional settings such as hospitals or prisons, or those who are homeless (Vartanian 2011)

What is the level of data aggregation?

Data may be provided at the disaggregated (individual) or aggregate level. The level of data aggregation or disaggregation refers to the extent to which the data are broken down. Disaggregated data provide information such as age, gender and geographical region on each individual case in the dataset. As a result, these data are generally more informative and useful than aggregate data. They allow for more extensive analysis, as the researcher can study associations between the characteristics of each case and so it is usually preferable to get individual-level data. Aggregate data are data which combine broad groups or cohorts of participants but it is not possible to distinguish the properties of individuals within those groups or cohorts (McCaston 2005). For example, geographical data may be grouped by spatial units such as county, or age data may be presented in age groups. Analysing breast cancer outcomes by age group is an example of aggregate data use; the researcher can compare cohorts but not individuals. While it may be preferable to obtain disaggregated data, this may not always be possible. For ethical or privacy reasons, particularly in relation to datasets that contain personal health information, data holders or owners may be reluctant to provide researchers with disaggregated data and the researcher may have to 'make do' with aggregate data (Trzesniewski et al. 2011).

What data-cleaning procedures have been applied to the data?

The quality of the data should be assessed before undertaking analysis. The two traditional measures of quality are reliability and validity. Reliability simply asks whether the survey measures things consistently. It addresses how the data were collected and coded for entry into the database and whether the data were arranged in an accurate and consistent manner that is replicable. Validity is concerned with the degree to which the dataset contains all of the variables required to address the research questions being examined (Pollack 1999; Groves et al. 2009).

What sampling procedures were used?

Sampling is an important component of any survey because of the significant impact it can have on the quality of the results. There are two types of sampling – probability and non-probability sampling. With probability sampling (including simple random, stratified and cluster sampling), all people in the population have some opportunity of being included in the sample, and the mathematical probability that any one of them will be selected can be calculated. This reduces the potential for human bias in the selection of cases to be included in the sample. As a result, probability sampling provides a sample that is highly representative of the population being studied, assuming that there is limited missing data. The advantage of probability sampling is that sampling error can be calculated. Sampling error is the degree to which a sample might differ from the population. When inferring to the population, results are reported plus or minus the sampling error (Korn and Graubard 1999; Groves et al. 2009).

Conversely, non-probability sampling methods (including quota, convenience and snowball sampling) are not based on probability. With these methods, a sampling frame is defined in advance of data collection and a sample is chosen from this list, but not at random. Surveys may employ quota sampling as it is cheaper, quicker and easier to carry out. With quota sampling, the researcher first identifies the strata or demographic groups and their proportions as they are represented in the population. People are selected on the basis of their ease of access or availability, and are assigned by the researcher to demographic groups based on variables like age and sex. This differs from probability sampling, where the strata are filled by random sampling. When the quota for a given stratum or demographic group is filled, the researcher will stop recruiting subjects from that particular group. In non-probability sampling, as the selection of participants to be included in the sample has not been chosen using random selection there is the possibility of sampling bias. It also means that it is not possible to make generalizations or statistical inferences from the sample to the population, which can lead to problems of external validity. When reporting the results of secondary data analysis, the sampling procedures used in the original study should be clearly described, as the sampling will have an effect on the results and their generalizability (Groves et al. 2009).

Random error is another form of sampling error. It relates directly to the size of the sample – and is basically a predictor of precision. In general terms, as sample size increases, random sampling error decreases. However, a carefully selected small sample can be more accurate than a less carefully selected large sample. The secondary data analyst must determine whether the sample size is large enough to be precise. An adequate sample size is determined by three factors: the estimated prevalence of the variable of interest, the desired level of confidence, and the acceptable level of precision (margin of error). The World Health Organization published a practical manual on sample size determination in health studies (Lwanga and Lemeshow 1991) that provides tables of the minimum sample size required for various study calculations.

Analysing secondary data

Statistical analysis of secondary data should be approached in the same way as analysis of primary data (Garmon 2007). Secondary datasets may be quite complicated and are often provided in SPSS, SAS or Stata formats, so the researcher will need expertise in at least one of these programs. Most datasets will require some recoding, combining and constructing variables and extracting data for particular years or subgroups. This requires some degree of database management skills using one of the above-mentioned programs (Vartanian 2011).

As a first step, a copy of the original dataset should be made and kept separate from the data file that will be worked on. This ensures that if any errors are made with recoding etc. then there is a clean copy to work from. If it is a large dataset it may also be useful to delete the variables that are not needed, which will make the dataset more manageable. The codebook provides a listing of all the variables in a dataset and includes the exact wording of each question, which will make it easier to determine what variables will be required, and it will also give information on how each variable is coded. It is useful to run simple descriptives and frequencies at the outset to check for data quality and completeness. This also helps the researcher to form an overall impression of the data before doing more complex analysis. Cross-tabulations should be conducted to check for logical errors in the data. For example, a male should not be recorded as having any previous pregnancies, or the percentage of the sample that report smoking in the last year should not be higher than the percentage that report any lifetime use (Boslaugh 2007).

It can take time to clean up and organize the dataset before starting the analysis but this will make the data more manageable and easier to analyse. Almost all datasets include some missing data, and is important to note the extent of missing data and to determine whether this will adversely impact the results (Trzesniewski et al. 2011). A syntax file should be created as this will help the researcher keep track of what recoding has been done, and will be useful if the analysis has to be repeated for any reason. When new variables are being created, filling in the variable labels properly will make the outputs easier to decipher.

Data collected from survey respondents are usually weighted, which simply means that the raw survey data are adjusted to represent the population from which the sample is drawn, to alleviate the impact of any biases arising from the differences between sample and population. Weighting can be done on the basis of gender, age and other demographic characteristics, and is usually described in the survey's documentation. When the analysis is being undertaken these weights will have to be applied to the data. The weighting should already have been done by the primary researchers and a weighting variable should be in the dataset. The secondary data analyst must ensure that their analysis is done on the weighted rather than the unweighted data, as this reduces bias (Vartanian 2011).

Datasets, particularly those from large national surveys or administrative databases, often contain huge numbers, both in terms of the number of cases and the number of variables. Although a large sample size is an advantage, it can also be a problem as vast quantities of data can be daunting to manage. With large samples there is a greater likelihood of obtaining results that are statistically significant. When a statistic is significant, it simply means that you are very sure that the statistic is reliable. It doesn't mean the finding is really meaningful or that any clinical decisions or policy changes can be based on it (Huston and Naylor 1996). Therefore, statistically significant results should be interpreted with caution, and the effect size should also be calculated as this emphasizes the size of the difference rather than the sample size.

A common pitfall is to underestimate the overall length of time needed to conduct a study using secondary data. Although the actual data collection and organization required to undertake secondary data analysis takes less time than with primary research, the secondary researcher must identify the dataset, negotiate access to and develop a plan for analysing the data, all of which can consume a great deal of time (Castle 2003). A researcher who collects their own data understands more clearly than the secondary data analyst the data-collection methodology, its completeness, the documentation and the data structure itself. Gaining familiarity with an existing data source can be time-consuming and challenging (Vartanian 2011).

Box 19.1 Examples of secondary datasets that can be used for health care research

- In Ireland the Irish Social Science Data Archive (ISSDA), based at University College Dublin, holds a number of key Irish and international comparative datasets that may be used by secondary data analysts interested in health research. All data disseminated by ISSDA have undergone rigorous checks to ensure that they have been fully anonymized, thus protecting the individual data confidentiality. They can be converted to SPSS, Stata and CSV formats. Some of these datasets are described in further detail below. ISSDA also provides the relevant study documentation for each survey, including the sample design, the questionnaire, codebooks and reports based on the survey's data. Further information may be accessed at http://www.ucd.ie/issda/

- The Growing Up in Ireland study is a national longitudinal study of children. The study is following the progress of two groups of children: the child cohort, which includes 8,500 9-year-olds born in 1997–98 who were interviewed again at the age of 13; and the infant cohort, which includes 11,000 9-month-olds born in 2007–08, who were interviewed again at the age of three. The child cohort dataset contains variables on each child's health, use of health services, diet and exercise, and emotional health and well-being. In addition, it contains variables on their parents' health and lifestyle as well as sociodemographic information. The infant cohort dataset contains variables on the child's health and development, daily routines and childcare arrangements, and their parents' health and lifestyle. Waves one and two have been completed; data from the first wave are available for research purposes, while data from the second wave of the infant cohort will be available from March 2013 and data from the second wave of the child cohort will be available in the second half of 2013. Further information may be accessed at http://www.growingup.ie.

- The Irish Longitudinal Study on Ageing (TILDA) aims to study a representative cohort of at least 8,000 people aged 50 and over and resident in Ireland, charting their health, social and economic circumstances over a ten-year period. The survey collects detailed information on all aspects of their lives, including the economic (pensions, employment, living standards), health (physical, mental, service needs and usage) and social aspects (contact with friends and kin, formal and informal care, social participation). Both survey interviews and physical and biological measurements are utilized. The first wave of data from the project is now available on request. Further information may be accessed at http://www.tcd.ie/tilda.
- SLÁN (Survey on Lifestyle and Attitude to Nutrition) is a series of surveys of adults aged 18 and over that were designed to produce baseline information for the on-going surveillance of health and lifestyle behaviours in the Irish population. Three surveys have been conducted to date – in 1998, 2002 and 2007 – with sample sizes ranging from 5,992 to 10,364. Datasets are available for each. The survey contains variables on general health (including self-reported height and weight), self-reported physical and mental health and well-being, tobacco, alcohol and illegal substance use, and dietary habits. Further information may be found at http://www.ucd.ie/issda/data/surveyonlifestyleandattitudestonutritionslan/.

Conclusion

Analysis of secondary data sources can provide a quick and cost-effective means of generating data that can provide a cheaper alternative to the collection of primary data. However, as the researcher has no control over the way the data were initially collected, it is essential that they can evaluate the quality of a secondary dataset and assess its usefulness. Statistical analysis of secondary data should be approached in the same manner as statistical analysis of primary data, and the time and expertise required to do this should not be underestimated. Ultimately, secondary data analysis can be a practical, appropriate and cost-effective research process that can be used to answer important clinical and policy questions.

Key concepts

- Analysis of secondary data sources can provide a quick and cost-effective means of generating data that can provide a cheaper alternative to the collection of primary data.
- As the researcher has no control over the way the data were initially collected, it is essential that they can evaluate the quality of a secondary dataset and assess its usefulness.
- Statistical analysis of secondary data should be approached in the same manner as statistical analysis of primary data.
- Depending on the extent of data aggregation, it may be feasible to conduct trend analysis and monitor change over time.
- Secondary data analysis may be particularly useful when combined with primary data analysis.

Key readings in secondary data analysis

- S. Boslaugh, *Secondary Data Sources for Public Health: A Practical Guide* (Cambridge: Cambridge University Press, 2007)
  This guide provides an introduction to secondary data and issues specific to its management and analysis.
- J. Kiecolt and L. Nathan, *Secondary Analysis of Survey Data,* Sage University Paper Series on Quantitative Applications in the Social Sciences, Series no. 07-001. (Beverly Hills: Sage Publications, 1985)
  This book provides a good overview of the advantages and limitations of secondary survey analysis. It provides guidance on how to locate appropriate data and how to make effective use of existing survey data.
- K. Trzesniewski, B. Donnellan and R. Lucas, *Secondary Data Analysis: An Introduction for Psychologists* (Washington, DC: American Psychological Association, 2011)
  This book provides an introduction to secondary data analysis and provides information on available datasets and the different methodological techniques that can be used when undertaking analysis.
- T.P. Vartanian, *Secondary Data Analysis* (New York: Oxford University Press 2011)
  This book provides an introduction to secondary data analysis, its advantages and disadvantages, and how to determine the feasibility of using secondary data. It also gives examples of datasets used in social work.

Examples of the use of secondary data analysis in health care research

- H. Cooper, C. Smaje and S. Arber, Use of health services by children and young people according to ethnicity and social class: Secondary analysis of a national survey, *British Medical Journal,* 317 (1998), 1047–51
- M. Goldacre and S. Roberts, Hospital admission for acute pancreatitis in an English population 1963–98: Database study of incidence and mortality, *British Medical Journal,* 328(7454) (2004), 1466–9
- I. Hajjar and T. Kotchen, Trends in prevalence, awareness, treatment, and control of hypertension in the United States, 1988–2000, *Journal of the American Medical Association,* 290(2) (2003), 199–206
- D. Leon and J. McCambridge, Liver cirrhosis mortality rates in Britain from 1950 to 2002: An analysis of routine data, *Lancet,* 367 (2006), 52–6

References

Boslaugh, S. (2007) *Secondary Data Sources for Public Health: A Practical Guide.* Cambridge: Cambridge University Press.

Bowling, A. (2002) *Research Methods in Health: Investigating Health and Health Services,* 2nd edn. Buckingham: Open University Press.

Castle, J. (2003) Maximising research opportunities: Secondary data analysis, *Journal of Neuroscience Nursing*, 35(5): 287–90.

Economic and Social Research Council (2012) *The Research Ethics Guidebook: A Resource for Social Scientists*. Available at http://www.ethicsguidebook.ac.uk [Accessed 12 January 2012].

Garmon, S. (2007) Issues associated with secondary analysis of population health data, *Applied Nursing Research*, 20(2): 94–9.

Groves, R., Fowler, F., Couper, M., Lepkowski, J. and Singer, E. (2009) *Survey Methodology*, 2nd edn. New Jersey: John Wiley & Sons.

Hanney, S., Gonzalez-Block, M., Buxton, M. and Kogan, M. (2003) The utilisation of health research in policy-making: Concepts, examples and methods of assessment, *Health Research Policy and Systems*, 1(1): 2, doi: 10.1186/1478-4505-1-2 PMC151555.

Hearst, N., Grady, D., Barron, H. and Kerlikowske, K. (2001) Research using existing data: Secondary data analysis, ancillary studies, and systematic review, in S. Hulley, S. Cummings, W. Browner, D. Grady, N. Hearst and T. Newman (eds) *Designing Clinical Research*, 2nd edn. Philadelphia: Lippincott Williams & Wilkins, pp. 195–215.

Huston, P. and Naylor, C. (1996) Health services research: Reporting on studies using secondary data sources, *Canadian Medical Association Journal*, 155(12): 1697–709.

Kiecolt, J. and Nathan, L. (1985) *Secondary Analysis of Survey Data*, Sage University Paper Series on Quantitative Applications in the Social Sciences, No. 07-001. Beverly Hills: Sage Publications.

Korn, E.L. and Graubard, B.I. (1999) *Analysis of Health Surveys*. New York: Wiley-Interscience.

Lowrance, W. (2003) Learning from experience: Privacy and the secondary use of data in health research, *Journal of Health Service Research Policy*, 8(Supp. 11): 2–7.

Lwanga, S. and Lemeshow, S. (1991) *Sample Size Determination in Health Studies: A Practical Manual*. Geneva: World Health Organization.

McCaston, K. (2005) *Tips for Collecting, Reviewing, and Analysing Secondary Data*. USA: Partnership and Household Livelihood Security Unit, CARE. Available at http://pqdl.care.org/Practice/DME%20-%20Tips%20for%20Collecting,%20Reviewing%20and%20Analyzing%20Secondary%20Data.pdf [Accessed March 2013].

Nicoll, L. and Beyea, S. (1999) Using secondary data analysis for nursing research, *AORN Journal*, 69(2): 428–33.

Pollack, C. (1999) Methodological considerations with secondary analysis, *Outcomes Management for Nursing Practice*, 3(4): 147–52.

Safran, C., Bloomrosen, M., Hammond, W., Labkoff, S., Markel-Fox, S., Tang, P. and Detmer, D. (2007) Toward a national framework for the secondary use of health data: An American Medical Informatics Association White Paper, *Journal of the American Medical Informatics Association*, 14(1): 1–9.

Trzesniewski, K., Donnellan, B. and Lucas, R. (2011) *Secondary Data Analysis: An Introduction for Psychologists*. Washington, DC: American Psychological Association.

Vartanian, T.P. (2011) *Secondary Data Analysis*. New York: Oxford University Press.

20   Presenting your research findings

Emma Stokes

Chapter topics
- Presenting research findings in a dissertation or thesis
- Presenting research findings in poster presentations
- Presenting research findings in oral presentations
- Practical advice and suggestions for using visual aids in each of the three presentation methods

Introduction

The aim of this chapter is to discuss a number of key issues relating to the presentation of your research findings. It focuses on the presentation of results in your dissertation and at conferences rather than in written formats such as those used for peer-reviewed publication. The chapter begins by considering how to present your research findings in a results chapter in a thesis or dissertation. It then explores why the dissemination of research findings at conferences is important. Thereafter, the chapter provides some suggestions for preparing both oral and poster presentations.

Presenting research findings in a dissertation or thesis

It is likely that you will write your findings for two different audiences. Prior to writing your dissertation or thesis you may have written up parts of your research findings for submission to a peer-reviewed journal, but for the purposes of submitting your thesis or dissertation for examination your findings will form one or more chapters of the final document. The presentation of quantitative findings in a dissertation is the focus of this section of this chapter.

The purpose of your findings chapter is to demonstrate to the examiner the outcome of the investigations you have undertaken in search of the answers to your research questions (Hardy and Ramjeet 2005). As will be discussed in subsequent sections, knowing your audience is very important in the preparatory stages. In preparing a dissertation, it is important to remember that the examiner may be correcting a number of dissertations or may not read the total dissertation in one sitting from start to finish, hence making the findings chapter easy to read but comprehensive in its articulation will benefit the reader (Easterbrook 2005). From the outset, it is helpful to rehearse the aim and research questions of the research study. If you have not done so already, there is a need to set out any a priori hypotheses. If you have one set of findings, it is likely that these will be presented in one chapter, to be followed by your discussion chapter. In some instances, however, the findings and discussion may be combined into one chapter. This may occur when there are discrete sections in the research that are best discussed together.

Suggestions for presenting research findings

When presenting your findings in a dissertation, a combination of narrative text and illustrations are commonly used. A description of, and justification for, the statistical analysis chosen would have been given in the methodology chapter, so there is no need to repeat this information in your findings chapter. In general, descriptive statistics are presented initially and, where appropriate, followed by inferential statistics. At the outset, the attributes of your sample are described including, where relevant, the results of your recruitment process or the response rate to an invitation to participate. Thereafter, you must address each of your research questions and describe in written format what results you recorded and the results of your statistical analyses. You should keep this section as short, clear and concise as possible (CETL-AURS 2012). Tables, graphs or figures can be used when describing your results but they should not be simply presented in the chapter without linking them to explanatory text. They are tools that can be used for describing your research findings, and are used because visual representations of data can be clearer and more concise than text in some instances. It is not normal practice to present the same data in both a graph and a table, so it is advisable to use one or the other, but not both. Moreover, there is no requirement to repeat in the text what is illustrated in the table, figure or graph. Data commentary usually has the following elements (Swales and Feak 2004):

- a location element – text that tells the reader which table or figure is being referred to
- a summary of the information presented in the figure or table
- a highlighting statement to point out what is significant in all the data presented, such as trends, patterns, results that are more important than others

Figures and tables

Figures are used to illustrate data in a number of ways. For instance, pie charts are useful to show proportions, scatter plots are helpful to understand the degree of association between two variables, bar charts can illustrate changes in quantity over time, as can line graphs, while horizontal bar charts can be used to compare differences between groups (Reynolds 2005). Excel and other software programs may offer a range of options for figures and graphs, but the general rule is 'the simpler the better'. Although 3-D graphs look impressive, this can make differences between interventions harder to interpret. Frequently there is a temptation to generate your figures or graphs in a statistical package and simply copy and paste them into your text file. However, CETL-AURS (2012) suggest the following points should be considered when creating your figures or graphs, since they may not always remain consistent when an illustration is imported from one software program to another:

- **Size** – the labels and legends within the figure must be large enough to be clear to the reader but not so large that they dominate the page.
- **Scale** – software programs often generate default scales for the axes notwithstanding your largest value. You may wish to modify the scale of the axis to make the figure or graph more meaningful to the reader, but if you are comparing different graphs they should all have the same scale.
- **Gridlines** – these are helpful to the reader because they can be a reference to where data points lie on a scale, but too many of them can make the figure unclear.
- **Colour** – if you plan to use colour for figures or graphs you will need to print those pages in colour for your final version, but if your work will be printed in black and white, use patterns to distinguish between groups or interventions rather than different shades of black, grey and white.
- **Labelling and legends** – figures and graphs are introduced in the text but they should be clear enough to be read as a stand-alone illustration, so it is important to ensure that the descriptors on the axes make sense and the legend is informative: short but descriptive.
- **Statistics** – if you are using percentiles, error bars, medians or outlier points in your figures or graphs, make sure the reader knows what they are.

Tables are normally used to present datasets that are too large for figures, but as with figures the tables must be clear and have sufficient clarity in their headings and labels to be comprehensible to the reader. Tables are often used to summarize the results of a number of statistical tests, and should include all relevant data such as measure of central tendency, variance within the data, t-values, F-scores, degrees of freedom, confidence intervals and p-values as appropriate. When presenting percentages in tables, it is helpful for the reader to be provided with an indication of the total sample size from which the percentages were drawn. Normally, data are presented in either a table or a figure/graph, but it is not usual to present the same data in both.

Presenting research findings at conferences

There are a variety of reasons for presenting your research findings at conferences and other meetings like journal clubs and in-service lectures. The most obvious is the opportunity to tell your audience what you have discovered. For many researchers, it is part of professional development: the publication of an abstract and an entry in your curriculum vitae. But the presentation itself, a poster or an oral presentation, represents the outcome of a process that is very valuable for a variety of different reasons. By giving a conference paper the researcher develops other skills and gains valuable insights. Preparing a paper for a conference encourages the presenter to consider and reflect on the meaning of the research findings and the audience for which it is intended. Any subsequent feedback from the audience could be used to inform future research development.

Normally, the presentation of your research findings begins with an abstract – a précis of your work in approximately 250 words. Giving an oral presentation provides an opportunity to develop and practise public speaking and presentation skills. Reducing the size of your research report and its findings into a concise set of points or concepts focuses your mind on the essentials you wish to present. Furthermore, it allows you the opportunity to synthesize your work, contextualize it within your field and develop the message you wish to communicate. The process of creating a focused presentation – whether oral or poster – is one that requires reflection, and as such may help you to consider the implications or future directions of your work.

Giving presentations at conferences offers an opportunity to introduce your research to an audience. You may be presenting your research or preliminary results as a *work in progress*, which hopefully will generate discussion and feedback that could be incorporated into your dissertation or future presentations or research directions. If the audience includes key researchers in the field, the opportunity for constructive feedback can be invaluable, for example by offering an alternative perspective, one that you may not have considered, or perhaps new questions that may improve the quality of the research study. If you are a graduate student, the questions asked and the feedback received during your presentation may be very valuable when preparing for a viva or public defence of your thesis at a later stage. Presenting to a lay audience, for instance to a patient or client support group, provides an invaluable opportunity to review your findings in the light of what they may mean to the group of individuals for whom the research may have the ultimate personal impact. In creating a presentation using non-scientific language, you have to focus on the essence of the translational aspect of your research – what will this mean for the individual who is the focus of the research question?

Perhaps the most important reason for presenting your research findings is the public dissemination of your work. The audience may be a small group of colleagues, a wide audience of researchers or a lay audience. The purpose of the presentation may be part of a job interview, but more commonly it is about informing an audience about your research and the relevance of the findings for clinical practice or further research. The purpose of research is to create new knowledge but its value is only achieved when that knowledge is disseminated and incorporated into practice. It has been suggested that it can take up to 20 years for the findings of research to be actually incorporated into practice (Green 2008), hence the message for your audience must be communicated clearly and succinctly.

Presentation formats – traditional and novel

Is a poster worth the effort? Posters can often be considered a less valuable format for disseminating research findings than an oral presentation, but if managed well by the conference organizers and presenters they can be an excellent opportunity for researchers to present findings and engage with an audience in a less formal way than an oral presentation session. They provide an ideal opportunity to make contacts and network with other researchers and practitioners who have similar interests (Hardicre et al. 2007a). Before you decide to submit an abstract for a poster session or agree to a poster session, you need to find out about the timing and positioning of the poster sessions. It may be worth asking if there is a designated time on the programme for the posters or whether they are scheduled to run in a concurrent session with other oral presentations. Moreover, the following questions may focus your mind on the *value* you and others will place on agreeing to a poster presentation:

- Will this format provide me with an opportunity to share my ideas with a relevant audience? Or will I be competing against other sessions?
- Will conference delegates participate in the presentation? Will I be in a position to share and/or receive feedback on my work from relevant individuals?
- What will I learn from developing and presenting a poster?

Poster walks and chaired or guided poster sessions, where conference delegates move through a themed poster session facilitated by a chair or moderator, are exciting opportunities to actively engage with the poster presenters and the conference attendees. These may require the poster presenter to prepare a two-minute presentation on the key findings from their study. Exciting developments such as virtual poster halls – for example the American Diabetes Association Scientific Meeting – provide delegates with year-round access to all posters presented at the meeting. In addition, each poster has a 2-D bar code, and scanning this into a smartphone allows the reader to access additional details about the research (American Diabetes Association 2012).

Presenting research findings for poster presentations

Academic poster presentations are a widely used medium to communicate research findings, but they have limitations if used in a traditional format (two-dimensional, page-limited format) (Goodhand et al. 2011; Rowe and Ilic 2011). Miller (2007) described posters as a *hybrid form* – the interaction between the presenter and the audience is less structured than an oral presentation, where the presenter determines the flow. With a poster presentation, the audience may focus on varying aspects of your poster depending on their interests (Miller 2007). The design of a poster will be paramount to both the engagement of the reader and the memorability of the content– that is, the more attractive and clear your poster is, the more a reader will be drawn to it and the more likely they are to remember what they read. Posters are a visual representation of your research; the key points on a poster are the tools by which you engage your audience, which is why you should be clear about the nature of the poster session at which you will present. Hess et al. (2010) have an excellent website giving guidance – http://www.ncsu.edu/project/posters. In essence, the authors say, a 'poster shows, not tells'.

To be successful with posters, the following are worth considering carefully.

Planning

- *Know your audience and your message:* Key to engaging your audience is to know who they are and to create a poster that will be relevant for them. The poster you created for a previous meeting may not match the expectations of this audience. Knowing your audience will help you decide what information may need to be presented as background or contextual information – an audience with detailed knowledge will need less information and you can focus more on your methods and results. The consistent message for posters is to focus on two or three key messages.

- *Familiarize yourself with the poster requirements:* Be clear about the dimensions and the orientation – landscape or portrait. You may also have a format you are required to follow (for instance, the conference organizers may have stipulated that posters should include certain headings). Consider what institutional information you may need to include, such as organizational logos, and check that you are using the most up-to-date and approved version. Check if you need to supply suspension materials such as Velcro.

Design

- *Eye-catching:* You want the poster title and construction to draw the readers to you so that you can engage with them on the substantive ideas.
- *Focused:* As discussed above, a short presentation or poster is a distilled version of your research. Consider the key message you want readers of your poster to take away.
- *Imagery:* Use imagery and graphics rather than large blocks of text. You can supplement details through discussion or a short handout.
- *Signposts for readers:* Use clear headings or numbering to guide the reader over your poster. Visual grammar is the 'graphic hierarchy that helps readers identify the most important parts of your poster' (Hess et al. 2010).
- *Font:* Use a font that is easy to read and a size that is legible from a distance of approximately 1 metre. Bear in mind that readers may not view it one by one but as a group. Suggested font sizes are 100 points for the main text, 50 points for subheadings and 25 points for the body of the text (Hardicre et al. 2007a).

Optimize the experience

- *For you:* Decide what you wish to achieve from the presentation. Maybe you wish to engage with researchers in the field – if so, distribute business cards and request one from interested researchers who come to view your poster. Rehearse the narrative to support your key messages on the poster so that you have a way of engaging with each viewer or with a group of researchers who may visit your poster as part of a structured poster session. Have questions ready for your audience if you would like to receive specific feedback on your poster presentation.
- *For your audience:* At conferences, there may be large numbers of posters and other presentations. Make it easier for your audience by preparing copies of your abstract or a one-page summary of your work with more details than those provided on the poster. In addition, provide your contact details in case the reader may have any future queries or questions. Try not to overload the poster with details that can be supplied by discussion or with supplementary reading.

Presenting research findings for oral presentations

Once you have had an abstract accepted for oral presentation, a different journey to that of creating a poster begins. There are a variety of considerations, described as the 'four P's', as follows:

- Preparation: both initial and then immediately before the presentation.
- Presentation development: to include decisions on structure and content.
- Practice: of the presentation, alone and with others.
- Performance: includes considerations of your delivery of the presentation.

Preparation

The acceptance of your abstract and an invitation to present your research findings is not a rite of passage. It is the result of a peer-review process and may be very competitive; hence, preparation in advance of the day as well as on the day is important, no matter how experienced a speaker you are (Hardicre et al. 2007b). In advance of the conference, especially if you have not attended or presented at it before, talk to colleagues who have presented to get an understanding of the nature and 'culture' of the event, as well as the audience likely to attend. Knowing your audience is essential to the preparation of your presentation. A very knowledgeable audience or fellow researchers may not require significant background material but may wish you to provide a detailed account of your findings, whereas with a more clinically focused audience you may wish to focus on the clinical rationale for the research as well as any specific information that could be used to change practice. In addition, you may wish to ascertain the type of room in which you will present – the conference organizers may be able to provide you with information about size and lighting, both of which are important for the design of your presentation. Once the conference programme is finalized, spend some time finding out with whom you are presenting and where your presentation may fit into an overall session profile. If you are starting off the session you may need to spend some time contextualizing your work, but if you are midway through or towards the end of the session much of the introductory information may have been previously presented and you may not wish to repeat it, thus allowing you more time for the description of your methods, results and conclusions (Gifford and Ireton-Jones 2010).

In the more immediate time before your presentation, when you have arrived at the venue where you will present, it is helpful to check in with the team managing audio-visual support. You may have already sent your presentation to the conference organizers or uploaded it to a computer in a speakers' lounge, but it is advisable to bring a back-up version on a memory stick or flash drive. Check that the slide format, graphics and colour have not altered in the transfer from your computer to another. Familiarize yourself with the room where the presentation will take place. Consider its orientation: will you have to manage possible interruptions during your presentation due to later arrivals entering through a door at the front of the room? Is the lighting suitable for your presentation? Two versions of the same presentation, one with a light background and dark text and another with the opposite, can accommodate for an unexpectedly dark or bright venue. Take some time to introduce yourself to the Chair and the other presenters. Familiarize yourself with any timing devices or signals that may be used during your presentation to notify you of the time, and finally ensure that you will have a glass of water near you when you are presenting. Table 20.1 provides a checklist.

Table 20.1 Pre-presentation checklist

	Pre-presentation checklist
Room	• Location • Orientation – podium • Glass and water • Lighting
Technology	• Timing devices • Laser pointer • Microphones
Presentation	• Copy of presentation on flash drive • Notes or aide-memoires • Final view of slides for format
Session	• Introduce yourself to session Chair • Provide biography details if required • Meet other presenters

Presentation development

Reflect on your message: All too frequently the first step in preparing a presentation is to open a presentation software program such as PowerPoint. Wright (2009) describes how, 40 years ago, the main presentation aids were chalk, blackboards and books – discussion without visual or audio support played a far greater role in the presentation and discussion of research findings. Nowadays, the use of presentation software programs is ubiquitous. Nonetheless, it is widely advocated, if not necessarily commonly practised, that when preparing for a presentation, an analogue approach should be employed (Reynolds 2005; Chandra 2009). This is often called the storyboard technique – the idea of 'starting with the end in mind' and using a pen and paper or a whiteboard to sketch out the presentation you want to give, bearing in mind that you should be designing a message for a particular audience in the time you have been allocated. Figure 20.1 illustrates the use of a storyboard technique. The storyboard enables you to take a view of what your overall plan will be for your presentation. Then, for each section, you need to decide what details need to be included, given the time you have for your presentation. Starting out by creating a set of slides has been likened to a film director starting to film without the cast of actors and the script. Even when the structure of the presentation is traditionally prescriptive, the value of beginning with what your message for the audience will be is an excellent

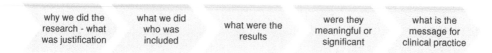

Figure 20.1 Example of a storyboard.

way of focusing your mind on what should be included in the presentation, especially when you have more data than the presentation time will allow.

Presentation format: The slides you prepare are the visual aids for your presentation: your presentation, including the style of your delivery and your narrative, is the *main act*. If the audience simply wanted to know the information about your research, they could read the abstract or subsequent publications. Table 20.2 outlines

Table 20.2 Suggested tips for oral presentations

Theme	Suggested tips
Font size	• The font size must be sufficiently large to be seen at the back of the room • Font size of 24 at least is advised
Font type	• Avoid serif fonts such as Times New Roman; they are designed for text that is to be read in documents • Use sans serif fonts such as Arial or Gill Sans
Colour	• Avoid slides with fussy watermarks in the background, e.g. images of your institution • Choose colours for contrast, e.g. dark font on an off-white or light background or a light colour on a dark background • Avoid reds and greens as people who are colour-blind may have difficulty reading these slides • White backgrounds are very stark and can be hard on viewers
Content	• Try not to use too many words or bullet points • The slide is a guide, not the full presentation text • Diagrams and images can break the monotony of text slides • Use figures carefully to illustrate results – what is legible on paper may not be in a slide or from a distance
Distractions	• Animation, transition effect and sounds should be used sparingly as they can simply become distractions
Images	• Permission is required from study participants for use of their image • Images are useful to illustrate a message – they are good for connection with the audience • Try to use high-quality graphics • If the image is free and easily available, it is likely that it has been seen by many in the audience and so may have less impact
How many slides?	• The rule of thumb is one slide per minute of the overall allocated time for the presentation • If you wish to discuss detail in each slide, you may wish to allocate up to three minutes per slide • If presenting to an audience in a language that is not their first language, it is best to opt for fewer slides • Practice sessions will be informative in terms of the number you need

Table 20.3 Suggested slide outline

Component	Number of slides	Content
Title	1 slide	
Introduction Background	1 slide	• Tell the audience what you will describe and the rationale for why this is important. • If you know that the speakers before you will provide general background information to the study, you may focus more on your particular area. • Try to avoid repetition of contextual information. If the information on your introductory slide has been presented by a previous speaker, link the detail to that speaker – e.g. 'as the previous speaker mentioned, stroke is a leading cause of disability' – and then move on to your particular focus. • Include the aims and objectives you will describe.
Details/methods	2–3 slides	• Describe an abbreviated version of the research methods – just the key points. • What is the most important aspect of your methods that you wish to impart to the audience?
Results	4–6 slides	• Present the main findings relevant to this audience. • Depending on time, choose key findings. • You may have the chance to expand on findings in the question and answer session.
Conclusion	1–2 slides	• You may wish to consider any limitations of your work. • What is the 'take home' message you have for your audience? • Maybe this is how your results will inform practice.
Acknowledgements	1 slide	• List of acknowledgements, especially participants and funding agencies.
Questions and answers		

a series of suggestions that is consistently reported in the literature about the use of software to aid presentations (Hardicre et al. 2007b; Chandra 2009; DeSilets and Dickerson 2009; Gifford and Ireton-Jones 2010; Longo and Tierney 2012).

Table 20.3 outlines a traditional structure for presenting research findings (Hardicre et al. 2007b; Gifford and Ireton-Jones 2010), including a suggestion for slide numbers for a 15-minute presentation (Zerwic et al. 2010).

Practice: To become more confident and comfortable as a speaker, practice is essential, especially for a novice presenter. Initially you may wish to practise on your own, maybe in front of a mirror, but practising with peers will enable you to develop and change your presentation with feedback. Practising the narrative to accompany your slides provides an opportunity to establish whether the presentation flows as you planned, and if the key messages are clear. It provides an opportunity to familiarize yourself with the technology you may be using, including the use of a laser pointer and microphones or any aide-memoire you may use, such as cue cards.

When getting feedback from others, ask about verbal tics – the sounds we use to fill gaps in sentences and speech patterns – that may become obvious when we present, for example frequent use of 'I suppose', 'basically', 'essentially' (McConnell 2009), or physical actions that may be manifestations of stress but which will be distracting to an audience, such as tucking your hair behind your ear, touching your face, throat clearing. When attention is drawn to these behaviours, we become more aware of them and can take action to minimize them when presenting. Recording your own presentation during practice will provide you with an opportunity to hear how you sound, and can be very helpful in gaining insights into your delivery style. When you practise, time yourself to be sure you are within your set time for the presentation. The impact of exceeding your time may result in a disregard for both you as a presenter and your topic. Finishing a little early is better than speaking over your allocated time.

Performance: It would be surprising not to be nervous before your presentations; even experienced presenters feel nervous before giving an important talk, but the more frequently you present, the easier it becomes. Longo and Tierney (2012) suggest that it is worth spending some time before you begin with the 'ABCs' of *affirming* (yes, I can), *breathing* and *composing yourself*. From the outset of your presentation, it is vital that you get the audience's attention, so if there is noise or chatting in the audience it may be best to pause and wait for silence before you begin.

In preparing for the presentation, you may have decided to use an aide-memoire. While it may be tempting to include your notes in a 'notes pages' facility in your presentation software, large sheets of paper can be difficult to manoeuvre at a podium and may be distracting for the audience. Small cue cards are useful for recording key headings you wish to address during your presentation. If you decide to write the text word for word, use this as the basis for your presentation but do not read it out. Written and spoken words are constructed differently – reading a prepared text may sound stilted and overly formal, and it limits eye contact with your audience (DeCoske and White 2010). Your cue cards should be written in a large font and numbered, just in case you drop them in a moment of anxiety before your presentation. As you become more practised, the need for speaking notes becomes less. Making and maintaining eye contact with your audience also becomes easier with experience but is vital for engaging with your audience (Hardicre et al. 2007b). There is a tendency to look straight ahead, but remember to look both to your left and right to draw in those members of your audience rather than focusing on just one or two members of the audience.

MacKay (2011) describes how the voice can be used to facilitate access to your presentation through projection, pitch, pace and pauses, and clear pronunciation.

Accuracy in your presentation is important, and this does not only refer to the obvious requirement for your research data but also to pronunciation and names. If you think an author you will quote in your presentation is well known to the audience, or indeed may be part of the audience, ensure you pronounce his or her name correctly. Pitch, power and pace can be altered to emphasize a point and to draw in a flagging audience. The use of pauses – which are very powerful, underutilized, but get easier with experience – can cause the audience to reflect on the last statement you have made, drawing their attention to a key point in your presentation. They can also refocus attention and interest (DeCoske and White 2010).

Finally in performance, it is best to expect the unexpected (Longo and Tierney 2012). Unexpected events can be technical in nature (e.g. audiovisual equipment), environmental (e.g. external noise) or in the audience. The latter, for instance side conversations or a question delivered to you in an inappropriate manner, should be managed by the Chair of your session, but may not be. As considered above, you will have checked the audiovisual supports before your presentation, but should a problem arise, signal to the Chair and seek assistance from the technician, who should be able to help. Noise from sources outside the room, if brief or as part of conversations, can often be managed by pausing. The challenging questioner becomes less of a challenge with experience, and if you have prepared for questions then you should be able to answer most questions, but if not, it is best to have a diffusion answer prepared, such as 'thank you for your very interesting question/comment, it's certainly a matter for future consideration'. If the questioner is truly an expert, you might wish to suggest that you have an opportunity to discuss the question further after the session and then follow up with such a discussion.

Audience with whom you do not share a first language: Potgieter (2011) suggests the following key points to remember when presenting to an audience with whom you do not share a first language:

- speak slowly
- use humour carefully
- work with your interpreter
- do not use jargon, colloquialisms or idioms
- be sensitive to the nuances of language and culture
- use local terminology

Conclusion

Whether you are presenting your research findings in a thesis or at a conference, it is important to remember that this aspect of your work is part of the story of your research journey. Guidelines and specific requirements on how to present your findings in a thesis/dissertation or at a conference presentation may already exist, and it is important that these are always followed. Visual aids such as figures, tables, slides and posters can be used to communicate and illustrate research findings and enhance the story of your research journey. For both, setting aside time for preparation and practice are key to ensuring a high-quality final product.

Key concepts

- Presenting research findings is part of the research cycle. Dissemination is important for transforming new knowledge into practice.
- Imparting information in meaningful ways will aid in its uptake by end-user groups. These groups can vary from members of the general public to specialists from different fields, and it is important to ensure that your presentation is prepared to match the audience.
- Knowing your reader or your audience is key to your preparation and delivery.
- Visual aids such as figures, tables, slides and posters are just supports, nothing more. They do not replace the substantive text in a thesis/dissertation or presentation at a conference.

Key readings on presenting research findings

- A.A.M. Nicol and P.M. Paxman, *Presenting Your Findings: A Practical Guide for Creating Tables*, 6th edn (Washington, DC: American Psychological Society, 2010)
- A.A.M. Nicol and P.M. Paxman, *Displaying Your Research Findings: A Practical Guide to Creating Figures, Posters and Presentations*, 6th edn (Washington, DC: American Psychological Society, 2010)

Useful websites

- http://www.slideshare.net/brianchandra
- http://www.speakingaboutpresenting.com/audience/foreign-audience/
- http://www.garrreynolds.com/Presentation/slides.html

References

American Diabetes Association (2012) *72nd Scientific Sessions*. Available at http://professional.diabetes.org/Congress_Display.aspx?CID=85274 [Accessed 25 March 2013].

Centre for Excellence in Teaching and Learning in Applied Undergraduate Research Skills (CETL-AURS) (2012) *Writing about Your Results*. Available at http://www.engageinresearch.ac.uk/section_4/writing_about_your_results.shtml [Accessed 04 June 2012].

Chandra, B. (2009) *Presentation Designs*. Available at http://www.slideshare.net/brianchandra [Accessed 12 June 2012].

DeCoske, M.A. and White, S.J. (2010) Public speaking revisited: Delivery, structure and style, *American Journal of Health-System Pharmacy*, 67(1): 1225–7.

DeSilets, L.D. and Dickerson, P.S. (2009) Graphic design principles for audiovisual presentations, *Journal of Continuing Education in Nursing*, 40(1): 12–13.

Easterbrook S (2005) *How Theses Get Written*. Available at http://www.cs.toronto.edu/~sme/presentations/thesiswriting.pdf [Accessed March 2013].

Gifford, H. and Ireton-Jones, C. (2010) Taking your message to the street: Presentation and publication, *Support Line*, 32(6): 16–19.

Goodhand, J.R., Giles, C.L., Wahed, M., Irving, P.M., Langmead, L. and Rampton, D.S. (2011) Poster presentations at medical conferences: An effective way of disseminating research?, *Clinical Medicien*, 11(2): 138–41.

Green, L. (2008) Making research relevant: If it is an evidence-based practice, where is the practice based evidence?, *Family Practice*, 25(Supp. 1): i20–4.

Hardicre, J., Devitt, P. and Coad, J. (2007a) Ten steps to successful poster presentation, *British Journal of Nursing*, 16(7): 398–401.

Hardicre, J., Devitt, P. and Coad, J. (2007b) Ten steps to successful conference presentation, *British Journal of Nursing*, 16(7): 402–4.

Hardy, S. and Ramjeet, J. (2005) Reflections on how to write and organise a research thesis, *Nurse Researcher*, 13(2): 27–39.

Hess, G.R., Tosney, K. and Liegel, L. (2010) *Creating Effective Poster Presentations*. Available at http://www.ncsu.edu/project/posters/ [Accessed 07 May 2012].

Longo, A. and Tierney, C. (2012) Presentation skills for the nurse educator, *Journal for Nurses in Staff Development*, 28(1): 16–23.

MacKay, J. (2011) Take command of the stage, *Nursing Standard*, 25(38): 63.

McConnell, L. (2009) Effective oral presentations: Speaking before groups as part of your job, *The Health Care Manager*, 23(30): 264–72.

Miller, J. (2007) Preparing and presenting effective research posters, *Health Services Research*, 42(1): 311–28.

Potgieter, L. (2011) *7 Tips to Ensure You're Understood when Speaking to a Foreign Audience*. Available at http://www.speakingaboutpresenting.com/audience/foreign-audience/ [Accessed 28 June 2012].

Reynolds, G. (2005) *Top Ten Slide Tips*. Available at http://www.garrreynolds.com/Presentation/slides.html [Accessed 05 June 2012].

Rowe, N. and Ilic, D. (2011) Poster presentation – a visual medium for academic and scientific meetings, *Paediatric Respiratory Care*, 12(3): 208–13.

Swales, J.M. and Feak, C.B. (2004) *Academic Writing for Graduate Students: Essential Tasks and Skills*, 2nd edn. Michigan: The University of Michigan Press.

Wright, J. (2009) The role of computer software in presenting information, *Nursing Management*, 16(4): 30–4.

Zerwic, J.J., Grandfield, K., Kavanaugh, K., Beeger, B., Graham, L. and Mershon, M. (2010) Tips for better visual elements in posters and podium presentations, *Education for Health*, 23(2): 1–6.

Index

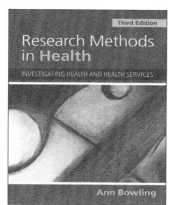

RESEARCH METHODS IN HEALTH
Investigating health and Health Services

Third Edition

Ann Bowling

9780335233649 (Paperback)
2009

eBook also available

This bestselling book provides an accessible introduction to the theoretical concepts and descriptive and analytic research methods used in research on health and health services. The third edition has been thoroughly revised throughout to include updated references and boxed examples, with additional information on key methodological developments.

Key features:

Health technology assessment
• Patient based outcome measures
• Systematic reviews

www.openup.co.uk

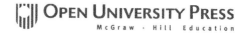

OPEN UNIVERSITY PRESS
McGraw - Hill Education

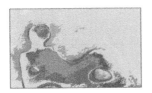

**HANDBOOK OF HEALTH RESEARCH
METHODS**
Investigation, Measurement and Analysis

Ann Bowling and Shah Ebrahim (Eds)

9780335214600 (Paperback)
2005

eBook also available

This handbook helps researchers to plan, carry out, and analyse health research, and evaluate the quality of research studies. The book takes a multidisciplinary approach to enable researchers from different disciplines to work side-by-side in the investigation of population health, the evaluation of health care, and in health care delivery.

Key features:

- Which research method should I use to evaluate services?
- How do I design a questionnaire?
- How do I conduct a systematic review of research?

www.openup.co.uk

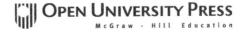

OPEN UNIVERSITY PRESS
McGraw - Hill Education

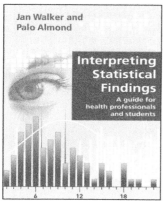

INTERPRETING STATISTICAL FINDINGS
A Guide for Health Professionals and Students

Jan Walker and Palo Almond

9780335235971 (Paperback)
2010

eBook also available

This book is aimed at those studying and working in the field of health care, including nurses and the professions allied to medicine, who have little prior knowledge of statistics but for whom critical review of research is an essential skill. This book offers guidance for students undertaking a critical review of quantitative research papers and will also help health professionals to understand and interpret statistical results within health-related research papers.

Key features:

- A worked example of a published RCT and a health survey
- Explanations of basic statistical concepts
- Explanations of common statistical tests

www.openup.co.uk

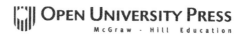